Accident & Emergency Nursing

Accident & Emergency Nursing

A New Approach

Third Edition

Mike Walsh

PhD BA RGN PGCE DipN (Lond)
*Head of the Department of Nursing Studies,
University College of St Martin,
Lancaster*

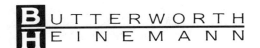

Butterworth-Heinemann
Linacre House, Jordan Hill, Oxford OX2 8DP
A division of Reed Educational and Professional Publishing Ltd

$\mathcal{R}$ A member of the Reed Elsevier plc group

OXFORD   BOSTON   JOHANNESBURG
MELBOURNE   NEW DELHI   SINGAPORE

First published 1985
Reprinted 1987, 1989
Second edition 1990
Reprinted 1992, 1993, 1994
Third edition 1996
Reprinted 1997

British Library Cataloguing in Publication Data
A catalogue record for this book is available from the British Library

Library of Congress Cataloging in Publication Data
A catalogue record for this book is available from the Library of Congress

ISBN 0 7506 2443 4

Printed and bound in Great Britain by
Biddles Ltd, Guildford and King's Lynn

CONTENTS

Acknowledgements   vi
Preface   vii

Section I   The Environment
1 The Sociology of Trauma and Illness   3
2 Patients, People and Nurses—Psychology in A & E   16
3 The Role of the Nurse in A & E   33

Section II   Critical Care
4 Nursing Care of the Critically Injured Patient   55
5 Nursing Care of the Critically Ill Patient   89

Section III   Nursing Care of the Injured Patient
6 Fractures and Dislocations   119
7 Plaster of Paris Application   138
8 Soft Tissue Injury   151
9 The Burnt Patient in A & E   171
10 Eye Complaints and Emergencies   184
11 ENT and Dental Emergencies   195
12 Children in A & E   206
13 Elderly People in A & E   220
14 Women's Health Problems in A & E   230
15 Major Disaster Planning and Radiation Casualties   243

Section IV   The Patient with Behavioural Problems
16 Deliberate Self-harm   255
17 Substance Misuse   266
18 The Mentally Ill Patient in A & E   279
19 The Difficult Problems that Nobody Else Wants   290
20 Sexual Problems in A & E   304

Section V   The Research Base for A & E Nursing
21 Nursing Research in A & E   315

Index   325

ACKNOWLEDGEMENTS

Earlier editions of this book have acknowledged the debts I owe to my old training school at the West Cumberland Hospital and to Barbara Vaughan as my tutor when she ran the old JBCNS A & E course in Oxford, not to mention all the staff I was lucky enough to work with in the Bristol Royal Infirmary A & E Department. However, my debt of gratitude bears repeating again, so thank you one and all!

Since the last edition I have moved back to my northern roots and on into a more educational role at the University College of St Martin's College, Lancaster. It is worth saying a thank you to colleagues at St Martin's for being such a pleasure to work with and to our students for being such a pleasure to teach. A major thank you is due to the library staff at both our Lancaster campus and our Borders outpost in Carlisle and to Ruth for help with proofreading. A major acknowledgement must be made to the nursing profession; it is only sad that those in government who run the NHS do not seem to appreciate the value of nursing in the same way.

Finally, thank you to absent friends, Maggie and Anne Kathryn.

Mike Walsh
Lancaster

PREFACE

We live in rapidly changing times, so although it is only a little over five years since the second edition of this book, a third edition is now essential. Developments such as new drugs, changes in resuscitation protocols and the relentless march of AIDS compete for the A & E nurse's attention alongside the tragic sequence of events that stretches from the Bradford City fire in 1985 to the most recent major disaster.

Nursing itself has been subject to an intense period of change and challenge, from Griffiths to Project 2000, and now major government proposals which are fundamentally changing the very nature of the NHS. All of these developments affect A & E and must be addressed in a book of this type.

And finally, what of the author? I have moved on from being an A & E charge nurse to a primarily teaching role, though still with a substantial clinical involvement in A & E. My own views on individualized care and the Orem nursing model have evolved on from where they were in 1990, but the fundamental philosophy of the 1990 edition remains constant. I maintain that we must treat each A & E patient as an individual human being, acknowledging his/her physical, psychological and social needs, and striving to give integrated, individualized and rational care that attempts to meet *all* such needs. I am grateful for the chance to share such views with you the reader.

The Environment

1   The Sociology of Trauma and Illness
2   Patients, People and Nurses—Psychology in A & E
3   The Role of the Nurse in A & E

Chapter 1

THE SOCIOLOGY OF TRAUMA AND ILLNESS

Each year 11 million people pass through the doors of A & E departments in the UK—a number approximately equal to the population of Australia. It can be said then that A & E nurses deal annually with a population equal to that of a major country. This implies that in their work A & E nurses will meet the full range of human society in terms of class, age, religion, ethnicity and culture. It is important, therefore, to place A & E nursing in its sociological perspective, as it is from this extensive and varied tapestry of the human condition that our patients originate and to which we will return them.

In every tapestry, certain colours dominate and characteristic shapes and patterns are discernible as individual fibres are woven into the final complex picture. So it is with the sociological make-up of a typical day's patients in an A & E department. There will be certain accident patterns that dominate (e.g. alcohol-related accidents, motorbike accidents, assaults) and the patterns will shift and change with the time of day. Furthermore, a large number of patients will have factors in common, such as occupation, age and class. These factors will give the A & E picture a characteristic social colouring. Looked at this way, therefore, A & E patients constitute a group from which striking sociological patterns emerge. These patterns demand the attention of the nurse if nursing care is to be carried out in the patient's best interest.

A discerning nose in A & E after 10 p.m. will detect the smell of alcohol on the breath of most patients. To what extent is alcohol a causative factor in trauma, especially late at night?

A glance through the register of any A & E department will show that certain districts or streets crop up with remarkable frequency. Is there a link between where people live and, therefore, their wealth, social class and their health record? Walsh (1990a,b) has shown that strong linkages do exist.

The woman with a bruised and battered face, the baby with a broken arm, the overdosed teenager vomiting in a cubicle, the junkie and the depressed middle-aged alcoholic person are all familiar figures in A & E. They may seem to have very different problems, but could the root cause be the same? Could it be the breakdown and disintegration of normal family and interpersonal relationships?

The alert A & E nurse will quickly perceive these sorts of patterns. They represent only a few strands, however, of the sociological pattern that goes to make up A & E. Furthermore, while a tapestry is a permanent picture, A & E is a dynamic scene that changes with the passage of time in response to changes within society. The rest of this chapter will attempt to pick out some of these themes and patterns.

Accidents, Emergencies and Social Class

It is thought that there are two main causes of accidents—the environment and the behaviour of the individual. Both these causes are closely linked to social class. This link was explored as part of a much wider-ranging enquiry into health and society carried out under the chairmanship of Sir Douglas Black. This study, known as the Black Report, concluded that where you are in the social scale plays a major part in determining your health: 'Gender and class exert highly significant influences on the quality and duration of life in modern society' (Townsend and Davidson, 1982).

One important finding of the Black Report was that, in the age range 16 to 64, the death rates for men of all social classes are nearly twice as high as the death rates for women. Clearly there are social forces at work that make being male in some ways more unhealthy than being female.

In order to see how mortality rates vary between social classes, it is necessary to define social class. The definition chosen in the Black Report was that of the Registrar General which is based upon occupation.

The Black Report showed that Social Class V (unskilled) has two and a half times the death rate of Class I (professional). Whitehead (1988) has followed up this work into the 1980s and shown that these inequalities persist as strongly today as they did in the 1970s for all types of ill health and accidents, with mortality rates for 1983

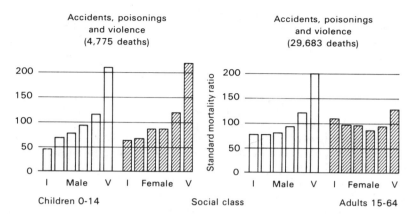

Fig. 1.1   Occupational class and mortality for children aged 0–14
and adults. (Source: Occupational Mortality, England and Wales
1970–72, HMSO, 1978)

running twice as high in Class V as Class I. Whitehead also describes much research showing that unemployment, one of the major social problems of the 1980s, has had a disastrous effect on health.

The mortality statistics relating to accidental death are shown in Fig. 1.1, and reveal a similar gradient, both for children and adults. Fig. 1.1 shows that social class exerts a major influence over the chances of any individual (child or adult) dying as a result of an accident. Children in Social Class V have over four times the likelihood of dying in accidents than children of Social Class I. Similar graphs to Fig. 1.1 can be plotted for other emergency conditions commonly seen in A & E such as cardiovascular, respiratory and genito-urinary diseases. The poorer social classes have the cards heavily stacked against them in terms of a more dangerous environment to live and work in, less health education, and fewer resources with which to look after their health.

This environmental effect is most clearly seen in the statistics for children, among whom in the UK and the rest of Europe, accidental death is the greatest single cause of death. Children in Social Class V have ten times the death rate from falls, fire and drowning, and five to seven times the death rate from road accidents than Social Class I children. Black states that 'While the death of a single child may appear as a random misfortune, this overall distribution indicates the social nature of the phenomenon.' Several factors can explain this difference: the lack of safe play areas in the poorer parts of towns and cities, the more dangerous types of household heating and furnishing which tend to be found in poorer homes, the lack of health knowledge among poorer groups, and the lack of parental supervision which is often due to situations where a single parent cannot take or is not granted time off from work to look after children who are on school holiday or absent from school ill.

Social class determines where a person lives and to a significant degree the amount of stress in a person's life. There is plenty of evidence, in addition to the Black Report, to show how these factors affect the likelihood of a person becoming an A & E patient.

A survey by the Road Research Laboratory (Clayton et al., 1977) found that in urban areas where the housing dates from the 19th century, there is a road traffic accident rate two to three times greater than in areas of post-1919 housing, while the casualty rate among children from road accidents is twice as high in the areas of older type of housing than in the newer housing areas.

The effects of stress are shown by the work of Brown and Harris (1978) who studied mental health problems among working class women in Camberwell, London. Their conclusions were that 'The mother's psychiatric state and the presence of a serious long term difficulty or a threatening life event were related to increased accident risk to children under 16. These factors were more common among working class children and in so far as they are causal, they go a long way to explain the much greater risk of accidents to working class children.' Further evidence of the effects of the inner urban environment on child trauma comes from the work of Maclure and Stewart (1984) who showed that children from deprived areas of Glasgow were nine times more likely to be admitted to hospital than from the rest of Glasgow.

Nurses are by definition Class II and are therefore likely to be from a different social class than that of many of their patients in A & E. But as individualized patient care can only be achieved by considering the social background of the patient, the nurse must be able and willing to bridge that social gap. In planning care the A & E nurse must be able to see the problem through the eyes of a single parent mother living on social security or a casual labourer who has lengthy spells on the dole in between jobs. Environment and class must be considered in nursing care as they affect the resources and health knowledge available to the patient on discharge from A & E.

Patients are people and people are products of their environment, and it is that environment which is a major determining factor as to who attends A & E and why.

Age, Gender and Accidents

In writing his famous passage about the Seven Ages of Man in *As You Like It*, Shakespeare seemed to have one eye on a future A & E unit, for A & E units span the whole human age range. In one cubicle there will be the person in 'second childishness and mere oblivion; sans teeth, sans eyes, sans taste, sans everything', while in the next cubicle will be 'the infant mewling and puking in the nurse's arms'. This has significant implications for A & E nurses.

The dramatic increase in the elderly population has serious implications for all aspects of health care, including A & E units. In 1971, 1.3 million people were aged 80 or over in the UK. By 1989 this figure had risen to 2.1 million and is projected to rise to 2.5 million by 2001 (CSO, 1993). The elderly are prone to accidents by virtue of failing faculties, degenerative changes in the musculo-skeletal system and the increasingly poor conditions that many elderly people are forced to live in. This compounds the other health problems associated with ageing leading to the elderly being a very important group of patients in A & E who have special needs (Chapter 13).

Road traffic accidents are undoubtedly a major factor in accounting for the high number of young people seen in A & E and the marked bias towards males. Fig. 1.2 shows a comparison of numbers of deaths in RTAs in 1982 and 1992.

The role of motorbikes in causing this tragic waste of young lives is well documented. Motorbikes are involved in more than eight times as many accidents as motor cars and 25 times as many deaths per kilometre travelled (*Social Trends*, 1993). A total of 3484 males and 1414 females died from motor vehicle accidents in 1990 (CSO, 1993). If male behaviour explains the higher mortality figures in large part, it is therefore interesting to note this extends to pedestrians also. In England and Wales the 1990 mortality statistics show 1009 male pedestrian deaths compared to 632 female (OPCS, 1991).

The work of McCoy et al. (1989) sheds interesting light on RTA fatalities. They studied 131 road deaths in a two-year period in Oxfordshire and found that in the age group 15–20 there were more

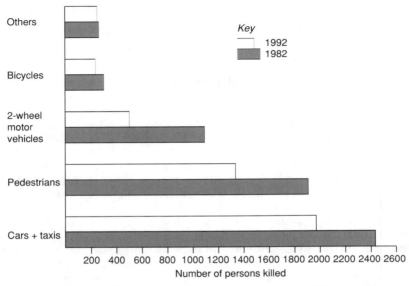

Note: 29.4% of all persons killed or seriously injured in RTAs are aged
between 15 and 24 and a further 25.6% between 25 and 34.

*Fig. 1.2   Persons killed in RTAs in the UK 1982–92 (Source: C.S.O.,
1994, Social Trends)*

than twice as many deaths as in any other 5-year age group. Of the
fatal accidents, 63% happened in daylight, 87% on dry roads and
59% on main A class roads. The most common causes of death were
head injury (45 cases) followed by intrathoracic haemorrhage (33),
multiple injuries (18), combined head and chest injury (11) and
spinal injury (8). One-third of the victims died on their way to
hospital or in hospital. It is also worth noting the findings of Storie
(1977) who demonstrated that while there was no difference between
accident rates for male and female drivers, male drivers had far more
serious accidents.

The much higher male attendance rate at A & E in the under 64
age group can be partly explained by the more hazardous nature of
male work and sport. However, the tendency to aggression and
assertiveness that is revealed by Storie's study undoubtedly underlies
much male trauma leading as it does to more dangerous behaviour
on the roads, increased alcohol consumption and violence. As male

children are socialized into this aggressive/assertive role from child-hood, nurses may speculate on how many accidents would be, in fact, preventable if we had different child-rearing practices, and it should be remembered that the victims of male aggression are not always male.

Families, Women and A & E

Marxists see traditional families as a tool of capitalist oppression as they create a large pool of cheap female labour. Feminists, on the other hand, see families as trapping women and denying them equal rights. The traditional role of women in the family is under attack from all sides, and the trebling of the divorce rate between 1966 and 1976, one symptom of the changing role of women, has led to many women now being the lone heads of families. Of these lone mothers, only 18% are in full-time employment, although 78% have to cope with the burdens of living alone rather than with families.

In the many families where the woman is the head (18% of families with children in 1991 had a lone mother as their head, OPCS, 1991) there are special problems when either the woman or her children become A & E patients. First, it is very difficult for a lone mother to supervise her children; the stress involved takes its toll on the mother—if she is ill, she may have to make special arrangements for someone to look after other young children, or the A & E unit will have to step into the breach on a temporary basis. Alternatively if one of the children is ill, the only way that the mother can accompany the child to A & E is to bring the rest of the children along as well. This requires that the A & E unit be able to look after well children as well as injured or ill children. Second, after unemployment, single parenthood has been the major cause of poverty in the 1980s, while the median single woman's wage in 1987 was only 60% of the married man's (CSO, 1989).

One further problem faced by women in the context of the family is that of violent partners. It is important for A & E nursing staff to realize that a woman's injuries may be due to violence from her partner, even though she may not admit this at first. Stark and Flitcraft (1985) reported that assault is the single biggest cause of injury amongst women, while Walsh (1990c) found women more likely to attend A & E as a result of assault than an RTA. A reluctance to leave the A & E unit after treatment for minor injuries suffered as a result of a 'fall' may be understood better in this light and A & E nurses should be alert for tell-tale signs of anxiety and inappropriate injuries when compared to the story of how they occurred. The existence of women's refuges should be known to the nurse together with the knowledge of how to contact one if needed. A battered woman may be more prepared to talk about her problems to a female nurse than to a male doctor. She is most unlikely to involve the law.

Another traditional role of the woman in the family is to look after aged relatives. However, increased family mobility, increased numbers of women in work, and the decline of the extended family have led to a decline in the numbers of women able to play this role. Elderly parents are left behind as their adult children move around the country. Distance weakens emotional ties; one week at Christmas does not compensate for 51 weeks apart and finally, after 20 to 30 years, children and parents may become strangers to each other.

A & E units face then a dual problem—an increasing number of elderly people living alone and who are therefore more accident prone, and fewer situations where an elderly patient can be discharged home with someone to look after them. Relatives of elderly patients who are unwilling to look after them (possibly for very good reasons) may feel very guilty, with the result that the wrong attitude by the nurse or an inadvertent word may lead to serious difficulty, which will be of no benefit to the patient and can lead to a serious deterioration in relationships between family and hospital. The A & E nurse should be non-judgemental at all times, and never more so than when dealing with the relatives of an elderly patient who refuse to take the patient home because they cannot look after him or her. The need is to see the problem from the family's perspective.

Culture, Ethnicity and A & E

The UK is fortunate in that it is a multiracial society and as a result has a rich and diverse cultural heritage and ambiance. If the A & E nurse is to give individualized patient care, then the ethnic and cultural background of the patient must be a major consideration. This in turn requires A & E nurses to familiarize themselves with cultural factors. It is a mistake for the nurse to judge the patient's beliefs against his or her own which usually will be Caucasian Christian. Such an ethnocentric approach will lead to a failure in individualized care.

It is strange to talk of individualized care when many nurses do not know the patient's correct name, a situation that often arises with the Asian community. In the case of Sikhs, Singh merely indicates male and Kaur female; either title will be preceded by a personal name and followed by the name of the subcaste which is borne by the whole family (equivalent to a surname): for example, Mohinder Singh Sandhu or Gurmit Kaur Sondh would be correctly addressed as Mr Sandhu or Mrs Sondh. Sometimes the last name is dropped, and only then is it correct to talk of Mr Singh or Mrs Kaur. Hindus use one or more personal names followed by the subcaste name (equivalent to a surname) but do *not* use the titles Singh or Kaur.

The Muslim naming system is more complex as there are many titles that are not names, for example, Abdul, Mohammed, Shah, Syed; other titles such as Ahmad, Ahmed and Rahman can become names when combined with other titles, for example, Abdul Rahman. Khan and Choudhery are common names in Pakistan but these too are titles rather than names, while Bibi, Begum and Khatoon all signify that the bearer is female and do not act as true names. It is quite usual for members of the same family to have different names, with no common family name.

Human behaviour is largely learnt rather than innate, therefore the response to pain and illness will be environmentally determined. In other words, it will be a product of cultural background. This should lead the A & E nurse to realize that in dealing with patients from a different cultural background to the nurse, there will be significant differences in how the patient responds to illness and pain. Such differences are not to be interpreted as signs of weakness but rather as a normal learnt behaviour pattern. The whole concept of what is illness itself varies from ethnic group to ethnic group, and from class to class within any group (Helman, 1990). That which is defined as illness by one group may be considered normal by another, thus illness becomes socially constructed; its perception and how you respond to it are relative to where you are in society. Little is absolute!

Alcohol-related Accidents and Emergencies

Alcohol-related problems will be considered in depth later in the book. However, at this stage, the A & E nurse should recognize the role of alcohol as one of the major causative factors leading to the front door of A & E. The effect of alcohol on drivers is well known,

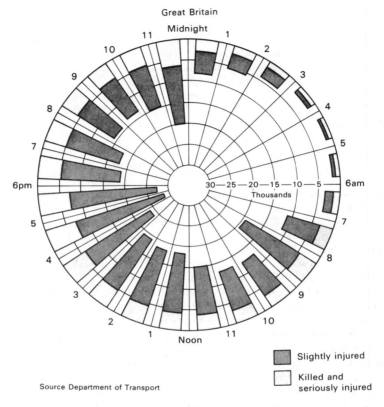

*Fig. 1.3   Road accident casualties: by hour of the day and severity
of injury, 1982. (Source: Department of Transport)*

but it is also a major factor in pedestrian trauma. A study in the
West Midlands by Clayton et al. (1977) found that 22% of all fatally
injured pedestrians had a blood alcohol level above the legal limit
for driving. At blood levels two and a half times the legal driving
limit (about 5 pints of beer), the chances of being killed were 23
times greater than that of a control group. The social profile of the
drink-impaired pedestrians who died was young to middle-aged,
semi-skilled to unskilled (Social Class IV or V), divorced, separated
or single.

There is an overwhelming volume of statistics which shows the effects of alcohol on drivers: Storie's survey found that alcohol was the greatest single impairment factor in accidents, that alcohol-impaired drivers were almost exclusively male, and that alcohol was involved in 35% of accidents where male drivers were to blame. The recent work of McCoy et al. (1989) confirms these findings as 33% of fatally injured pedestrians had significant alcohol levels in their bloodstream. More recently, it has been shown that, in 1991, 22% of drivers killed in RTAs had blood alcohol levels over the legal limit (*Social Trends*, 1993).

Alcohol is frequently associated with acts of self-harm such as over-dose and self-inflicted injury, while the depression of inhibition effect of alcohol leads to many acts of violence and other behaviour which results in trauma. The depression of inhibition may also result in behaviour which makes it impossible to treat a patient, and alcohol consumption will also delay the giving of an anaesthetic.

Individualized Nursing Care and Social Factors

The first step in nursing care is assessment. Social factors such as class, age, gender, housing, and cultural and ethnic backgrounds will all affect the A & E nurse's assessment of the patient. Furthermore, without these factors being considered in all stages of nursing there can be no individualized nursing care. This task is made more difficult by the fact that often the patient will be from a very different sociological grouping than the nurse. Therefore, it is necessary for the nurse to try to see things from the patient's point of view and level of understanding. Only if the nurse and patient are looking at the same problem in the same way is there hope for understanding and cooperation; the patient's perspective on a problem, because of class, gender, age, family, culture, religion and ethnicity, may be very different from the nurse's.

During assessment, an open-minded, non-judgemental attitude will help to bridge what may be a very wide gap between nurse and patient.

In planning care, nurses have to plan for what is possible and for what the patient sees as the problem. What is possible will be partly determined by the factors discussed so far; what the patient sees as the problem will be the result an interaction between his or her previous life experience and beliefs, and what the nurse can explain and teach.

Our patient may have a beautifully applied plaster or burns dressing in the A & E department, but what are we sending him or her home to? Can a single mother look after two young children with a burns dressing on her hand? Does she understand what will happen if she removes the dressing and the hand becomes infected? Can an elderly lady look after herself (and her even more dependent elderly husband) with her leg in a below knee walking plaster? Is it reasonable to expect a family living 60 miles away with three young children to take on the care of a confused, incontinent elderly father who has not lived with his daughter for 20 years and who has a fractured humerus? Should we be surprised if an Asian lady will not allow intimate procedures to be performed by a male doctor?

The point is that in planning and carrying out care we have to plan for what is *socially* possible, and be prepared to include a large amount of education and teaching in our care package, and make sure that the patient understands fully the importance of what is being done. After all, it is not what is taught that is important, it is what is learnt.

When we evaluate the success of our care, we must consider whether the goals set were socially attainable and realistic, and we must be prepared to alter our goals in accordance with experience and home environment.

In conclusion, the A & E nurse needs to realize how important environmental factors are in both the causation and care of the victims of trauma and sudden emergencies, and he or she needs to be prepared to take a leaf out of community nurses' book in giving due care and attention to the home and social circumstances of the patient.

References and Further Reading

Brown G., Harris T. (1978). *The Social Origins of Depression*. London: Tavistock.

Clayton B., Booth A. C., McCarthy P. E. (1977). *A Controlled Study of the Role of Alcohol in Fatal Adult Pedestrian Accidents*. Transport and Road Research Laboratory.

CSO (1989). Key Data. London: Government Statistical Service.

CSO (1993). Key Data. London: Government Statistical Service.

CSO (1993). *Social Trends* 25, London: HMSO.

CSO (1994). *Social Trends* 26, London: HMSO.

Helman C. G. (1990). *Culture, Health and Illness*, Oxford: Butterworth-Heinemann.

McCoy G., Johnstone R., Nelson I., Duthie R. (1989), A review of fatal road accidents in Oxfordshire over a 2 year period. *Injury*, **20**:2, 65–68.

O'Neil P. (1983). *Health Crisis 2000*, London: Heinemann Medical Books.

OPCS (1991).

Stark E., Flitcraft A. (1985). Spouse abuse. In *Surgeon General's Workshop on Violence and Public Health: Sourcebook*. Atlanta Centers for Disease Control, US Public Health Service, SA1-45.

Storie V. J. (1977). *Male and Female Car Drivers, Differences Observed in Accidents*. Transport and Road Research Laboratory.

Townsend P., Davidson N. (1982). *Inequalities in Health*. Harmondsworth: Penguin.

Walsh M. (1990a). Social factors and A & E attendance. *Nursing Standard*, **5**:9, 29-32.

Walsh M. (1990b). Geographical factors and A & E attendance. *Nursing Standard*, **5**:8, 28-31.

Walsh M. (1990c). Why do people go to A & E? *Nursing Standard*, **5**:7, 24-29.

Whitehead M. (1988). *The Health Divide*. London: Health Education Council.

Wilson H., Herbert G. W. (1978). *Parents and Children in the Inner City*, London: Routledge & Kegan Paul.

Chapter 2

PATIENTS, PEOPLE AND NURSES— PSYCHOLOGY IN A & E

Paul Simon once sang of 'Hearts and Bones'; he could have been singing about A & E however, as there is more to A & E nursing than physical problems such as broken bones. There are emotional and mental problems as well. An understanding of psychology is essential for good nursing practice, for how can we truly individualize care unless we consider the mental processes of our patients? This chapter aims, therefore, to familiarize the reader with some of the areas of psychology that are most relevant to A & E and to show how psychological insights can make a real and beneficial impact on patient care.

Emotion

In A & E, nurses work in an emotion-charged atmosphere. They come into contact with depression and sadness, happiness and joy, and guilt and anger—in fact, with the full range of human emotion. The suddenness with which many patients are taken ill and the media image of the A & E department—as a place full of wailing sirens, flashing blue lights and life-saving heroics—combine to make sudden illness in the A & E department a highly emotional and anxiety provoking experience for the general public.

Nurses sometimes overlook the emotional content of a patient or a relative in A & E, because they do not know what they are looking for. However, there is a useful body of research on the psychology of emotion that can be applied to the A & E department to improve nursing care and to prevent problems arising out of emotional behaviour.

In reviewing various classic experiments and theories of emotion, Atkinson et al. (1991) consider that emotion is triggered by an arousing event which leads to autonomic arousal. The emotional experience that follows is determined by a process known as cognitive appraisal. This term means the way we interpret the event, and early work by Schachter and Singer (1962) suggests this is heavily influenced by previous experiences and cues from the surrounding environment.

The sudden onset of illness or trauma followed by the rapid movement to A & E will certainly act as an emotionally arousing event leading to autonomic stimulation. Similarly, when a family is told that their relative has been 'rushed to hospital', their emotions will be aroused.

When the patient and the family arrive in the A & E, together or apart, the nurse will be one of the most potent sources of emotional cues. Schachter's work suggests that much of the patient's emotional behaviour will depend on the nurse's behaviour. If the nurse is anxious and hostile, the patient may well be anxious and hostile. Conversely, if the nurse is calm and confident, this manner will help bring a distressed patient to a clearer and calmer state of mind. The same applies to the nurse's interaction with the family.

In addition, nurses should remember the effect of previous experience on emotion and consider that a patient's apparently unreasonable emotions may have their origins in some previous unhappy experience. Furthermore, the experience undergone by patients today will have an important effect on their reaction to future hospitalization; this is especially true of young children and their fears of hospital.

A potent source of such cues will be A & E staff who are therefore in a good position, by their own emotional behaviour, to reduce anxiety, fear and anger among patients and relatives.

Grief and Bereavement

Today some two-thirds of all deaths occur in institutions, with a high proportion of sudden deaths occurring in A & E departments. It is the suddenness of death in A & E and the age range involved that makes coping with death and the bereaved family and friends one of the most difficult aspects of A & E work.

Most nurses will have witnessed death before coming to A & E, but these deaths will usually have been the result of a lengthy illness so that the act of dying is expected and fits well into Saunders' moving description of terminally ill patients (1959).

They were not frightened nor unwilling to go, for by then they were too far away to want to come back. They were conscious of leaving weakness and exhaustion rather than life and its activities. They rarely had any pain but felt intensely weary. They wanted to say goodbye to those they loved but were not torn with longing to stay with them.

In contrast, the dead person in the A & E department is often the cheerful child last seen by his mother setting off to school, the baby found in its cot, the husband and father collapsing at work or the teenager who never came home from a party. It is the stunning suddenness of this most final act of all that lends such a devastating dimension to the problem of caring for the bereaved in A & E.

The grief reaction consists of a cultural and an individual component. Nurses in A & E should remember that the cultural background of the bereaved may be very different from their own and, therefore, not to be surprised if the relatives' behaviour is different from that which nurses expect as a result of their own cultural upbringing.

Descriptions of grief include shock, denial, anxiety, depression, guilt, anger and a wide range of somatic signs linked to anxiety. However, these manifestations should not be thought of as a strict succession of stages. Regression is also common.

It is a long walk from the resuscitation room to the relatives' waiting room when a patient has died. How can the above comments help the nurse who has to make that walk with bad news to impart at the end? The response of relatives will vary with culture and individual factors, therefore their response may lie anywhere in a wide range of behaviours—from stunned unbelieving silence through to collapse and a flood of emotion and on to stoical acceptance. The nurse should not be fooled by the stoical response, the grief is there and it has to be worked through in the long term. Stoicism certainly does not convey a lack of care for the dead person or an easy acceptance of the death.

The nurse must be prepared for many questions. 'Why me?' 'Why her?' 'Couldn't anything be done?' 'It's all my fault, isn't it?' These questions do not have answers in this context. A denial response may be observed with the relative simply refusing to believe the person is dead. This denial has to be overcome as an essential part of the grief work, if acceptance is to be reached. The relative should be shown the body and allowed to touch and feel the deceased in order to help with the grief work. This is especially true of mothers of children and infants who have died (particularly cot death infants). The mother should be encouraged to hold the dead baby in her arms to help her overcome the denial mechanism so that she may more readily come to terms with the death of her baby.

A single bereaved person should never be left alone in the department or left to go home alone. Somebody must sit with them until a relative or friend can be found. Providing human company at this most difficult hour of a person's life is a nursing responsibility. In providing that company, nurses provide the person with an opportunity to verbalize their grief and they protect the person from possible harm. If in the process of doing this, nurses themselves feel moved to tears, there is nothing wrong in that. It is an expression of human empathy, not inadequacy.

One important practical point concerns the identification of the deceased. Friends can mistakenly identify a person they have known for years under the stress of an A & E resuscitation room and in the aftermath of a resuscitation attempt on a badly injured patient. The result may be that the wrong relatives are informed.

If nurses find that they are upset by a death in A & E, they should know that this is a normal reaction to a very stressful event that is rather different from death in other hospital areas. Nurses in A & E can take comfort in the fact that although sometimes we do lose a life, there are times when we win as well. And most of the time, our work lies somewhere in between—we simply help people through their present problems.

How We Perceive Others

How do patients perceive nurses and how do nurses perceive patients? Research into person perception suggests that the answer may be that they perceive each other very differently and that neither's perceptions may be very accurate. Nurses need to look carefully at how misperception occurs, for misperception may radically alter their assessment of the patient—and accurate assessment is central to the process of nursing.

One view of perception sees it as depending heavily upon previous experiences, with judgements being inferred from the information available. In addition, however, we have systems of rules by which we understand what we perceive. These association rules are based on experience and culture. Some may in addition be unique to the individual. These rules create mental sets that act as pigeon holes into which perceived information can be conveniently filed and rapidly understood.

We expect people to behave in certain ways because they conform to stereotypes. These are defined by Leyens and Codol (1988) as theories of personality that a group of people share about their own group or another group. Common to all stereotypes is that they deny the person's individuality.

The nurse who treats all elderly patients as deaf, confused and incontinent is not nursing people but stereotypes. That nurse is failing to deliver individualized nursing care. Unfortunately, there is a large amount of evidence that nurses do stereotype the elderly in this way in both the USA (Caporeal et al., 1983) and the UK (Coupland et al. 1988). Quality nursing depends upon accurate assessment and that means we must look beyond the clothes a person wears, or the number of wrinkles in a person's skin, and treat each as an individual avoiding the short cut of pigeonholing them as 'a typical . . .'.

One final aspect of perception is the old cliché that 'first impressions count'. Luchins (1957) carried out research which showed that there is a great deal of truth in this statement. In forming impressions of people, we do allow our first impression to control much of what follows, often leading to serious errors in perception. Atkinson et al. (1987) have summarized a mass of research data which confirms Luchin's original findings. If A & E nurses are aware of this trap, they will find it easier to put first impressions to one side and to spend time talking to patients, trying to get to know them a little better, before making an assessment. Their assessment will be more accurate for the time spent.

It should also be remembered that the same mechanisms which cause misperception are also at work in the patient who will be working with a stereotype of you as a nurse. Impressions of you will be formed based on the first minute of your interaction.

Accurate patient observation and assessment therefore depends upon the nurse being aware of factors which influence perception. In making observations of people and their behaviour, the nurse is inevitably led into seeking to explain that behaviour. The nurse therefore makes attributions or inferences about causality and in doing so, as psychologists have demonstrated, makes all sorts of mistakes or attribution errors (Atkinson et al., 1991).

The original work on attribution theory stems from Heider (1958) who proposed that humans tend to attribute behaviour to either factors within the individual (internal attribution) or situational, environmental factors outside the individual (external attribution). The fundamental attribution error that people make seems to be to overemphasize the importance of internal attribution (Ross, 1977). Consequently, in explaining behaviour, we tend systematically to ignore a range of possible environmental explanations and locate the reasons for behaviour within the individual. Internal attributions are linked to the notion of intent; in making such an attribution we also tend to assume that the person knew the likely consequences of their actions. A further key element of attribution theory is the suggestion that the more socially undesirable the consequences of an action the more we tend to attribute to the individual a disposition to behave in that way—an internal attribution is therefore made (Hewstone and Antaki, 1988).

In assessing A & E patients, attribution theory suggests nurses should be wary of how they interpret and explain observed behaviour. It seems as though we may consistently ignore the importance of the strange A & E environment and other situational factors in our assessment, attributing patient behaviour to a pathological cause or to their personality and hence making erroneous judgements about the type of person they are. We are also prone to assume that the patient knew the consequences of his or her actions. This is particularly true of the patient whose behaviour may be seen as antisocial such as a homeless person, a drug user, or a person who has committed an act of self-harm such as self-poisoning. Apart from underlining the importance of not making judgements about patients and consequently displaying attitudes lacking in the essential caring qualities that help define nursing as a profession, attribution theory should remind us to tread carefully and approach patients with an open mind in attempting to understand any behaviour displayed in A & E.

How We Perceive our Environment— Sensory Deprivation in A & E

When a person is deprived of meaningful sensory input, they are said to be experiencing sensory deprivation. After a period of only a few hours, sensory deprivation can produce hallucinations, anxiety, fear and other mental disturbances.

Let us think of a typical A & E cubicle where a patient can remain for several hours. What sensory input does a patient have in that situation? There is no clock to tell the time. Often the patient cannot even tell if it is day or night. The walls are blank. Loose curtains block off the view beyond the end of the trolley. Overhead there is the ubiquitous neon strip lamp in an equally bare ceiling. If the patient has no friends or relatives present, and no nurse has the time to chat with her, how will she be able to assess the passage of time? We have put our patient into a state of sensory deprivation. How much apparent 'confusion' in elderly patients has its origins in the sensory deprivation of an A & E cubicle? To take the case a step further, what if the patient is deaf or wears spectacles and the hearing aid or spectacles are at home? The sensory deprivation will be even more acute.

The patient will probably also be suffering from perceptual deprivation as we may be exposing her to stimuli that are meaningless: the X-ray machines, the ECG monitors, the strange sounds and the mysterious jargon of modern hospitals mean very little to most people. All this adds up to the patient being deprived of meaningful perceptions.

Many sudden mood changes and cases of apparent confusion, therefore, may be the result of the A & E environment depriving the patient of meaningful sensations and perceptions. If a patient is likely to be in A & E for any length of time, reality orientation must be a vital part of the care plan. Leave the curtain at the end of the cubicle pulled back a little so patients can see what is going on. Tell them the time. Talk to them. Make sure spectacles and hearing aids are worn and working. Explain the sounds and sights of the A & E department so that patients have meaningful perceptions of it (the nurse as the interpreter of the hospital experience). Above all, give the patients some meaningful stimulation. Nurses may even want to consider having quiet piped radio in the A & E to help while away the time.

In short, A & E nursing staff need to be aware of the risks of sensory deprivation to their patients.

Learning and Behaviour

Why do we behave the way that we do? This is a vast field that lies in the province of psychology, however a few simple ideas are presented here as they are of relevance to the work of A & E nurses.

The Behaviourist School which had its origins in the experiments of Thorndike and Skinner in the early years of this century is one major approach.

The main thrust of behaviourism is that human behaviour is a product of learning experiences and of the environment and that it is not due to pre-programmed activity or instinct. This implies, therefore, that behaviour can be learned and can be changed. As nurses, we often need to do just that, change behaviour. Hence the importance of behaviourism to learning—and to nursing care.

Let us first of all consider learning through operant conditioning. If an act is followed by desirable experiences, it is more likely to be repeated; the desirable consequences act as positive reinforcement. If an act is followed by punishment, the effect is to suppress the behaviour, but not to eliminate it—for when the punishment is removed, the behaviour will reappear.

A more effective way of eliminating behaviour is by *extinction*. In this case, positive reinforcement is withheld. This leads to a long-term removal of the behaviour.

These three ideas can be illustrated with a familiar example in A & E. A disturbed young woman with a disordered personality is a regular attender at A & E. She comes in regularly with self-inflicted minor lacerations on the arms, accompanied by attention-seeking and disruptive behaviour. The attention that follows such actions acts as a positive reinforcement leading to repetition of this behaviour. If, however, the attention that the woman receives and the disruption that she causes with each visit are denied to her—if we simply ignore her behaviour—then the extinction effect will be expected to lead to the patient reducing her self-harming and attention-seeking behaviour. On the other hand, a punitive response—for example, calling the police to remove the patient—will lead to further disruption and more positive reinforcement. In the long run, court proceedings will not usually have much effect on this sort of situation. The punitive approach simply rewards the patient with attention that they want and leads to more disruptive behaviour.

A further form of learning that comes under the heading of operant conditioning is negative reinforcement. In this case, behaviour leads to the removal of unpleasant or adverse situations. Alcohol abuse is a good example of negative reinforcement; the patient drinks to avoid the difficult realities of everyday life. The difficult behaviour of some patients can also be explained in terms of avoiding

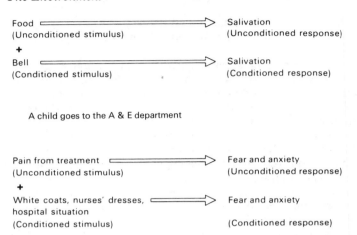

Fig. 2.1   Pavlov's classic experiment and an A & E example: the unconditioned and conditioned stimulus become paired together to produce a conditional response.

problems of living by getting other people to perform various tasks for them.

Positive reinforcement is potentially a powerful tool for the nurse who seeks patient compliance and for the nurse who wants to teach and motivate junior staff. In teaching a patient how to use crutches or how to do the essential finger exercises for an arm in plaster, we must reward correct actions with praise (positive reinforcement) if we want those actions to be repeated. Similarly, if a junior member of staff is being taught a skill or a junior nurse performs an intelligent or thoughtful piece of nursing care, then we should praise the nurse and say 'well done'. Such positive reinforcement will produce a more caring, better motivated and more skilful nurse. Ignoring good work will produce extinction of that good work, while merely telling the nurse off for poor work (punitive reinforcement) will not bring about good care.

Having discussed operant conditioning, it now remains to look at classical conditioning, the origins of which lie in the famous work of Pavlov and his dogs (Fig. 2.1). Pavlov presented food to a dog (unconditioned stimulus) and obtained a response of salivation (unconditioned response) which was a reflex action. If he rang a bell at the same time (conditioned stimulus), he found that after a while the dog associated the bell with the food and salivated to the sound of the bell only. Salivation had become a conditioned response.

This form of learning has been demonstrated in humans. Consider the example of the small child taken to A & E after an accident. The combined efforts of the nurses and a casualty officer may do a very good job of stitching his scalp back together, but this can be a very frightening experience for the child. The strange environment and those funny strangers in white coats and dresses will become associated with the pain and discomfort involved in having a wound stitched. The result will be that the next time the child has to attend hospital, white coats and nurses' dresses will act as a conditioned stimulus to produce the conditioned response of fear and anxiety. It is thought that the origins of many irrational fears and phobias lie in this mechanism, where the response to one stimulus is transferred onto another stimulus by classical conditioning. Examples range from fear of injections through to phobias about spiders and on to sexual fetishes.

The implications of Pavlov's work for the A & E nursing of children is clear: if we want to prevent children developing fears about hospitals, the unconditioned stimulus must be reduced by reducing pain and discomfort to a minimum; children's experience of A & E must be made as pleasant as possible; on the other hand, we can also try to remove the conditioning stimulus of white coats, nurses' uniforms and all the other hospital paraphernalia. Ideally there should be a special children's section in the A & E department with toys and a play area, where staff should be in ordinary clothes and where the hospital environment should as far as possible be minimized.

One other method of learning behaviour that needs discussion is learning by imitation. Bandura (1973) originally showed that children learn violent behaviour by copying adults. Subsequent work in this area of modelling led Bandura (1986) to propose that modelling can influence behaviour in adults in a wide range of ways. In nursing, more senior nurses act as models for junior staff all the time; imitation or modelling has been shown to be a very potent way of learning practical skills. The power of modelling as a means of learning behaviour is so potent that it is not surprising that the student copies what he or she has seen in the clinical setting, which sets up tensions if very different things are taught in college. The nurse

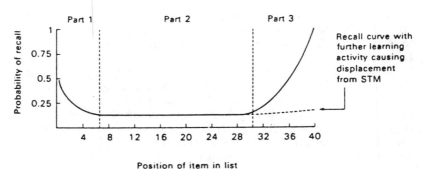

Fig. 2.2   Free recall curve. (Murdock, 1962)

smelling of a recently extinguished cigarette should also consider the health behaviour she is modelling for A & E patients to follow.

Memory

How do we remember information? What can we do to improve recall? These two questions deserve our attention if we are to ensure optimum results from teaching patients prior to discharge about their dressings, exercises, plasters and other aspects of care. A patient who has had a Colles fracture reduced and plastered has enough problems to contend with. However, if s/he forgets the importance of exercising the fingers, maintaining the arm in a sling, looking out for signs of discoloration, excessive swelling or symptoms such as a tingling sensation, then all manner of neurovascular complications may arise.

Similar comments apply to a whole range of treatments, drugs and instructions with which we discharge patients every day from A & E. Nurses, therefore, need to know something of the work that has been done in the field of memory, for not only will it benefit patients, but, incorporated into teaching, it will improve the way that student nurses learn.

Insights into memory can be gained from the early work of Murdock (1962). He gave people a series of words to remember and later tested them to see which could be recalled. The results were plotted as a serial position curve as shown in Fig. 2.2. On this graph, the frequency of successful recall of any word is plotted against its position in the series of words given.

The curve that Murdock plotted can be explained as follows (Atkinson et al., 1991). Memory is thought of as consisting of two components, long-term memory (LTM) and short-term memory (STM). The short-term part of memory can only retain about seven items which are then either lost from STM by displacement by new items to remember or are passed on into LTM after appropriate rehearsal. If we study the curve, it becomes apparent that the high success rate at the end of the curve (Part 3) is due to short-term memory. However, if we give the person another learning activity to perform immediately afterwards, the effect is greatly to reduce the recall (dashed line) due to items being displaced out of short-term memory by the new learning activity.

The high success rate in Part 1 of the curve reflects the working of LTM and is called the primacy effect. However, LTM will diminish (Part 2) due to emotional upset and interference, where similar items get in the way of what we are trying to recall. Improvements in LTM can be brought about by repetition of what is to be remembered and by the provision of cues to enable us to access information more readily in LTM.

How then can the A & E nurse apply some of these insights into memory to improve care? Murdock's work shows us that a patient will recall best what is said first and last. Therefore, we must put the most important information first and last. To help patients to remember what is said in the middle (and there has to be a middle), we can use repetition of key points coupled with cues to help memory; at the same time, we should try to avoid introducing spurious information which will only interfere with what has to be remembered, especially if it is similar in content. Emotional upset will interfere with memory also, so there is not much point expecting someone who is very anxious or distressed to remember detailed instructions—their emotional state has to be stabilized first. Finally, given the fallibility of human memory, consideration should be given to simple pre-printed instruction cards for such things as care of plaster of Paris, wounds, anti-tetanus follow-up and so on.

The points made in this section can be applied with equal validity when considering how best to help student nurses to remember what they have been taught.

The Psychology of Ageing

Important psychological changes occur with ageing, both in childhood and old age. A discussion of these changes has been left, however, to the relevant chapters later in the book which look at the problems of children and the elderly in the A & E department.

Pain

Pain is a subjective, psychological experience known only to the patient and often associated with fear. Research by Walsh (1993) has demonstrated the widespread prevalence of pain and anxiety amongst ambulatory A & E patients. He asked a sample of 200 adults who walked into a typical busy urban A & E unit to assess their pain and anxiety levels using a simple scale of 0–5 where 0 indicated the absence of pain or anxiety and 5 indicated the most severe pain or anxiety the person could imagine. Only 10% of patients stated they were pain free whilst 52% rated their pain as 3, 4 or 5. A total of 15.5% stated their anxiety levels were 5 while 50% rated their anxiety as 3, 4 or 5. Only 11.5% gave a zero score.

When the anxiety levels of those patients with low pain scores (0–2) were compared with high scoring patients (3–5), statistically significant differences emerged indicating that the higher the pain level reported, the higher the degree of anxiety that the person was experiencing. Greater anxiety levels were also associated with longer delays in deciding to attend A & E compared with those patients who reported lower levels. This effect was also found in the time taken actually to present to A & E once the decision to attend had been made.

Pain and anxiety are therefore common problems in A & E patients. It is unfortunate therefore that there is a strong body of evidence to show that nurses and doctors are very bad at assessing pain (Walsh and Ford, 1989). A common mistake is to ignore the personal and subjective nature of pain which means it often bears little resemblance to the degree of damaged tissue. Thus the amount of pain a patient is in cannot be assessed reliably from physical signs such as the extent of trauma, raised blood pressure, pulse rate or even facial expression. However researchers such as Jacox (1979) and Saxey (1986) found that these were precisely the signs that nurses used in preference to verbal reports.

Different cultures express pain in different ways and within any one culture there are different rules for male and female. The familiar phrase 'Now be a brave boy and don't cry' that is heard in A & E tells us a lot about our culture's views: it is permitted for females to cry but not males.

A classical piece of research by Hayward in 1975 showed that the greater a patient's anxiety, the more pain they reported and their morale was lowered accordingly. Hayward also showed that, by giving patients information, it was possible to reduce anxiety and pain.

The nurse cannot know what the patient is feeling. It is a unique experience to that individual and the most reliable guide to a patient's pain is what the patient says it is. This must be a fundamental principle in A & E nursing. In assessing a patient we start with the vital signs of ABC (p. 55). The very next step must be to assess pain and to remember to reassess at various stages in the patient's progress through A & E. As Walsh and Ford (1989) have discussed, patients are very unwilling to initiate requests for pain relief—they need to be asked by the nurse. It is sad that some nurses still see patients' requests for pain relief as attention seeking, undesirable behaviour or use stereotypes (p. 20) to decide on pain relief, i.e. 'If it's a Colles fracture, the patient should have . . .' rather than look at the individual person.

Individualized Nursing Care and Psychology

It remains to try to pull together some of the aspects of psychology touched upon in this chapter and show their importance to nursing in A & E.

If we start at the assessment stage, we are largely involved with obtaining information from and about the patient. The ease with which an assessment interview is conducted, and to some extent the physical signs that are displayed (for example, pulse and blood pressure), will be affected by the emotional state of the patient. We have already seen that nurses can act as a major controlling influence upon emotion by the cues they provide to the emotionally aroused patient and relatives. Some knowledge about human perception should make the nurse aware of the pitfalls that lie in wait for us in our perception of others: nurses need to beware stereotypes and first impressions, take into account the patient's environment and its likely effect upon his or her behaviour, and avoid the temptation to make judgemental assessments. Finally, the nurse should remember that people have different ways of using English depending upon their class background, with the result that a meaning that may be perfectly clear to the nurse may be completely baffling to the patient. The reverse situation also applies.

In planning patient care, there is a need to consider how best to avoid creating fears and phobias, especially in children, by inadvertent classical conditioning. The use of modelling or behaviourist techniques such as positive reinforcement and extinction should be considered in modifying behaviour both with staff or patients. In planning for maximum recall of information, the various aspects of memory theory have an important place. One final area of planning where psychological knowledge is of importance is in planning for the care of bereaved relatives.

A major problem in A & E is pain. As we have seen this must be assessed in terms of what the patient says it is, rather than what we think it ought to be. A pain scale could be used, with patients asked to rate their pain from 0 (no pain) to 5 (most severe imaginable). This permits reassessment of the effectiveness of our pain relief. While there will be many physical interventions discussed in this book that can relieve pain, we should remember that keeping the patient informed about what is happening, and other measures to reduce anxiety, will have a very beneficial effect in reducing pain levels.

In evaluating the effectiveness of our nursing interventions, we need to take into account again the misperceptions and language problems that can arise from code usage being different in patient and nurse, as well as from the 'jargon-speak' that the patient cannot understand. Evaluation of effectiveness in pain reduction must take into account differences of culture—it would be a mistake to judge non-Europeans by European standards, or South Europeans by North European standards and so on.

This chapter has looked at some of the aspects of psychology that may allow the A & E nurse to see patients in a different light, and to understand better the sometimes odd ways in which people behave when under the twin stresses, on the one hand, of acute illness and pain and, on the other hand, of the strange and unfamiliar environment of hospital. It is not the nurse who is ill and to the nurse the hospital is a familiar environment. It is from this dysjunction of experience that many problems arise in A & E that could be resolved with a little consideration of the psychological processes involved.

References and Further Reading

Atkinson R., Atkinson R., Smith E., Hilgard E. (1991). *Introduction to Psychology* 19th edn. New York: Harcourt Brace Jovanovitch.
Bandura A. (1973). *Aggression: a Social Learning Analysis*. Englewood Cliffs, NJ: Prentice-Hall.
Bandura A. (1986). *Social Foundations of Thought and Action*. Englewood Cliffs NJ: Prentice-Hall.
Coupland N., Coupland J., Giles H., Henwood K. (1988). Accommodating the elderly: invoking and extending a theory. *Language in Society*, **17**.
Hayward J. (1975). *Information: A Prescription Against Pain*. London: RCN.
Heider F. (1958). *The Psychology of Interpersonal Relations*. New York: Riley.
Hewstone M., Antaki C. (1988). Attribution theory and social explanations. In Hewstone M., Stroebe W., Codol J., Stephenson G. (eds) *Introduction to Psychology*. Oxford: Blackwell.
Jacox X. (1979) Assessing pain. *American Journal of Nursing*, **79**, 895–900.
Kübler-Ross E. (1973). *On Death and Dying*. London: Tavistock.
Leyens J. P., Codol J. P. (1988). Social cognition in introduction to social psychology. In Hewstone M., Stroebe W., Codol J. P., Stephenson G. (eds) *Introduction to Psychology*. Oxford: Blackwell.
Luchins A. (1957). Primacy-recency in impression formation. In Houland C. I. (ed.) *The Order of Presentation in Persuasion*. New Haven: Yale University Press.
Murdock B. B. (1962). The serial position effect in free recall. *Journal of Experimental Psychiatry*, **65**, 482–6.
Ross L. (1977). The amateur psychologist and his shortcomings: distortions in the attribution process. In Berkowitz L. (ed.) *Advances in Experimental Social Psychology*, vol. 10. New York: Academic Press.
Saunders C. (1959). *Care of the Dying*. London: Macmillan.
Saxey S. (1986). Nurses response to post op pain. *Nursing*, **1**, 377–81.
Schachter S., Singer J. E. (1962). Cognitive, social and physiological determinants of emotional states. *Psychological Review*, **69**, 379–99.

Walsh M. (1993) Pain and anxiety in A & E attenders. *Nursing Standard*, 7:26, 40–42.
Walsh M., Ford P. (1989). *Nursing Rituals: Research and Rational Actions*. London: Heinemann.

Chapter 3

THE ROLE OF THE NURSE IN A & E

Nye Bevan, the man thought of as the founding father of the NHS, once said that the only difference between a rut and a grave was that one was deeper than the other. Traditional nursing practice has worn a large number of ruts, some of which must be very deep by now, and A & E nursing is probably not exempt from this problem. However, if we wish to prevent ruts from turning into graves containing a nursing practice that is lifeless, then nursing needs to think anew about its role and rationale.

The aim of this chapter is to explore some new ways of looking at nursing and how such ideas can be of use in the A & E department.

Models of Nursing and their Application in A & E

Any profession must have well-established theoretical foundations. Nursing is no exception to this rule and vague notions about 'helping people get better' or 'assisting the doctor' are not adequate foundations. If nursing is to be taken seriously as a profession it must be able to answer the question 'What is nursing?' There should be a logical and coherent description of what is uniquely nursing, i.e. a model. The last two decades have seen a range of nursing models proposed but, as Walsh (1991) has argued, there is no one superior model that overrides the others. Rather it is about seeing models as loose frameworks that guide care delivery and choosing those which best suit the needs of the patients being cared for. Nurses may develop their own models or make up hybrids by synthesizing key components from differing models that are most appropriate to their own clinical area.

In A & E work, nurses are often confronted with a patient who will be going home from the department. This means that he or she will have to be responsible for *self-care* in conjunction with family and others. Patients may be thought of as being on a continuum of dependency: as they recover from their injury or illness, the amount of care that they need performing for them by others will decrease, while the amount of self-care that they can perform will increase. The model of nursing that most closely reflects the needs of A & E patients is, therefore, that due to Dorothea Orem (1991) which is based around the concept of self-care.

In normal circumstances Orem suggests human beings look after themselves in a variety of ways which she calls Universal Self-Care Demands, e.g. providing an adequate intake of air, fluids and food. She goes on to suggest though that we practise self-care in two other very important areas: development and growth, and coping with illness. These areas are known as Developmental and Health Deviancy Self-Care Demands. Assessment of patients therefore needs to consider whether they can achieve self-care in these areas and, where this is not possible, nursing care is required to help patients bridge their self-care gap or deficit.

Orem views nursing as moving from a wholly compensatory phase when the patient has no active role in meeting self-care demands, through to a partly compensatory phase, and on to a final educational-developmental stage where the nurse is providing advice and teaching to allow the patient to achieve full self-care. This view is very appropriate for A & E, as is Orem's inclusion, of the family and significant others in assisting the patient to meet self-care demands, given that the destination of most A & E patients is home.

Orem encourages nurses to anticipate potential problems and to include the family circumstances in care planning, and most important of all, she urges nurses to think about how the patient will manage *on their own at home* (or on the ward if they are to be admitted). Orem's model promotes the idea of nursing care in parallel to the normal process of recovery and rehabilitation from injury as the patient hopefully becomes less dependent with the passage of time. It gives a concise and relevant assessment model from which can be derived care that will help nurses to avoid the sort of pitfalls that are all too familiar in A & E—such as when the patient returns a few days later with their plaster of Paris or dressings in disarray, or when they fail to keep their appointment or to take their medication (e.g. antibiotics), or when they are brought back by the family as 'just unable to cope'. The common denominator for these sort of care failures is that the patient could not practise adequate self-care because either they were not given the information that was necessary in a way they could understand, or because the self-care targets that were set were unrealistic.

Orem's model will be used throughout the book in the hope that it will be possible to show how to avoid these sorts of self-care problems, and at the same time to have a sound theoretical basis for the process of nursing in A & E. Other nursing models may be used in A & E however and Sbaih (1992) has reported the successful use of Minshull's (1986) Human Needs Model which is derived from Maslow's work on motivation and human need (1954).

Care Planning in A & E

Ward-based staff will be familiar with the notion of the nursing process as a logical sequence of assessing the patient, working out patient problems, setting patient goals, writing down necessary interventions to achieve those goals and then evaluating care to assess its effectiveness. The aim is to provide individualized care for each patient. This has recently been allied to the notion of primary nursing whereby each patient has a nurse who takes total responsibility for planning his/her care. There is much more to primary nursing than that of course and the concept has been critically reviewed by Ford and Walsh (1994) who, while recognizing many strengths in such an approach, also point out significant problems, not least of which is the lack of research evidence that shows primary nursing makes any difference to the quality of care delivered.

The application of these two concepts to the A & E field is possible but only after careful thought and adaptation to suit the very different care environment that is A & E.

A typically busy A & E unit sees approximately 200 patients a day. To avoid confusion, therefore, it is essential that care is logically organized on an individual basis. The use of task-based care, e.g. having a 'stitch' nurse who does all the stitching, fragments care and leads to confusion over who has done what. The primary nursing approach requires the 'named nurse' to assess the patient on admission, plan and supervise his or her care throughout and ensure a satisfactory discharge.

Primary nursing is said to have many advantages: it improves communications and reduces the risks of parts of the patient's care being overlooked because 'I thought someone else was doing it'. It also gives the patient a feeling of security and should allow any changes in condition to be noted more readily.

The nurse who is accountable for an individual's care needs to have a method of planning that care and where necessary charting progress. The traditional, time-consuming, repetitive writing of care plans according to the dogma of the nursing process has been extensively criticized (Ford and Walsh, 1994) and is clearly not appropriate in A & E. This is confirmed by research carried out by Sbaih (1992) who found formal care planning in A & E far too time consuming.

There are two approaches to care planning and documentation in A & E. For many patients it is sufficient that the planning of care goes on inside the nurse's head with anything that needs writing down briefly noted on the patient's A & E notes alongside the medical notes. As professional staff, it is ridiculous to expect nurses to write down every single step in planning care for every single patient!

A typical example will illustrate the point. A young woman with a painful swollen ankle is diagnosed by the doctor as not having broken any bones, but she still has to get home and is in need of some pain relief. A quick assessment should reveal that she is walking with a painful limp, and it is 4 miles to home. Setting goals for the patient is the next step, and without recourse to paper, it is obvious that the goals are that the patient will get home and will experience relief of pain. The nurses plan and implement care around these two goals; they decide upon a tubular support bandage, coupled with advice about rest, analgesics and elevation to relieve pain, and offer the patient the use of a telephone to ring a friend to come and collect her or to book a taxi.

In setting goals, nurses must set a time limit for meaningful evaluation to occur (possibly, one hour and six hours respectively in this case), and in order for objective evaluation to be possible, the goals must be couched in terms of observable patient behaviour. By defining the nursing care goals in terms of patient behaviour and by setting time limits, evaluation has been made quite easy. For example, if the patient is still sitting in the A & E department two hours later, the part of the care plan concerning transport has failed; while if, after being instructed to return if the pain does not ease, the patient returns the following day, then either the instructions about rest and elevation were not properly understood, or something more substantial than a support bandage was needed, e.g. a plaster of Paris.

This common example shows how it is possible to *think* the nursing process and implement it without the need for documentation. Alternatively, the nurses could have noted the doctor's cryptic instruction 'DTG' (Double Tubigrip), not planned individualized care, bandaged the ankle in the same way that all sprained ankles are strapped up ('We always do it this way, why should she be any different?'), and left the patient limping precariously to the door clutching a shoe in one hand, with no idea of how she is going to get home or what to do about her still painful ankle when she gets there. Such an approach leads to poor care of an unacceptable standard.

Having seen that one way of looking at care planning in A & E is to see it as a way of thinking about nursing rather than a bureaucratic chore, it now remains to examine one other way of implementing planned care in A & E. If we consider the patient with more substantial problems (e.g. burns, chest pain, a fracture), then it is clear that some documentation of care is needed. The time involved in writing out an individual care plan in each such case in a busy A & E unit is prohibitive. However, it is possible to recognize many similarities in the care requirements of groups of patients with the same complaint such as a burn or chest pain. This led to the idea of *standardized care plans*, drawn up in advance and based on the common elements that are expected to be found in the care of each complaint.

The Registered Nurses Association of British Columbia drew up a series of such care plans (1977), and noted that the time saved by having standard plans ready in advance permitted more time to be spent dealing with individual problems in each patient's case.

The advantages claimed for this standardized care plan approach also included giving new staff a framework of care to follow, a reliable assessment guide, improved communication with wards receiving patients from A & E while retaining space to deal with problems unique to the individual.

In recent years the concept of critical pathways has grown out of standardized care planning. Nelson (1993) has reviewed their use in A & E and describes a critical pathway (CP) as a chart showing the expected key stages in a patient's pathway through A & E, set within an expected time frame. Different CPs can be developed for different presenting conditions such as chest pain, acute respiratory distress or a fracture of the lower limb. Actual writing by the nurse is confined to charting by exception, i.e. documenting variations on that which is expected to happen.

Critical pathways should be developed by experienced nursing and medical staff meeting as a group and identifying the major, common, presenting conditions for which CPs are needed. They should then set down the ideal stages, with time limits, for treating a patient with a given condition. It is then necessary to review actual practice in the department and assign a realistic time frame to progress in order that the CP remains realistic. The CP then needs documenting in such a way that there is space to chart variations upon patient progress. An example is given in Fig. 3.1.

The CPs can in this way be written to meet the standards and expectations of staff locally as well as incorporating national protocols and guidelines. Examples of CPs will be used in the book as chapter summaries. The reader is invited to try and develop real CPs for their own department as a means of giving structure and planning to care while also providing a documentary record which does not consume vast amounts of nursing time. Critical pathways can also be incorporated into quality assurance work as they represent a powerful standard setting tool. Staff should however think carefully about the time targets that are set in order that idealism is tempered with realism.

The Expanded Role of the Nurse in A & E

As medical theory and practice have advanced over the years, there has been a steady pressure on nursing to keep pace with medicine, and for nurses to be prepared to learn and practise new skills. It was not that long ago, for example, that it was thought that only a doctor could take a blood pressure. Many nurses themselves are also pushing for the expansion and development of the nursing role. This was recognized by the UKCC with the publication of their Scope of Professional Practice document (1992) which has signalled a move away from the sterile extended role debates of the past. The key to nurses expanding their role lies in accountability for practice coupled with recognition by nurses of the limits of their own competence. Education must underpin this development and the UKCC document Post Registration Education for Practice (1994) clearly points the way to developing advanced nurse practice in A & E, supported by education reaching Master's Degree level.

	0–5 min	6–15 min	16–40 min
Documentation	Registration as A & E patient	Notes ready for CO to write in	Completed for transfer CCU
Assessment	See triage nurse BP, P, PR recorded as baseline	Undressed 12 lead ECG. CO exams patient Patient on ECG monitor Blood taken	Vital signs checked ECG monitor XR form written, to have portable CXR on CCU
Medication	–	IV diamorphine 5 mg IV prochlorperazine 12.5 mg	–
Treatment	–	Venflon sited heparinized Oxygen 40%	–
Nursing care	Welcome patient Psychological support	Explain procedures Psychological support Ensure patient comfort	Continue
Referrals	–	On call med reg contacted	Med reg sees patient
Family	Ask if family know patient's whereabouts		See patient if present Informed of admission to CCU
Discharge	–	–	CCU informed of patient admission Porters called Transfer CCU with nurse escort

Variation in care

Name   John Smith   *A & E No.* 12345
Date/Time of admission   April 7 1994, 1430 hrs

Time	Variance	Cause
1440	28% O_2 administered	Patient has history of chronic obstructive airways disease
1630	Transfer to CCU delayed 2 hrs from admission	No bed available on CCU

Fig. 3.1   Example of critical pathway for patient with chest pain of probable myocardial origin

Triage and the A & E Nurse

Patients attending A & E do so with a wide range of conditions. It is therefore essential that there is a system to ensure those who need immediate medical attention receive it. The converse of this is that those that can afford to wait may do so in order that people with urgent needs are seen promptly. Placing people in order of priority for treatment is known as triage and it has increasingly become a nursing responsibility. A typical quality standard might be that patients should be seen by a triage nurse within 10 minutes of registration, who will then assess them and decide priority for treatment. A private area for triage is essential rather than carrying out the assessment in front of a busy waiting room which may prove distracting and embarrassing for the patient

Evidence to support the feasibility of triage consists of studies such as that by James and Pyrgos (1989) who found that when experienced nurses (but without the benefit of any special training in assessment) assessed and prioritized a sample of 332 ambulatory A & E patients, their ratings agreed in 97% of cases with independently carried out medical assessments. Triage work is very stressful (Rock and Pledge, 1991) and consideration of the UKCC Scope of Professional Practice document (1992) makes it clear that nurses must receive suitable education before they can be expected to act in this role.

Mallet and Woolwich (1990) described triage as providing early patient assessment, first aid, priority rating, control of patient throughput, initiation of diagnostic measures and liaison with other health professionals. In investigating triage on their unit Mallet and Woolwich showed that 93% of patients were seen by a triage nurse within 11 minutes of registration. These authors then compared overall waiting times in their unit and showed that, as the severity category increased, average waiting time to see a doctor decreased, demonstrating that triage was working and ensuring that those patients whose conditions were most urgent were being seen first.

The triage nurse can also play a major role in defusing potential aggression in A & E. The fact that the patient has seen a nurse within a few minutes of registration is reassuring, while explanations about waiting times will also help dispel unrealistic expectations. The high levels of anxiety and pain experienced by many A & E patients (see p. 28) makes it essential that they receive this immediate attention and psychological support. A significant number of patients may be advised by the triage nurse to seek alternative help such as from a GP or practice nurse.

A worrying feature of A & E work is the proportion of patients who walk out unseen after registration. The triage system ensures all patients are assessed which greatly reduces the risk of a person with a serious health problem walking out because s/he would not wait any longer and did not appreciate the risk to their health. (The author recalls seeing one patient who had come to A & E complaining of toothache; he looked pale and breathless, rapid triage put him top priority and within 30 minutes he was on the coronary care unit!) Walsh (1990) has shown that, in a large urban A & E unit which did not practise a formal triage system at the time, 8.2% of ambulatory adult patients walked out unseen. This figure was closely correlated with how busy the department was, reaching over 12% (i.e. 1 in 8) in busy periods. Further research (Walsh, 1993) showed this group of patients did not differ significantly from those who stayed but only 64% subsequently saw a doctor with their problem. It is a worrying thought that, amongst the 36% who did not, there might be some significant ill health that has escaped medical and nursing attention. The triage nurse system could reduce this risk by a large amount.

The A & E Nurse Practitioner

The nurse practitioner is a nurse working independently of medical supervision who is fully accountable for his/her practice (Stillwell and Bowling, 1988). This autonomous role was originally pioneered in the UK in general practice (Stillwell et al., 1987, 1988; Salisbury and Tattersall, 1988) and clearly has great potential in A & E which is where the hospital service and primary health care meet. Woolwich (1992) considers the A & E nurse practitioner as making a vital contribution to the unit by seeing patients with a range of minor conditions and chronic complaints and offering treatment, advice, health education or referral on to other appropriate agencies including the person's own GP or to a casualty officer in A & E.

Some idea of how such a scheme may work may be gained from reading the account of Covington and Sellars (1992) who described how a system of nurse triage and the option of a 'fast track' to see a nurse practitioner rather than a doctor, greatly reduced complaints and walkouts, while resulting in high levels of reported patient satisfaction.

It is important to stress that the A & E nurse practitioner is not a cheap substitute for a doctor nor is s/he an assistant doctor. The person remains a nurse above all else, but practising independently as an equal member of the care team rather than a subordinate to the doctor (the obvious comparison is with the way midwives function). To develop this role in the future there must be close cooperation between medical and nursing staff with agreed protocols for treatment and assessment. Further education is essential and it should be at a minimum of first degree level. Agreement with other professional groups such as radiographers and pharmacists is needed concerning the way developing nursing autonomy impacts upon their sphere of activity. For example, the nurse practitioner should be able to order X-rays and prescribe from an agreed formulary. It is encouraging that in a sample of 48 A & E doctors and nurses drawn from two large but very different A & E units, Walsh (1993) found 98% of staff supported the notion of developing the A & E nurse practitioner role.

The A & E Nurse as a Communicator

How often is a failure in care explained away by statements such as 'nobody told me, so how was I supposed to know?' Communication is an essential ingredient in health care. Reference has already been made to how sociological and psychological factors can impair effective communication with patients and to how, therefore, these factors should be taken into account in planning patient care. Much patient non-compliance is explicable in terms of communication failure, rather than a patient's desire to be 'awkward'.

The development of communication skills is an essential part of nursing and, it could be argued, in no area is communication more important than in A & E. The majority of A & E patients leave A & E to go home, where nurses have no control over subsequent events. The use of a self-care focused model of nursing such as Orem's in conjunction with primary nursing will help minimize the risk of care failures, but effective communication is also essential if the patient is to understand what is required in terms of self-care after discharge.

A key aspect of communication is the nurse as interpreter of the hospital experience for the patient. For the majority of the general public, the hospital environment is strange and frightening and this is especially true for the elderly and the young. The nurse therefore has a vital role to play in interpreting this experience so that the patient can make sense out of what is being said and done. Patient compliance will tend to increase with patient understanding.

Moving outward from the patient, there are whole networks of communication involving other professional groups and agencies— for example, doctors, social workers, ward staff, the ambulance service and the police—that the A & E nurse will have to communicate with on the patient's behalf. Aids to communication within the unit include the use of a marker board system whereby each cubicle is numbered and, by having a similarly numbered marker board plan on the wall which is kept up-dated with each patient's progress, it is possible to keep track of any patient's progress, regardless of how busy the department may be.

An effective way of improving communication with the ambulance service is to send staff out with the ambulance service for experience while at the same time inviting ambulance crews to spend time in the A & E department. Similar exchanges of staff prove successful with community and practice nurses, while the setting up of liaison committees to discuss mutual problems at regular meetings with, for example, the police or psychiatric service, can prove very effective. In short, A & E nurses must realize that they do not work in isolation, but need the effective cooperation of various other groups of staff. It is in the patient's interests if nurses take the initiative in seeking improved communication and understanding with other agencies.

The A & E Nurse and the Law

The police are one agency with whom the A & E nurse will have many dealings, and such is the nature of police interest in some patients that there are going to be occasions when difficult dilemmas of confidentiality arise. On the one hand, it is essential to have a good working relationship with the police, but on the other hand, there is the question of patient confidentiality and police access to information.

If a patient feels that what he or she tells a nurse is genuinely in confidence, and will not be immediately repeated to the police, vital clinical information may be forthcoming that would otherwise be withheld. Examples are in drug use, where it may be essential to know what drugs have been taken, the route and timing of administration, and in wounding cases, where information about the real manner in which the injury was sustained may be withheld, leading to inappropriate treatment and nursing care.

Nursing and medical records have been traditionally held as confidential. This includes the A & E Register, which on occasion the police may wish to access. This should not be allowed without the consent of the hospital management. Where records have been computerised the close controls of the Data Protection Act also apply. Enquiries about the names and addresses of patients who have attended A & E are best passed on to management, although details of patients involved in a road traffic accident (RTA) may be released directly to the police as this is required under law. The police must also be immediately notified of incidents involving firearms and suspected terrorism.

On occasions staff may suspect that a patient has sustained injuries in the act of carrying out a crime which the police are either unaware of or are enquiring about. This is a most difficult situation (unless it involves firearms, terrorism or a RTA as mentioned previously) as the demands of patients' confidentiality are such that theoretically nothing should be said to the police. However the nurse is also a citizen and, as a citizen, has certain responsibilities before the law. As Dimond (1990, p. 281) points out, 'The professions owe a duty to society which takes precedence over the duty owed to the patient.' There can be no hard and fast rules and each case must be treated on its merits, but if there is a strong suspicion that an individual has been involved in criminal activity, then a nurse should discuss the case with the doctor responsible for the patient, and a joint approach should be made to a senior manager or the consultant in charge. The Police and Criminal Evidence Act permits the police in serious cases to compel the hospital to produce personal information and even samples of human tissue (Dimond, 1990).

An example will illustrate the point. A rather scruffy young man comes to A & E with a cut leg. There is a large laceration through the back of his right calf and also through his jeans. The wound is obviously fresh and still bleeding. The friend who is accompanying the patient disappears for coffee while the patient explains his injury in vague terms of 'falling through a hedge'. At this stage the nurse's suspicions are aroused as the wound and story do not match. Enter a policeman and a rather distressed young woman with the story that the woman has just come home to find two men burgling her flat. They broke a window in making their escape, and one of them cut himself in the process. The flat is only a few hundred yards from A & E and the police have followed the blood trail to the front door. Meanwhile a nurse is applying a dressing to the leg, the wound having been sutured. A decision is needed quickly. This real example was dealt with by checking that the woman felt able to identify the men in question, followed by the suggestion that if the police wanted to wait by the main entrance, discreetly out of view, the young woman may be able to identify the men in question in the next few minutes. This was acceptable to the police who easily arrested the two men.

This example shows that, by using initiative and common sense, an awkward situation may be resolved satisfactorily.

Collecting evidence is another area of police work that the A & E nurse will come into contact with. Patient clothing may contain vital evidence and every effort should be made to preserve it. In the resuscitation room, it is often cut off the patient, but if possible this should be done in such a way as to leave undisturbed existing tears or holes as these may give clues as to the weapon used in an assault, for example. Clothing offers clues in 'hit and run' cases as it may contain traces of paint from the offending vehicle, while in shootings there will be gunpowder stains on clothes if the gun is fired from a range of less than three feet. Such evidence is vital to corroborate verbal testimony. Even shoes offer potential evidence, for there may be footprints found near the scene of the crime.

All possessions and clothing must, therefore, be safely labelled and stored, for if such evidence is to be admissible in court, it must be possible to establish continuity, otherwise there is the possibility of the evidence being 'planted'. A & E staff will be required to make statements in order to establish continuity of evidence, so the nurse should make mental notes of what is done with clothing and patient possessions during the course of a resuscitation attempt if there is suspicion of foul play.

One problem that commonly occurs involving police is when they want to breathalyse a car driver injured in an accident. As in other cases, they must have the consent of the casualty officer before they can proceed to administer a breathalyser test. If the patient has suffered significant facial trauma, the doctor may refuse consent for a breathalyser if in their opinion the patient's injuries will interfere with the ability to give a full and proper breath sample. However the nurse should be aware that it is not unknown for patients in this situation to offer bribes to A & E staff in an attempt to persuade them to deny the police a breathalyser test. If blood tests are required by the police, a police surgeon will be called to the department to take the necessary samples.

It is essential that there should be a good working relationship between police and A & E nurses, and this relationship may be assisted by trying to see things from the other side's point of view.

Turning away from matters involving the police to more general considerations of legal matters, readers should note that the legal aspects of treating patients against their will are covered in Chapter 17. However, this only refers to the Mental Health Act (1983) and does not cover the situation where the patient is a child or young person under 18.

Young people aged 16 or 17 may give valid consent for any treatment but not for participation in a research project unless it can genuinely be considered to be part of the treatment (Dimond, 1990). For those aged under 16 the situation is no longer as clear cut as it used to be when it was assumed that parental consent was always necessary for treatment unless in an emergency. In 1985, the Gillick Case, cited by Dimond (1990), led to a ruling in the House of Lords that, in some cases, mature minors under 16 who are capable of understanding the situation, can give valid consent. The safest course of action for the A & E nurse appears to be always to act in the best interest of the child, whilst recognizing the need for parental consent to be obtained normally, unless in emergencies.

In the rare case where parents refuse to consent to treatment which is clearly in the child's interests, the hospital authorities may apply to the courts for an interim care order or to have the child made a ward of court in order for treatment to proceed. This covers objections to blood transfusion on religious grounds for example. The difficult area of suspected child abuse will be covered in Chapter 12; suffice it to say here that every A & E unit should have a clearly understood policy drawn up with the local social services department and the police to cover such cases.

The situation may also arise where an adult patient refuses treatment, even though their life may be endangered by so doing. An example seen in A & E is the patient who has deliberately taken an overdose of medication or other drugs and who refuses treatment or admission. Davis (1993) points out that, although patients are legally entitled to refuse treatment, this right is poorly protected in law as the issue of how rational the patient is in making such a decision allows medical and nursing staff the opportunity to override the patient's wishes. There are strong professional arguments that make nurses and doctors attempt to intervene to prevent suicide although Davis (1993) considers that if the suicidal patient is competent, then legally s/he could be left to die. Treatment which involves touching the patient without his or her consent, according to Young (1991), entitles the patient to sue for battery. Young (1991) considers that the law tends to support the patient's refusal of consent but without considering the nurse in such a situation negligent if s/he respects the patient's wishes.

Davis (1993) rightly considers the A & E nurse to be caught in a moral and legal minefield when considering various ethical principles, the law and the UKCC Code of Professional Conduct. She recommends that the A & E nurse tries to ensure that the patient fully understands the consequences of refusing treatment and assesses the patient's level of insight into the situation. In this way refusal of consent could be said to be a rational and informed act. However, if in doubt, Davis advises the nurse to err on the side of life and rely on the defence of necessity. It might be added that membership of a professional trades union will greatly assist such a defence in the event of an attempt to sue the nurse subsequently.

It is understandable that nurses are often concerned about the risk of legal action being taken against them for neglect or malpractice, i.e. being sued for damages. It should be noted that part of being a professional is being responsible for your actions. On many counts A & E nurses feel particularly vulnerable to legal action being taken against them, and certainly many general letters of complaint are written about A & E staff to hospitals, which contain a wide range of allegations. Although all the nursing trade unions will support their members, it is strongly recommended here that all A & E staff belong to the Royal College of Nursing in order to obtain the benefit of their professional indemnity insurance cover and also to ensure that if complaints are made at local level, they are well represented by an RCN steward. Such representation is essential if staff are to have a fair hearing. The RCN also has a very active A & E Association, a section formed specially for A & E nursing staff.

With regard to the problems of negligence, the legal view is that, provided a nurse behaves in such a way as could be *reasonably* expected for a nurse of that position, then whatever the outcome, they are not guilty of negligence. The whole issue hinges on the principle of the nurse's actions being *reasonable*: it is reasonable to expect a qualified nurse to recognize a patient in cardiac arrest, but not reasonable to expect a qualified nurse with no training in the skill to intubate that patient.

An argument that is frequently aired is whether a nurse who witnesses an accident or other emergency situation should stop to render first aid. The debate is about the nurse's competence in first aid. Castledine (1993) has rightly argued that the nurse must help in any way possible as s/he has a moral duty to do so and the UKCC Code of Conduct requires him/her to so do. Castledine cites the case of a nurse who walked past an accident and was reported to the UKCC for not helping. The UKCC found her guilty of professional misconduct and disciplined her, although not striking her off the register. It is incomprehensible that an A & E nurse could ignore an accident and not stop to help for fear of legal repercussions if something went wrong. Such an attitude is inconsistent with the caring ethic that underpins nursing. The author has had first-hand experience of such situations and is dismayed at the legalistic arguments of Beattie (1993) who took issue with Castledine's views. Beattie is however correct to call for all nurses to have more first aid training, but it is sad that she does not recognize that A & E nurses are the experts who can give such training. Application of the simple principles of first aid and basic life support are a moral and professional duty for all nurses, at all times, in all situations.

The situation can be summarized by saying that, provided the nurse adheres to the twin principles of acting in what is perceived to be the best interests of the patient (adult or child) and only attempting to do things which could be reasonably expected of her or him in the light of their experience and training, then, coupled with adherence to Trust policy and membership of the RCN, the nurse should stay out of any serious legal trouble.

Health Education and the A & E Nurse

The National Health Service has been criticized for being a National Ill Health Service, i.e. for emphasizing treatment and attempting to cure once a person is ill and for not paying enough attention to the *prevention* of illness.

At present in many parts of the western world, the demand for health care is growing faster than the resources available to meet that demand; the UK is no exception. It is therefore essential to pursue vigorously a policy of prevention in order to try to reduce health demands. It should be noted here, however, that the other side of the coin is campaigning for greater resources to be made available for health care, which means becoming involved in the political process. A dual approach is needed, and nursing as the major caring profession has a responsibility to be in the forefront of both aspects of the campaign for better health.

The government's Health of the Nation initiative (DoH, 1992a) is a commendable attempt to reduce ill health. One of the key areas identified is the need to reduce accidents. Particular groups targeted are children under 15, young people aged 15 to 24 and the over 65s where targets of reducing the death rate from accidents by 33%, 25% and 33% respectively have been set. The DoH handbook on accidents (1992b) stresses the role of A & E staff in helping with accident prevention work, whilst nurses are clearly crucial in their health education role with regard to all the Health of the Nation targets besides the field of accidents (e.g. sexual health, smoking-related diseases).

The A & E nurse is in a very advantageous position to carry out health education. He or she will come in contact with many more members of the general public in a day's work than will most other nurses. Furthermore, the people that A & E nurses are dealing with will tend to be motivated by the fact that they have just had a first-hand experience of illness or trauma; they will therefore in most cases be receptive to advice about health or accident prevention.

Simple first aid is one obvious area in which the A & E nurse can carry out health education. Patients still come to A & E with burns covered in butter or toothpaste, with fractured arms where there has been no attempt at splintage, with dressings that are effectively tourniquets that lead to blue hands, or even with tourniquets to control bleeding from simple lacerations. The sight of a patient vomiting the hot sweet tea and brandy that was poured down their throat by a well-intentioned person is still all too common. The nurse has a major responsibility in explaining to the patient about the need to complete a course of anti-tetanus vaccine commenced in A & E, while patients starting a course of antibiotics must have the consequences of not completing the course explained to them. In addition to advice about first aid and medication, there are many other areas where the A & E nurse has a real preventative role, such as in advice about smoking, alcohol and drug problems, contraception, obesity and how to make the best use of social services and GPs.

In the future, health care will become increasingly a matter of prevention and the A & E nurse, far from being merely a 'picker-up of pieces', should use the opportunities that present themselves daily to promote health. Health education is rightly emphasized by Orem as an essential part of the self-care approach to health.

References

Beattie J. (1993). Should nurses walk away from the scene of an accident? *British Journal of Nursing*, 2, 607.
Castledine G. (1993). Ethical implications of first aid. *British Journal of Nursing*, 2, 239–41.
Covington C., Sellars F. (1992). Implementation of a nurse practitioner staffed fast track. *Journal of Emergency Nursing*, 18, 124–31.
Davis J. (1993). Ethical and legal issues in suicide. *British Journal of Nursing*, 2, 777–80.
Dimond B. (1990). *Legal Aspects of Nursing*. London: Prentice-Hall.
DoH (1992). *The Health of the Nation*. London: HMSO.
DoH (1992). *Key Area Handbook: Accidents*. London: HMSO.
Ford P., Walsh M. (1994). *New Rituals for Old: Nursing Through the Looking Glass*. Oxford, Butterworth Heinemann.
James M., Pyrgos N. (1989). Nurse practitioners in the A & E department. *Archives of Emergency Medicine*, 6, 241–6.
Mallet J., Woolwich C. (1990). Triage in A & E departments. *Journal of Advanced Nursing*, 15, 1443–51.
Maslow A. (1954). *Motivation and Personality*. London: Harper and Row.
Minshull J., Ross K., Turner J. (1986) The human needs model of nursing. *Journal of Advanced Nursing*, 11, 643–9.
Nelson M. (1993). Critical pathways in the emergency department. *Journal of Emergency Nursing*, 19, 110–14.
Orem D. (1991). *Nursing: Concepts of Practice*. St Louis: C. V. Mosby.
Rock D., Pledge M. (1991). Priorities of care for the walking wounded. *Professional Nurse*, May 1991, 463–5.
Salisbury C., Tattersall M. (1988). Comparison of the work of a nurse practitioner and a general practitioner. *Journal of the Royal College of General Practitioners*, 38, 314–16.
Sbaih L. (1992). *Accident and Emergency Nursing: A Nursing Model*. London, Chapman and Hall.
Stillwell B., Bowling A. (1988). *The Nurse in Family Practice*. London: Scutari.
Stillwell B., Drury M., Greenfield S., Hull F. (1987). A nurse practitioner

in general practice: working style and consultation patterns. *Journal of the Royal College of General Practitioners*, **37**, 154–7.

Stillwell B., Drury M., Greenfield S., Hull F. (1988). A nurse practitioner in general practice: patient perceptions and expectations. *Journal of the Royal College of General Practitioners*, **38**, 503–5.

UKCC (1992). *Scope of Professional Practice*, London: UKCC.

UKCC (1994). *Post Registration Education for Practice*. London: UKCC.

Walsh M. (1990). Why do people go to A & E? *Nursing Standard*, **5**, 24–8.

Walsh M. (1991). *Models in Clinical Nursing: The Way Forward*. London: Baillière Tindall.

Walsh M. (1993). Patient' views of their A & E experience. *Nursing Standard*, **7**, 30–32.

Woolwich (1992). A wider frame of reference. *Nursing Times*, **88**, 34–6.

Young A. (1991). *Law and Professional Conduct in Nursing*. London: Scutari.

Critical Care

4 Nursing Care of the Critically Injured Patient

5 Nursing Care of the Critically III Patient

NURSING CARE OF THE CRITICALLY INJURED PATIENT

The arrival in A & E of a critically injured patient is potentially one of the most difficult situations that can confront an A & E nurse, especially as several patients often arrive together from the same incident. If the nurse in charge does not take a firm, confident grip on the situation at the outset, chaos and confusion can result.

The requirement, therefore, is for a plan of action, known to all members of the A & E team, which will identify and prioritize the major life-threatening problems and the interventions required around these problems. Such a plan involves the well-known ABC checklist of resuscitation—Airway, Breathing and Circulation—and continues with Consciousness (head injury), Spinal injury and Abdominal injury. A rapid primary survey must be carried out of these critical areas. At all times during resuscitation, the universal precautions for the prevention of blood-borne disease must be observed.

Airway

Pathology

If the patient's airway is obstructed, all other considerations are of secondary importance and immediate intervention to clear the airway is required. Common causes of obstruction are vomitus, blood, inhaled material such as food or dentures, and soft tissue trauma affecting the neck or respiratory tract. This trauma can be caused by the inhalation of flames or of hot or noxious gases leading to burns of the trachea, by insect stings in the upper respiratory tract, or by a blow to the neck. The unconscious patient will be far less able to protect his or her airway than the patient who is conscious.

Assessment

Airway obstruction is the first step in assessing the A & E patient. Obvious respiratory distress, cyanosis, stridor, the history of the incident and the patient's level of consciousness are all relevant facts in assessing airway patency. The sound of the patient's voice is also important. Is it hoarse? Laryngoscopy should not be performed as it may provoke spasm of the epiglottis or vocal cords. Shining a pen torch into the open mouth is the most appropriate way to examine the upper respiratory tract. Frequency and depth of respirations are important parameters for the nurse to record.

Intervention

The first intervention is to clear the airway for the patient. This can be done manually with the aid of forceps or a gloved hand or with the aid of a wide bore, rigid sucker (e.g. a Yankaur sucker). Dentures often cause obstruction. In the case of an unconscious patient, the airway can be readily cleared by the chin lift or jaw thrust method. This action will pull the tongue away from the posterior pharynx. In the event of an unsuccessful injury the team should assume a cervical injury until proven otherwise and the head and neck should be stabilized in a correct alignment. Watson (1991) cites evidence to indicate there is a 5 to 10% chance of cervical injury in cases of blunt trauma to the head region. This emphasizes the importance of immobilizing the neck.

In serious cases of trauma to the neck region leading to an airway obstruction not amenable to clearance by manual or suction methods (e.g. soft tissue swelling), the medical staff may require assistance with a needle cricothyrotomy. Needle cricothyrotomy involves making a temporary (and possibly life-saving) entry into the trachea with a large bore (e.g. 14 G) IV cannula attached to a 10 ml syringe which applies a gentle negative pressure. The point of insertion is about 3 cm below the laryngeal prominence (the Adam's apple). After air is observed to fill the syringe, indicating entry into the trachea, the IV cannula can then be connected via an IVI giving set to an oxygen source. Baskett (1993) advocates using a second needle to facilitate exhalation. Such a procedure can 'buy' the time needed to set up for a tracheotomy. The A & E resuscitation room should have the equipment ready to perform both procedures, and the A & E nurse must know where the equipment is and what is required.

Once the airway is clear, the next intervention is to maintain its patency. The unconscious patient can be turned into the lateral position. Great care, however, is needed if there is any suspicion of a spinal injury and, in such cases, patients are best left flat with other means used to maintain their airway. One simple means of doing this is the oropharyngeal airway which will keep the tongue clear of the airway and which will also allow pharyngeal suction to be readily carried out with a long flexible suction catheter. The airway is introduced 'upside-down' into the mouth and then rotated into the correct position as it is slid over the back of the tongue.

The most satisfactory way of maintaining the airway is intubation. In most hospitals, this is a medical task, although ambulance crews are now trained to intubate, and with the development of A & E clinical nurse specialists, it could easily become part of the nurse's role.

At present the A & E nurse must know how to assist with intubation (see Fig. 4.1 for equipment). The first requirement is a muscle relaxant drug, usually suxamethonium, which will be stored in a fridge. The endotracheal tube will often require cutting to length before insertion, so scissors should be kept ready. The laryngoscope blade is then passed on the right side of the midline with the neck extended. The blade is used to elevate the tongue and visualize the glottic opening by pulling forward the jaw at 45°, not by levering on the front teeth. The laryngoscope should be checked every morning to ensure it is working. The tube is introduced into the glottic opening by the right hand. If the tube is too long, there is a danger that it will be introduced into the right bronchus, leaving the left lung unventilated. The cuff of the ET tube must be inflated using a 10 ml syringe, and a Spencer Wells clamp is used to ensure the air stays in the cuff. Once inflated, the cuff protects the airway from aspiration, deep bronchial suction is possible and efficient Intermittent Positive Pressure Ventilation (IPPV) may be performed.

As the patient will now be unable to breathe, because of the effects of the muscle relaxant drugs given to permit intubation, the next need is to connect the ET tube to a bag/mask device (e.g. Ambu bag) and an oxygen source via an adaptor and a catheter mount. It is essential that the A & E nurse have the correct equipment to hand immediately, can connect it together promptly and if need be, can take over ventilating the patient. The nurse should not forget the need for tape to tie and secure the ET tube in place.

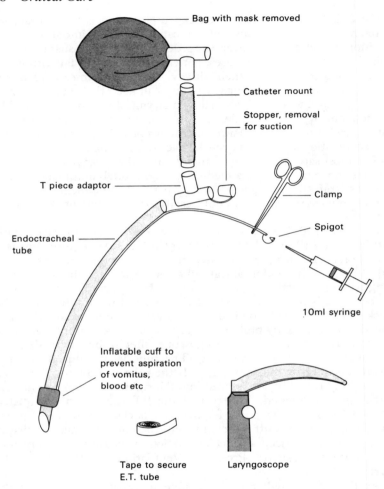

Fig. 4.1   Equipment for intubation and IPPV

Evaluation

Evaluation of the patency of the airway after intervention is crucial. The nurse should check the following. Does the patient's colour improve? What happens to the respiratory rate? Does the chest expand with ventilation in the case of an intubated patient? And is there air entry to both lungs?

Breathing

Pathology

Once the airway is cleared and maintained clear, the next questions are—can the patient breathe normally? And if not, how can the patient be helped to meet this most basic self-care demand? If the patient is making no respiratory effort, the procedure for respiratory arrest must be initiated at once with IPPV. However, the patient may be attempting to breathe but may be suffering from chest trauma which is interfering with normal respiration. If this trauma is serious, it may quickly prove fatal.

A common problem associated with serious chest trauma is pneumothorax in which air gains entry to the potential space of the pleura surrounding a lung. This will lead to the lung's collapse. A pneumothorax can arise spontaneously, without any trauma, due to the rupture of a weakness in the wall of the lung (Fig. 4.2A).

The most serious form of pneumothorax is a tension pneumothorax in which the hole into the pleura acts like a one-way flap valve, permitting air entry to the pleural space but prohibiting any escape of air (Fig. 4.2B). The result is a progressive build-up of pressure in the pleural space which will not only collapse the lung on the affected side, but will exert pressure on the uninjured side, leading to mediastinal shift, possible nipping of major blood vessels and collapse of the other lung.

If bleeding occurs into the pleural space, a haemothorax is said to be present. This too will prevent lung expansion, and often occurs in conjunction with a pneumothorax. The quantity of blood involved may be over one litre, so that in addition to serious respiratory impairment, there may also be hypovolaemic shock.

Rib fractures are an extremely painful condition—so painful that proper chest expansion and coughing will be severely restricted, greatly increasing the risk of chest infection. The very serious condition of a flail segment occurs if there are ribs with double fractures, as one segment of the chest wall will no longer be attached to the rest of the chest (Fig. 4.3). As a result, when there is a lowering of intrathoracic pressure (an essential step in respiration) brought about by expansion of the chest wall, the unattached flail

(a)

Simple hole
allowing air into
pleural space
leading to
collapse of
lung

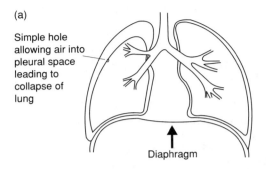

Diaphragm

(b)

Inhaled
air flows
out on
inhalation
into
pleural
space

Normal
pleura

Heart

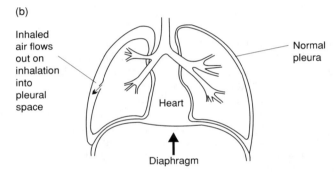

Diaphragm

Collapsed
lung

Tracheal
deviation

Flap closes
on exhalation
trapping
air in
pleural
space

Compression
of good lung
inhibiting
ventilation

Due to
build up
of pressure
from
injured side

Heart

Heart pushed
into normal
lung space,
leading to
kinking of vessels

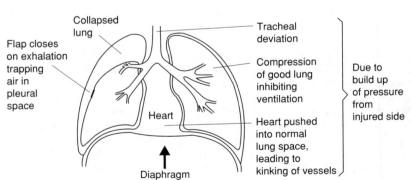

Diaphragm

Fig. 4.2   (a) Spontaneous pneumothorax. (b) Tension pneumothorax

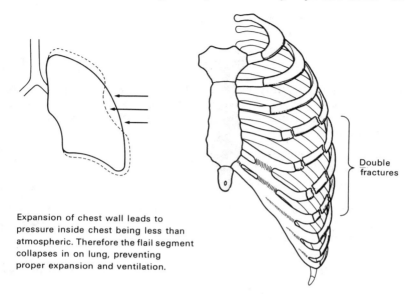

Expansion of chest wall leads to
pressure inside chest being less than
atmospheric. Therefore the flail segment
collapses in on lung, preventing
proper expansion and ventilation.

Double
fractures

Fig. 4.3   Flail segment

segment collapses inwards under atmospheric pressure, as the atmospheric pressure will be greater than the pressure within the thorax. The inward collapse prevents lung expansion. Flail chest can be readily observed as it results in what are known as paradoxical respirations, i.e. a section of chest wall collapsing inwards when the rest of the chest is expanding outwards. A flail segment constitutes a potential life-threatening emergency, especially as it is often associated with a haemo- or pneumothorax.

Within the lung tissue itself, trauma can cause respiratory impairment in several ways. Major blood vessels may be damaged due to penetrating injury or severe deceleration stresses. Lung tissue may be contused, leading to the extravasation of blood into the parenchyma which in turn will cause anoxia of the tissue. If a high pressure blast wave passes through the lung, the Spalding effect will produce what amounts to implosion of the alveolar walls leading to massive damage and pulmonary oedema which can be rapidly fatal. This effect must be looked for in all victims of explosions. Finally, there is the possibility of the inhalation of material deep into the lung tissue. This material can range from water in drowning victims to noxious gases in burns cases.

Assessment

The chest must be fully visualized for examination. If necessary, clothing should be cut off. The respiratory rate must be recorded, together with the depth and pattern of the respirations. The following should be watched for:

- Evidence of cyanosis.
- Notably shallow or deep respirations.
- The use of accessory muscles of respiration.
- Cheyne–Stokes breathing.
- Gulping, 'air hunger' type breathing (an indication of hypovolaemic shock).
- Stridor (an indication of airway obstruction).
- Pain (an indication of fractured ribs).

The chest wall should be examined for evidence of trauma, bruising and wounds. Crepitus, indicating rib fractures, may be inadvertently elicited while palpating for bony tenderness (the cardinal sign of a fracture). Surgical emphysema may be perceived as a crackling feeling. This is caused by air escaping into the tissues, typically into the upper part of the chest wall. Paradoxical respirations will usually be apparent if there is a flail segment.

Pulse oximetry is a widely used non-invasive monitoring procedure which measures arterial oxyhaemoglobin saturation (SaO_2) and therefore gives important information about the supply of oxygen to body tissues. It does not however provide the information about ventilatory status which might come from arterial blood gases, e.g. CO_2 tension or acid-base balance, and its acuracy is compromised by a range of factors such as patient motion, abnormal haemoglobin, dark skin pigmentation or nail polish (Durren, 1992). Adequate tissue oxygenation, according to Durren (1992), requires an SaO_2 of over 90% and adequate haemoglobin levels.

The medical staff's assessment will include the standard percussion and stethoscopic exam, chest X-rays (the area of lung collapse in pneumothorax is seen on an X-ray as a blank area without lung markings separating the lung margin from the chest wall) and arterial blood gases.

Intervention

If the patient is not breathing, IPPV must be commenced at once. Cardiac compression, however, should be withheld until an assessment has been made of cardiac output and the ECG. Using an oropharyngeal airway and a bag/mask connected to an oxygen supply, the A & E nurse should be able to ventilate the patient adequately. Watson (1991) suggests more effective ventilation occurs if a second person secures the mask on the face, as in this way a more airtight seal is achieved.

If the patient is exhibiting respiratory distress, 100% oxygen should be applied by mask at 6 l/min. If possible, the sitting-upright position should be adopted to assist respiration. Chest injuries are very painful; the nurse may relieve such pain by the administration of Entonox, which is 50% oxygen and 50% nitrous oxide.

If the patient is conscious, it is likely that he or she will require a great deal of psychological support as difficulty in breathing is a very frightening experience. It is suggested that such a patient should not be left alone at any time, for, in addition to the risk of deterioration going unnoticed, it may provoke great fear in the patient.

The need for pulse oximetry and continual monitoring of respiratory rate and effort cannot be overemphasized as this will give first warning of a deterioration in respiratory function. Cyanosis is a very late sign, and in a significant proportion of the population, i.e. the non-Caucasian population, it is an unlikely sign at all. In non-Caucasians, cyanosis can be seen in the mucous membranes. Drowsiness and confusion are associated with respiratory failure and are due to cerebral hypoxia. In multiple trauma victims, however, it may not be possible to differentiate between when these signs are caused by head injury and when they are due to respiratory failure.

The remaining area of nursing care for respiratory problems concerns supporting medical intervention. In the case of a pneumothorax or haemothorax, the requirement is for a rapidly introduced chest drain, together with an underwater seal, to drain off the air or blood that is compressing the lung (Fig. 4.4). Most of the equipment for this procedure should be ready in advance in the form of a CSSD pack in the resuscitation room. Great stress should be laid on asepsis during the procedure. Iodine in spirit is usually used as a skin preparation. Local anaesthetic will be administered around the area, followed by a small incision with a scalpel to facilitate the

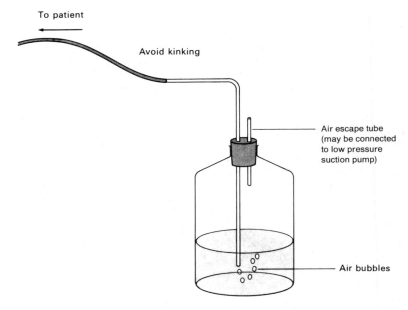

To patient

Avoid kinking

Air escape tube
(may be connected
to low pressure
suction pump)

Air bubbles

Fig. 4.4   Simplified diagram of chest drainage

introduction of the chest drain. The nurse should have the bottle
ready with a litre of sterile water and should ensure that the tubing is
connected the correct way, i.e. the drain coming from the patient
must be connected to the tube that ends underwater. Negative
pressure is usually applied to the system by means of a specialized
suction pump to facilitate drainage of blood. The chest drain will
be sutured in place and the area around it should be dressed with a
keyhole dressing secured with elastoplast. If it is correctly inserted,
the nurse should observe air or blood draining into the bottle, and
the fluid level in the drain will oscillate with the changes in intrathoracic pressure associated with the patient's breathing. The bottle
should never be raised above the level of the patient because, if
this is done, the contents of the bottle will syphon off through the
drain into the chest with catastrophic results. The traditional practice of clamping the drainage tube before moving the patient is not
necessary (Armstrong et al., 1991).
A dramatic improvement in the patient's condition often follows

chest drainage, the re-expanded lung being seen on a check X-ray immediately after the procedure. A nurse should accompany the patient during this X-ray, monitoring respiratory status and offering psychological support. If a haemothorax has been present, blood pressure and pulse need close observation because of the danger of hypovolaemic shock. The quantity of blood draining into the bottle needs to be recorded accurately.

In dealing with a large flail segment, it is likely that IPPV will be required, although the medical staff will not automatically resort to this measure; the patient's clinical condition is the key indication. The patient will require intubation for IPPV.

Evaluation

The effectiveness of interventions to improve breathing must be carefully evaluated. Simple mistakes can occur, such as having the oxygen mask connected to an oxygen point that is not turned on or to an empty cylinder. The chest drain can become kinked or blocked by clots and can therefore stop functioning. Patients may be placed in the correct position to help their breathing, but that is no guarantee that they will stay there. They have a tendency to slip down the trolley!

Airway and breathing problems are very dramatic and desperate situations. It is very easy, therefore, for some simple error to occur with potentially fatal results. Continual evaluation must be the rule to be absolutely sure that things are going to plan and that the patient is benefiting from our interventions to assist the self-care demand of normal breathing.

Circulation

Pathology

The next priority in the nursing care of the critically injured person is circulation. Here the principal concern is the possibility of cardiac arrest or of insufficient circulation leading to shock. Therefore, while attention is being paid to the patient's airway and breathing, a nurse should also be assessing the patient's circulation.

The pathology of shock is very complex and there remains much still to be learnt of its nature. However, the main common denominator in all types of shock is reduced cellular perfusion, i.e. insufficient

Table 4.1
Classification of shock by cause

Type of Shock	Cause
1. Hypovolaemic	
Haemorrhagic	Blood loss due to soft tissue bleeding, fractures, wounds, etc.
Burns	Loss of plasma in burn exudate.
Dehydration	Major body fluid loss, e.g. due to prolonged vomiting, diarrhoea, or metabolic disorders such as diabetic ketoacidosis.
2. Cardiogenic	Failure of cardiac pump leading to inadequate cardiac output although the blood volume is normal, e.g. after myocardial infarction.
3. Vasogenic	
Septic	Endotoxins from Gram-negative bacteria can cause massive vasodilatation in certain infective conditions.
Anaphylactic	Severe allergic reaction; histamine release increases capillary permeability and leads to dilatation of capillaries and arterioles.
Neurogenic	Loss of sympathetic control leading to dilatation of venules, capillaries and arterioles.

oxygen reaches the tissues of the body. If this condition is not corrected, it will eventually set in train a series of complex physiological changes which will result in irreversible shock and death. There are three main types of shock—hypovolaemic, cardiogenic and vasogenic—the causes of which are summarized in Table 4.1.

In hypovolaemic shock, the problem is that there is a loss of fluid from the circulation. In cardiogenic shock, there is a failure of the pump, although the blood volume is not affected. While in vasogenic shock, the blood volume is again not affected but rather the arterioles and capillaries dilate, leading to diminished venous return and hence diminished cardiac output, which in turn leads to decreased tissue perfusion, i.e. shock.

The body has compensating mechanisms against shock which come into operation after injury, and which can give rise to misleadingly normal blood pressures in the A & E patient. The main result of these mechanisms is vasoconstriction.

Decreased renal perfusion leads to the release of renin which in turn leads, via the plasma protein angiotensinogen to angiotensin, a powerful vasoconstrictor at the microcirculatory level. In addition, there is adrenaline and noradrenaline release, both of which are vasoconstrictors. This may allow patients to compensate for circulatory loss for some time with a normal blood pressure, especially if they are young and have, therefore, more elastic walls to their blood vessels.

Significant changes will occur in the urine output of the shocked patient. The reduction in circulating volume will reduce glomerular filtration and hence urine formation. Furthermore, the hormone aldosterone and the anti-diuretic hormone will be released as part of the compensatory effect, both of which will diminish urine output. In hypovolaemic shock, urine output may be less than 30 ml/h. This is a critical level since output below this value is indicative of renal failure. Hypovolaemic shock is therefore the major cause of acute renal failure.

Assessment

In assessing the patient's circulation, we first of all need to know if the heart is beating and if it is, whether it is producing an effective circulation. The A & E nurse needs, therefore, to take the patient's pulse, noting both rate and rhythm. The absence of a radial pulse indicates that systolic blood pressure is below 80 (Driscoll and Skinner, 1991). If the patient is unresponsive and making no apparent respiratory effort, the carotid pulse should be palpated and, if absent, a state of cardiac arrest assumed. The alarm should be raised first and then CPR initiated (European Resusc. Council, 1993).

If the patient has a cardiac output, the next step is to assess the risk of shock. Continual monitoring of blood pressure is required, and the nurse should bear in mind the possibility of compensated shock as outlined above. Blood pressure should preferably be monitored by the same nurse so that any differences will reflect real differences in blood pressure rather than different hearing abilities or any other subjective factors that can make blood pressure readings unreliable. Respiratory rate and pulse are other key parameters in the development of shock. Both will rise, the respiratory rate in response to the body's need to try to increase tissue oxygenation and the pulse in response to the falling blood pressure. The condition of the skin should be noted as the increased production of adrenaline and the resulting vasoconstriction will lead to a cool, pale and moist skin. The time for capillary refill to occur after blanching a digit by momentarily squeezing the extremity should be less than 2 seconds. A longer time is an indication of likely shock (Budassi-Sheehy, 1990).

If the patient is conscious or if witnesses are present, a history of the accident is required. The history will often indicate the risk of injuries that may produce hypovolaemia, e.g. trauma to the right upper quadrant of the abdomen will alert the nurse to the risk of liver damage.

The patient's mental state should also be assessed as psychological support is very important.

Intervention

If there is no cardiac output, CPR must be commenced immediately. After clearing the airway the patient's lungs should be slowly inflated twice with oxygen using a bag/mask device before chest compressions are commenced to produce an effective circulation. If a bag/mask is not available, 'mouth-to-mouth' expired air respiration should be commenced with two slow breaths. It should be remembered that there has been no demonstrated case of HIV transmission by this route and Zideman (1990) considers there is no realistic risk of AIDS infection as a result of mouth-to-mouth resuscitation, as long as blood is not present in the saliva. This view is supported by Baskett (1993).

The nurse should place both hands together on the sternum at a point some two fingers' width up from its lower end (xiphisternum). The fingers should be interlocked and the arms held straight, the aim being to use about half the nurse's body weight to compress the sternum by 4–5 cm. A rate of about 60 compressions per minute carried out correctly will give a cardiac output of between 33% and 50% of normal, sufficient to prevent cerebral damage and permit the medical staff to attempt various techniques aimed at restarting the heart (see below).

It is probable that the output produced in this way owes as much to a general rise in intrathoracic pressure and compression of the great vessels of the chest as it does to actual compression of the heart. For this reason, if equipment is available as it is in hospital, chest compression and ventilation may proceed independently as greater pressures will be generated in this way. A rate of 12–14 ventilations along with 60–80 chest compressions per minute should be aimed at although it is difficult to count precisely in the intense activity that surrounds a CPR attempt. Alternatively, a 5:1 ratio of compressions to ventilations is required in two person life support, or 15:2 in single person CPR.

The patient should be connected to an ECG monitor as soon as possible in order that cardiac activity may be monitored. The ECG and the presence or absence of cardiac output, as measured by a carotid or femoral pulse, will determine the medical treatment that follows. Effective CPR must be maintained at all times to ensure an oxygenated blood supply continuously reaches the patient's brain.

In a cardiac arrest the three most likely cardiac arrhythmias to be found are asystole, ventricular fibrillation or electromechanical disso-ciation. Other arrhythmias are discussed on p. 96. In asystole there is no cardiac electrical activity (straight line on the ECG) while in electromechanical dissociation the ECG looks normal except that unfortunately the heart is not responding and producing any contrac-tions; cardiac output is therefore nil. Ventricular fibrillation is a condition where there is uncoordinated electrical discharge through-out the ventricles and is the most common cause of cardiac arrest (Chamberlain, 1990). The result is that the myocardial muscle only quivers instead of carrying out its normal coordinated contraction and cardiac output effectively ceases. Giving an electrical shock, defibrillation aims to produce a simultaneous depolarization of all the myocardial cells, thus allowing them to repolarize at the same time and hopefully restore normal coordinated electrical and muscu-lar activity. Resuscitation guidelines are aimed at ensuring defibrilla-tion occurs at the earliest possible opportunity as prospects for success decrease at 5% per minute of CPR (European Resusc. Council, 1993).

Fig. 4.5 shows the three likely courses of action that will be followed, depending upon the ECG. Effective ventilation and chest compression must be maintained throughout, except during defibril-lation since the nurse would also receive the electrical shock!

In young children a different approach is required—the heel of one hand only for a small child, and two thumbs for a baby. The rate needs to be 80 to 100 compressions per minute, and the respiration rate correspondingly quicker but also more shallow.

The nurse will usually be responsible for drawing up and record-ing various drugs in a CPR attempt. It will greatly expedite the proceedings if nursing staff know what is likely to be asked for and have the drugs to hand.

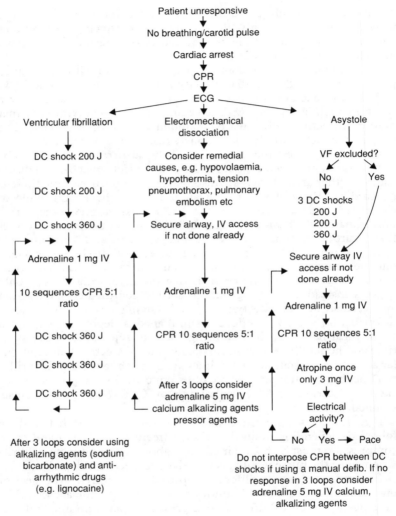

Patient unresponsive

No breathing/carotid pulse

Cardiac arrest

CPR

ECG

Ventricular fibrillation

DC shock 200 J

DC shock 200 J

DC shock 360 J

Adrenaline 1 mg IV

10 sequences CPR 5:1 ratio

DC shock 360 J

DC shock 360 J

DC shock 360 J

After 3 loops consider using alkalizing agents (sodium bicarbonate) and anti-arrhythmic drugs (e.g. lignocaine)

Electromechanical dissociation

Consider remedial causes, e.g. hypovolaemia, hypothermia, tension pneumothorax, pulmonary embolism etc

Secure airway, IV access if not done already

Adrenaline 1 mg IV

CPR 10 sequences 5:1 ratio

After 3 loops consider adrenaline 5 mg IV calcium alkalizing agents pressor agents

Asystole

VF excluded?

No   Yes

3 DC shocks
200 J
200 J
360 J

Secure airway IV access if not done already

Adrenaline 1 mg IV

CPR 10 sequences 5:1 ratio

Atropine once only 3 mg IV

Electrical activity?

No   Yes → Pace

Do not interpose CPR between DC shocks if using a manual defib. If no response in 3 loops consider adrenaline 5 mg IV calcium, alkalizing agents

NB Adrenaline and atropine can be given via ET tube providing double dose is administered.

Fig. 4.5   European Resuscitation Council (1993) Guidelines

Budassi-Sheehy (1990) describe how some of these drugs may be given via an endotracheal tube in a cardiac arrest. Lignocaine, atropine, naloxone and adrenaline are readily absorbed through the lungs, and this route should therefore be considered where an IV line cannot be readily established (e.g. in children). Doses should be doubled however. It should be noted that sodium bicarbonate and calcium chloride are not suitable for administration via this intrapulmonary route.

The nurse needs to know how to charge the defibrillator and to apply conducting pads to the chest in the correct positions (sternum and apex of the heart). If necessary, the nurse should be prepared to defibrillate if the nursing and medical staff have agreed to that being part of the nurse's role. The golden rule is to make sure that nobody is touching the trolley or else they too will receive a shock (200 to 360 Joules).

If CPR is successful in re-establishing cardiac output, continual ECG monitoring is required, and further drug therapy may be needed to stabilize the patient's rhythm.

Asystole does not respond to defibrillation, however Chamberlain (1990) points out the need to be sure asystole is correctly diagnosed and is not misread from the monitor as it may actually be very fine VF. If in doubt, defibrillation is recommended.

The most common cause of shock in the A & E department is hypovolaemia. Immediate nursing interventions should be to elevate the foot of the trolley to try to increase the volume of blood in the vital heart–lung–brain circulation, to administer high concentration oxygen to assist tissue oxygenation, to control any obvious bleeding with pressure dressings and to offer psychological support to the patient.

As hypovolaemic shock is the type of shock most commonly seen in A & E, and as it requires large-scale circulating volume replacement therapy, the nurse must be prepared to offer support to the medical staff in carrying out such potentially life-saving measures. Cannulation of the internal jugular or subclavian vein with a wide bore cannula will be carried out as well as establishing a peripheral line. Accurate fluid balance charts are required as there may be three drips running at once, together with CVP monitoring. Clear fluids alone, such as normal saline, are not satisfactory as they are easily excreted by the kidneys and can leak from damaged capillaries. Therefore, in resuscitating the hypovolaemic patient, colloidal solutions such as Haemaccel or Gelofusin are used as a temporary measure until whole blood is grouped and cross-matched. These IV solutions have such large molecules that they are not readily filtered out by the kidneys, and due to the osmotic pressure they exert, fluid is moved from the intracellular compartment into the circulation. Crystalloid solutions such as Ringer lactate may also be used to restore interstitial fluid loss (Baskett, 1991). An IVI warming coil should be available as such is the volume of fluid likely to be given that it may cause hypothermia if not pre-warmed to body temperature. To facilitate the giving of large volumes of fluid in short times, some form of pump is required. A simple device like a sphygmomanometer cuff can be inflated around the IVI bag to force the fluid in quickly.

A supply of O Rhesus negative blood should be available for emergency transfusion if one is needed while the patient's blood is being grouped and cross-matched.

Catheterization of the patient may be required in order to monitor urine output accurately on an hourly basis (see p. 67).

One form of effective treatment of shock used is MAST—Medical Anti-Shock Trousers. MAST is a cross between a pair of trousers and a sphygmomanometer cuff inflated with a foot pump. It is an inflatable pair of trousers that has the effect of splinting lower limb fractures, controlling lower limb bleeding and, most importantly, autotransfusing the patient with a litre or so of ready-warmed, compatible blood, by squeezing it out of the less essential lower limbs into the vital heart–lung–brain circulation. It is only a temporary device and needs very careful deflation, but MAST can bring about a dramatic improvement in a patient's condition in A & E. Randall (1986) described the use of MAST in A & E on seven patients suffering from leaking aortic aneurysm or multiple trauma who had no measurable BP. Their condition greatly improved in the short term and a BP became recordable. However, only two survived surgery. MAST in A & E can therefore be life-saving in some cases.

Evaluation

Continual monitoring of vital signs is essential to evaluate the progress of the shocked patient. Urine output must be carefully watched as acute renal failure is a grave sign (urine output less than 30 ml/h, Hudak and Gallo, 1994). If the patient is becoming more alert and the skin is feeling warmer, IV replacement therapy is likely to be improving the situation. Repeated checks should be made that the pressure dressing really is controlling bleeding. Is there another wound that has been missed at the first assessment, or is there evidence of internal haemorrhage? The nurse caring for the patient must be alert to these possibilities if care is to be effectively evaluated.

Head Injury

Pathology

The brain consists of relatively incompressible tissue. Therefore any force applied to it will be immediately transmitted through the tissue. This means that a blow delivered to one side of the head can produce brain injury on the opposite side, as the brain, which is independent of the skull, impinges on the inner surface of the skull.

The skull forms a closed box. The clinical implication of this is that if any bleeding occurs within the skull, raised intracranial pressure will result as there is nowhere for the haematoma to expand, other than to force the brainstem through the tentorial notch or foramen magnum. This condition is known as brainstem herniation.

Bullock and Teasdale (1991) estimate that head injured patients account for 10% of the workload of the A & E service. Despite this, the majority of head injuries seen in A & E are simple concussions. In concussion, after impacting on the inner surface of the skull, the brain suffers a brief interruption to the reticular activating system. This causes a short period of unconsciousness and amnesia. Bruising or contusion of the brain surface leads to more significant injury and neurological disturbance.

A much more serious injury occurs when a blood vessel is torn, leading to haemorrhage and haematoma formation in either an epidural (between dura and skull) or subdural (below the dura) location, or within the brain itself. North American studies have shown mortality rates for epidural haematoma of 25–50% and for subdural haematoma 70%, indicating the seriousness of these injuries (Budassi-Sheehy, 1990).

In such major injuries, there is often a short period of unconsciousness after which the patient regains consciousness. During this period of consciousness, the haematoma associated with the bleeding blood vessel develops, leading to a rise in intracranial pressure which will cause a gradual diminishing in the level of consciousness. This period of consciousness is known as the 'lucid interval', and the reason for observation of head injury patients is to try to detect evidence of a diminishing level of consciousness, associated with rising intracranial pressure, as early as is possible so that surgical intervention (burr holes) might relieve the pressure and improve the outcome.

Raised intracranial pressure or haematoma formation may manifest itself by compression of the third cranial nerve (oculomotor) which controls the iris and hence the size of the pupil. A sluggishly reacting or dilated pupil is evidence of compression of the oculomotor nerve if it is associated with diminished level of consciousness. There are a variety of other causes of unequal or nonreactive pupils unassociated with head injury. It must be emphasized that this is a late sign that will develop *after* a fall in the level of consciousness.

Skull fracture is not a very reliable guide to the seriousness of the injury, as many patients with a fractured skull have no significant neurological deficit, while other patients sustain serious brain damage without a fracture. Head injury, for example, is the leading cause of death in motor vehicle accidents; 2390 out of 4898 deaths in England and Wales in 1990 were due to head injury. However, in 28% of cases there was no skull fracture (OPCS, 1991).

Two types of skull fracture are important, however. Firstly, if the fracture is an open one, there is the risk of infection which may involve the skull itself (osteomyelitis) or the meninges surrounding the brain leading to meningitis. For an open fracture of the skull, there does not need to be a scalp wound as the fracture may be through the base of the skull, communication with the fracture occurring via one of the Eustachian tubes, the mouth or one of the ears. Secondly, if the skull fracture is depressed, the piece of bone pressing on the brain may act as an irritable focus and may cause fitting. A CSF leak may occur due to a tear in the meninges and as a consequence there is the risk of intracranial infection (Sinclair, 1991).

Assessment

After assessing airway, breathing and circulation, the next parameter to measure is level of consciousness and changes that occur in that level as this will give the first warning of rising intracranial pressure. It is essential to establish a baseline level of consciousness, and the

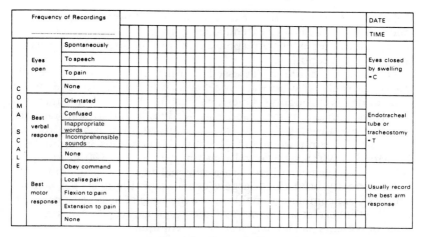

Frequency of Recordings				DATE
....				TIME
C O M A S C A L E	Eyes open	Spontaneously		Eyes closed by swelling = C
		To speech		
		To pain		
		None		
	Best verbal response	Orientated		Endotracheal tube or tracheostomy = T
		Confused		
		Inappropriate words		
		Incomprehensible sounds		
		None		
	Best motor response	Obey command		Usually record the best arm response
		Localise pain		
		Flexion to pain		
		Extension to pain		
		None		

Fig. 4.6   Coma scale

nearer that baseline is to the time of the accident the better. Witnesses, relatives, ambulance crew and policemen are all key personnel who can help nurses to estimate what the patient's level of consciousness was before arrival in A & E. The importance of level of consciousness as a guide to head injury progress cannot be overemphasized.

Such an assessment must avoid subjective terms like 'semiconscious' or 'drowsy' which mean different things to different people. The objective Glasgow coma scale is, therefore, recommended. On this scale, consciousness is assessed in terms of motor response, verbal response and minimum stimulus required to produce eye opening. Fig. 4.6 shows a coma scale. Alternatively, points can be allocated for each response on the scale starting from zero for no response up to 4 or 5 for the maximum response, the scores for each part of the scale being added together to produce a total. Proehl (1992) stresses the need for nurses to base their score on the patient's *best* responses in each category, while remembering that factors such as paralysis, intubation or periorbital swelling can invalidate all or part of the GCS assessment.

In assessing motor response to painful stimuli, the nurse is recommended to apply pressure to the nail bed of one of the patient's fingers with a pen or similar object and his/her own thumb (Proehl,

1992). Note whether the arm is withdrawn towards the patient's body (flexion to pain) or extended away from the body (extension to pain). This latter extensor response indicates brainstem compression, a very serious condition.

Orientation should be assessed in time and space with simple questions such as 'Where are you?' and 'What day is it?' and 'What time of day is it roughly?' Questions such as 'Do you know that you are in the Royal Infirmary and it is Wednesday afternoon?' are not helpful. An answer 'Yes' to this type of question is not proof of anything! The importance of objective observations is highlighted by Morris (1993), who found that, in a sample of 100 head injury referrals by casualty officers to a regional neurosurgical unit, only 30% correctly used the Glasgow coma scale. Eighteen per cent of doctors were completely unable to use the scale. The biggest problem area was incorrect assessment of the response to painful stimulus; 56% of patients had an inappropriate technique used.

In order to determine if the patient lost consciousness, in the absence of witnesses, the nurse should ask the patient to recall the accident. A gap in recall indicates the strong likelihood of unconsciousness, although this period may not be as long as the period of amnesia. Retrograde amnesia refers to a period of amnesia before the accident, while post-traumatic amnesia refers to amnesia after the accident.

In assessing pupil size and response, light of the same intensity should be used in each eye. The nurse should also be checking that when light is shone in one eye, the other responds as well. Unequal pupils in an alert, orientated patient are highly unlikely to indicate any head injury pathology as unequal pupils are a late sign following diminished level of consciousness due to raised intracranial pressure.

Physical signs that should be looked for include scalp wounds. Scalp wounds should alert the A & E team to the possibility of open fractures of the skull and of hypovolaemic shock which can be greatly exacerbated by profusely bleeding scalp wounds, if not primarily caused by such wounds, especially in the elderly. An important sign to look out for is bruising around the eyes (periorbital ecchymosis)—often called 'raccoon eyes'; this indicates an intraorbital fracture or basilar skull fracture. Bruising appearing 12 to 24 hours after injury, behind the ears in the mastoid area, is known as Battle's sign and also indicates basilar skull fracture.

Further evidence of a fracture of the base of the skull is provided by CSF leakage from the nose (rhinorrhoea) or the ear (otorrhoea). Bleeding from within the ear also indicates a fracture of the base of the skull. If there is fluid leaking from the nose, the patient should not be allowed to blow the nose as this could cause contamination of the meninges.

The development of any obvious limb weakness should be reported as this suggests damage to the motor centres in the brain. The nature and duration of any fits must be carefully documented, and medical attention drawn to their presence immediately.

In monitoring the vital signs, respiratory rate is vital, as brain damage may involve the respiratory centre leading to disturbance of both depth and rate of breathing. Respirations may become progressively more shallow and gradually fade away. The temperature regulating centre is thought to be adjacent to the hypothalamus and damage in this region can lead to hyperthermia (temperatures over 40°C). The patient may however be hypothermic as a result of lying still for a period of time after the injury in a cold environment. An accurate baseline temperature is therefore required, taken rectally where appropriate.

A late sign of serious head injury is a rising BP and a slowing pulse. This is explained in terms of the raised intracranial pressure making the heart beat more strongly as blood has to be forced into the brain in order to overcome capillary resistance. Baroreceptors that are situated in the carotid arteries monitor blood pressure and in response to a rising blood pressure act via the cardiac centre in the brain to slow the heart rate. This is the same mechanism responsible for increasing the heart rate when the blood pressure falls.

Assessment of children after head injury requires the nurse to allow for the varying stages of cognitive development. Information from the parent about normal behaviour is invaluable if the nurse is to observe abnormal behaviour. As Harrison (1991) states, the normal observation of adult head injured patients requires adaptation to suit the needs of children and her paper gives a good account of such procedure.

Intervention

Airway and breathing must be main priorities in intervention. Administration of high concentration oxygen to head injury patients is beneficial because it reduces cerebral CO_2 levels, and high levels of

CO_2 in the brain cause cerebral oedema, thereby raising intracranial pressure further.

In handling and moving head injury patients, the nurse must realize the possibility of spinal injury. Unconscious patients must be assumed to have a spinal injury until proven otherwise, and great care should be taken even if the patient is conscious.

The absolutely vital role of the nurse is the scrupulous monitoring of the level of consciousness, and the maintenance of the patient's airway and respiration.

One final word of caution concerning the nursing management of head injury—many apparently unconscious patients have surprisingly accurate recall of events that occurred and of words that were spoken while they were 'unconscious' in hospital. Perhaps a more accurate description is to say they are 'unresponsive' but possibly aware or 'conscious' of what is said in their presence. Nursing staff should bear this in mind while looking after such patients and talk and behave at all times as if their patient can hear every word they say, because they just might.

Medical interventions that will require nursing support include intubation and ventilation of the patient in order to ensure adequate oxygenation of the brain and airway management, a detailed neurological exam, X-rays, possibly CAT (Computerized Axial Tomography) scanning to define areas of bleeding in the brain accurately (this may be done under general anaesthetic), anticonvulsant or antibiotic therapy as required, and possibly in extreme cases, burr holes which will be drilled in the skull to relieve intracranial pressure and allow clot evacuation. An osmotic diuretic, mannitol, may be given to try to shrink the brain by reducing oedema. This requires catheterization but may help as a temporary measure pending transfer to specialist neurosurgical care (Sinclair, 1991).

The administration of powerful opioid analgesics in multiply-injured patients is not advisable if there has been head injury, as they have a depressing effect on the level of consciousness. The mistake may be made of assigning a decreased level of consciousness to the effect of the drug, when in fact it is due to rising intracranial pressure. Entonox should also not be used with confused patients or where a serious head injury has occurred (Baskett, 1993).

The vast majority of patients seen in A & E will fortunately have only suffered minor head injury and will be discharged home. Medical criteria for admission or neurosurgical consultation may be found in Sinclair (1991). Symptoms such as dizziness, headaches, irritability, poor concentration and memory loss may last for days afterwards and a study by Lowdon et al. (1989) reported that among a sample of 114 such patients, 90% reported these symptoms lasting up to two weeks after injury. It is important that the nurse discuss these symptoms with the patient and a friend or relative, and also stress the need for the patient to be brought back to hospital if they persist or worsen.

Evaluation

It is essential that senior nursing staff ensure that junior staff understand fully the reasons why they are performing the repeated observations that they are carrying out on the head injury patient. If junior staff do not understand fully, the observations will not be performed accurately and the significance of some vital change will go unreported. Senior staff should monitor the accuracy of their juniors' observations, doing so discreetly and using such a process as a teaching tool.

Spinal Injury

Pathology

The spinal cord is enclosed in a canal extending through the vertebral column with nerves branching off (motor) or entering (sensory) via openings in the vertebrae. The soft nature of the spinal cord makes it very vulnerable to injury with potentially disastrous consequences.

Injury occurs when either a vertebra is fractured and/or spinal ligaments (whose function is to hold the vertebrae in alignment) are ruptured which allows subluxation of the vertebrae. The result will be either compression of the cord or a partial or complete transection. All injuries should be assumed to be unstable until proven otherwise.

The forces causing the injury can be either flexion, extension or rotation, or any combination of these forces. For example, the injury known as a 'whiplash', which is seen in car occupants whose vehicle has been struck from behind, is an extension/flexion injury. Flexion/rotation injuries are seen in accidents in sports such as rugby or gymnastics. These tend to be cervical injuries. The lumbar spine is typically injured in falls where the person lands feet first and a lumbar vertebra is either crushed or, if there if flexion as well, wedged. Alternatively, however, in this case, the vertebra may shatter and produce a burst fracture. The thoracic spine is commonly injured by a direct blow such as a roof collapse in mining or when a person falls, landing on his, or her back.

Complete transection of the cord is fortunately rare and, as Folman and Masri (1989) point out, it is very difficult to demonstrate clinically, citing studies of patients with apparent complete cord transection where some 10 to 20% made some degree of recovery. These authors have looked at a series of 70 patients with incomplete transection between the 4th cervical and 10th thoracic vertebrae and can find no better indicator of recovery than the amount of sensation and function present after the first few days. They urge A & E staff not to jump to conclusions about recovery based on a rapid assessment in A & E, particularly when the patient may be suffering the immediate effects of head injury and other trauma. A careful assessment carried out after a few days is the best indicator of recovery.

The difficulty of predicting outcomes is shown in a study of 410 patients with major blunt trauma carried out by Ross et al. (1992). The only significant predictors of unstable cervical injury were loss of consciousness, neurological deficit on assessment and neck tenderness. A total of 13 patients in this sample had an unstable injury, i.e. 6.1%.

Assessment

Complete transection of the cord produces a flaccid paralysis. It may also lead to spinal shock due to loss of vessel tone (an example of vasogenic shock). Sensation will also be lost. Male patients may display an erection in cord transection. If the injury is incomplete, there will be a mixed picture of sensory/motor loss. The nurse should, therefore, be looking for any weakness or any complaint by the patient of unusual sensations, tingling or numbness. The best way to assess weakness in the upper limbs is to ask the patient to hold the arms out in front of the body for a period of time. If there is any motor weakness, the affected limb will be seen to fall away gradually after a few seconds. To assess lower limb weakness, the patient, lying flat, should be asked to push the nurse away while he or she presses against the soles of the patient's feet with the palms of the hands. Weakness may be perceived in one or both of the limbs.

It is important in the case of neck injury to note how the patient is behaving, as there will be considerable muscle spasm involved in a serious injury. The patient will tend to hold their neck with both hands. Such behaviour in a patient should act as a warning sign of significant injury.

Intervention

All head and multiply-injured patients must be assumed to have an unstable spinal injury until proven otherwise. This requires minimal movement of the patient, and then only in a carefully controlled way. In transferring them to the A & E trolley, the ambulance scoop should be used if one is available. Otherwise at least four people must make the lift with a fifth person supporting the head and neck to prevent movement of the cervical spine. The head should be immobilized with sandbags where practicable, and a cervical collar applied. The soft foam type are less than 100% effective in immobilizing the neck and, therefore, either a rigid splint or a vacuum suction splint should be used. Research by Ferguson et al. (1993) has measured a wide range of tissue interface pressures beneath different types of collars, some of which might be expected to cause jugular venous obstruction and hence raised intracranial pressure. They recommend the use of a moulded cervical collar which supports occiput, mandible and shoulder girdle, as these produced the lowest tissue interface pressures. Soft collars are again contraindicated by this research and staff are encouraged to think carefully of the dangers of applying collars too tightly.

The patient should be kept flat at all times, turning being accomplished using the log rolling technique. The principle of this is to move the patient in such a way that the spine remains in a straight line and no part of the spine moves relative to another. This will need four people to perform properly. The person in charge of the movement is the person who is bridging the injured part of the spine with their hands. As the patient is being cared for in a flat position, there should be a nurse with the patient at all times, and suction equipment must be immediately available in case of vomiting.

If the patient is conscious and aware of the possibility of spinal injury, the nurse must be prepared for anxious questions from the patient and also from the family. Such questions are very difficult to deal with, but they must be answered honestly and realistically. The patient will need a great deal of psychological support in this sort of situation.

In the A & E department the aim is to prevent any further worsening of the situation by not allowing displacement to occur in a potentially unstable injury. The immediate aim of the medical treatment after a detailed neurological exam and radiography will be to stabilize the spine. This may involve traction applied in the short term, while long-term options include operative fixation or the patient may be immobilized in halo traction. The use of the halo brace after stabilization of the injury permits early mobilization and is now becoming common (Hudak and Gallo, 1994).

For the spine-injured patient, there will be many long-term problems involving bowel and bladder training, chest and urinary tract infections, pressure sores, rehabilitation, and social and psychological trauma.

There has been a major increase in less serious neck injuries over the last twelve years. The term acute neck sprain is more accurate than 'whiplash' as this latter term is only strictly applicable in a small number of RTA cases. Galasko (1993) has charted a rise in neck sprain injuries from 7.7% of RTA victims in 1981 through to 45.6% in 1991 and suggests this is related to driving standards and traffic flow patterns rather than seatbelt wearing. It should be remembered that many patients will have painful symptoms from neck sprain injury many years after the accident. Robinson and Cassar-Pullicino (1993) reported that 86% of patients in a sample of 21 followed up over 10 years later still had painful symptoms from acute neck sprain after an RTA.

Abdominal Trauma

Pathology

The seriously injured patient can have an almost infinite variety of abdominal lesions. They can be due to blunt trauma such as a severe blow, to crushing, or to deceleration forces associated with high velocity road accidents. Alternatively, there can be a penetrating injury due to stabbing, impalement or bullet or shrapnel wounds.

The major life-threatening pathology associated with abdominal injury is hypovolaemia, due to either a leaking major blood vessel or the rupture or laceration of a vascular organ such as the spleen or liver. For example, a correctly restrained car occupant in a high velocity collision may sustain a tear of the aorta due to the deceleration forces involved; a person falling from a ladder or a motorbike may take the brunt of the fall with their abdomen, leading to the rupture of the spleen. Penetrating injuries may lacerate major blood vessels as well as the viscera.

A second major area for concern is peritonitis, caused by the rupture of an organ such as the bowel or gall bladder. It can be either an infective or a chemical peritonitis.

Damage to the diaphragm is a serious problem due to the interference that will occur with respiration, and it should always be considered as a possibility in abdominal trauma.

Assessment

In undressing the patient, the abdomen should be carefully examined for external evidence of trauma such as bruising, wounds or 'tattooing'. The phenomenon of tattooing is found where a very high pressure has been applied to the skin through clothing, resulting in the pattern of clothing being transferred to the skin. Examples are commonly found on the chest and abdomen due to seat belts restraining a patient in a high velocity accident, or in victims of assault who have been kicked or struck with an object such as a billard cue. The relationship of such external markings to the organs of the abdomen should be considered in assessing possible injury.

Small puncture wounds may conceal very serious damage in cases of stabbing. It is very important to try to obtain an estimate of the depth of the wound and the direction of entry in order to assess the seriousness of the injury. Contrary to common belief, the entry and exit wounds of bullets are usually both small, even with high velocity bullets, yet they may conceal catastrophic damage, especially in the case of high energy missiles due to the shock wave and cavitation effects of supersonic projectiles (see p. 152). Bullets which explode on impact such as those used by Ryan in the Hungerford Massacre of 1987, or a short range shotgun blast, can produce huge and grossly contaminated wounds.

Close monitoring of the vital signs is required in order to detect signs of hypovolaemia as early as possible. Abdominal girth may be expected to increase with haemorrhage. However, its measurement is so unreliable that it is of no value and nursing staff should not waste precious time with a tape measure when a sphygmomanometer will allow for a much more accurate assessment of patient progress (Walsh and Ford, 1989).

The appearance of one or two drops of blood at the external

urinary meatus is evidence of rupture of the urethra. Patients who are suspected of having urethral damage should be asked to try to avoid passing urine, while the advice of a urologist is sought. All other patients, however, should be asked to provide a specimen of urine to test for haematurea, which may indicate trauma to the kidney. It is unusual for the bladder to rupture unless it is full, which unfortunately it often is in the case of late night road accidents.

Vaginal bleeding (other than menstrual) indicates that significant gynaecological trauma may be expected.

The detailed examination of the abdomen is the province of the medical staff; however, the A & E nurse should be able to recognize bowel sounds, or their absence which indicates paralytic ileus. Nurses should also be able to recognize the guarding sign associated with peritonitis; the patient holds their abdomen tense, lying flat on the trolley, unwilling to sit or bend at the waist as it is too painful.

The recognition of such signs is essential in the initial nursing assessment if the patient is to be correctly prioritized by the nursing staff.

Intervention

Prompt surgical intervention is required after stabilization of the patient's circulatory status. Nursing staff will be fully involved in IVI and vital sign monitoring, in ensuring that the patient is kept nil by mouth, and possibly in passing a nasogastric tube. The usual hospital protocols concerning any patient going to theatre must be observed as far as is possible.

If there is an impaling object *in situ*, it is best left there until it can be removed under controlled conditions in theatre while the wound is carefully explored. It is conventional surgical wisdom that the track of any penetrating injury must be fully explored.

All patients who are to undergo surgery need psychological support and explanations of what to expect, both before and after surgery. This applies especially to the patient who is to be operated upon in this kind of emergency situation.

One diagnostic test that may be carried out in A & E and that will require nursing support is peritoneal lavage. The aim of this is to discover if there is blood in the peritoneum, which is a strong indication of the need for laparotomy. The test consists of running 10 ml/kg of Ringer's lactate or normal saline via a peritoneal dialysis

	0–5 min	6–15 min	16–60 min
Documentation	Registration as A & E patient	Notes ready for writing in. ID tag applied to patient	Completed for admission to ITU
Assessment	Triage as top priority with multiple trauma. Primary survey of life-threatening problems (ABC)	BP P RR T ECG PaO$_2$ GCS commenced. Secondary survey obtained history from patient. Take bloods. Monitor peripheral circulation in injured limbs. Pain	Continue vital signs monitoring. Peritoneal lavage XR: comes after resuscitation
Medication	–	Analgesia for pain. Other urgent drug therapy as required (e.g. in CPR)	Analgesia. Adsorbed Tet Tox. Other drug therapy as required
Treatment	Commence CPR if needed, secure airway, ventilate	Commence therapy as soon as need for intubation, ventilation, circulatory support identified. O$_2$ therapy MAST	Catheterize. Chest drains if needed, IV therapy continues for low BP. Resusc. Continues until VS stable, consider urgent surgery
Nursing care	Begin undressing patient. Obtain history from ambulance crew	Undress patient. Give psychological support, assist medical team in resusc. Dress wounds (NB Universal Precautions apply). Immobilize injured limbs/neck. Prevent harm to patient e.g. cot sides	Maintain psychological support, be with patient at all times. Maintain IV document fluid balance
Referrals	–	Senior medics see patient in A & E	Arrange transfer to theatre/ITU
Family	Direct to private waiting room	Offer use of phone psych. support, try to obtain history	Keep informed of progress, allow to see patient
Discharge	–	–	Transfer ITU, theatres or specialist unit

Fig. 4.7 Critical pathway example: the patient with multiple trauma

catheter and an ordinary IVI giving set into the patient's peritoneum, allowing it to drain off by syphonage and, most importantly, assessing the fluid that returns. If there is no trauma, it should be clear. Frank blood or evidence of 100 000 red cells per mm^3 is taken as evidence of intra-abdominal bleeding (Baskett, 1993). Research by Driscoll et al. (1992) suggests that qualitative 'rule-of-thumb' estimates are unreliable and the only way of determining the concentration of red cells is by quantitative measurement. Strict asepsis should be followed, and the skin should be prepared with iodine in spirit. The procedure is carried out under local anaesthetic and the small incision is made with a scalpel.

The blood loss may be so severe in some cases that circulatory resuscitation in A & E is not possible and immediate surgical intervention is needed as a life-saving measure. In such extreme cases, the A & E team should be able to get a patient, if necessary, from the resuscitation room onto the operating table within 5 minutes.

Evaluation

It is essential to evaluate whether the patient understands what is being explained—both explanations about what is happening in A & E and those concerning what will happen in theatre subsequently. Psychological support revolves around patient understanding.

In dealing with hypovolaemia, steps such as elevating the foot of the trolley, IVI administration and MAST application can be evaluated by BP and pulse monitoring.

Abdominal trauma may be very painful, analgesia being withheld until the surgical team are sure of a diagnosis. Once analgesia is given, however, its effectiveness in relieving pain should be evaluated. (See Fig. 4.7 for Critical pathway example: the patient with multiple trauma.)

Trauma Scoring Systems

Such are the complex possible permutations of injuries in dealing with multiply-injured patients, that attempts have been made to devise simple scoring systems which will indicate those patients at most risk of death in order to prioritize treatment. Much of this work originated in the USA and has recently aroused interest in the UK, particularly with reference to audit work. Davies (1993) has provided a good introduction to this subject and shows that the Revised Trauma Scoring system, based upon the systolic BP, respiratory rate and GCS, correlates well with the probability of survival. There are drawbacks with this approach, not least of which, as Davies points out, is the validity of importing a North American system with its very different patterns of trauma to the UK.

References

Armstrong R., Bullen C., Cohen S., Singer M., Webb A. (1991). *Critical Care Algorithms*. Oxford: Oxford Medical Publications.

Baskett P. (1991). Management of hypovolaemic shock. In Skinner D., Driscoll D., Earlam R. (eds) *ABC of Major Trauma*. London: BMJ.

Baskett P. (1993). *Resuscitation Handbook* 2nd edn. London: Wolfe.

Budassi-Sheehy S. (1990). *Manual of Emergency Care*. St Louis: C. V. Mosby.

Bullock R., Teasdale G. (1991). Head injuries. In Driscoll P., Skinner D., Earlam R. (eds) *ABC of Major Trauma*. London: BMJ.

Chamberlain D. (1990). Ventricular fibrillation. In Evans T. R. (ed.) *ABC of Resuscitation*. London: BMJ.

Davies S. (1993). Trauma scoring. *Accident and Emergency Nursing*, 1, 125–31.

Driscoll F., Hodgkinson D., Mackway-Jones K. (1992). Diagnostic peritoneal lavage: it's red but is it positive? *Injury*, 23:4, 267–9.

Driscoll P., Skinner D. (1991). Initial assessment and management. In Skinner D., Driscoll P., Earlam R. (eds). *ABC of Major Trauma*. London: BMJ.

Durren M. (1992). Getting the most from pulse oximetry. *Journal of Emergency Nursing*, 18:4, 340–42.

European Resuscitation Council Working Party (1993). Adult advanced cardiac life support: the European Resuscitation Council guidelines 1992, *BMJ*, 306, 1589–93.

Ferguson J., Mardel S., Beattie T., Wytch R. (1993). Cervical collars: a potential risk to the head-injured patient. *Injury*, 24:7, 454–6.

Folman Y., Masri W. (1989). Spinal cord injury: prognostic indicators. *Injury*, 20:4, 92–3.

Galasko C. (1993). Neck sprains after RTA: a modern epidemic injury. *Injury*, 24:3, 155–7.

Harrison M. (1991). The minor head injury. *Paediatric Nursing*, Dec 1991, 15–19.

Hudak C., Gallo B. (1994). *Critical Care Nursing*. Philadelphia: J. B. Lippincott Co.

Lowdon I., Briggs M., Cockin J. (1989). Head injury. *Injury*, 20:4, 193–4.

88   *Critical Care*

Morris K. (1993). Assessment and communication of conscious level: an audit of neurosurgical referrals. *Injury*, **24:**6, 369–72.
OPCS (1991). *Mortality Statistics England and Wales*. London: Government Statistical Service.
Proehl J. (1992). The Glasgow Coma Scale; do it and do it right. *Journal of Emergency Nursing*, **18:**5, 421–3.
Randall P. E. (1986) MAST: a review. *Injury*, **17:**6.
Robinson D., Cassar-Pullicino V. N. (1993). Acute neck sprain after RTA: a long term clinical and radiological review. *Injury*, **24:**2, 79–82.
Ross S. et al. (1992). Clinical predictors of unstable cervical spine injury in multiply injured patients. *Injury*, **23:**5, 317–19.
Sinclair M. (1991). *Nursing the Neurosurgical Patient*. Oxford: Butterworth-Heinemann.
Walsh M., Ford P. (1989). *Nursing Rituals: Research and Rational Action*. Oxford: Butterworth-Heinemann.
Watson D. (1991). Management of the upper airway. In Skinner D., Driscoll P., Earlam R. (eds) *ABC of Major Trauma*. London: BMJ.
Zideman D. (1990). AIDS, hepatitis and resuscitation. In Evans T. R. (ed.) *ABC of Resuscitation*. London: BMJ.

Chapter 5

NURSING CARE OF THE CRITICALLY ILL PATIENT

Care of the Patient with Chest Pain of Cardiac Origin

Pathology

Ischaemic heart disease (IHD) is the most common serious cause of chest pain seen in A & E departments, accounting for some 150 000 deaths per year in England and Wales. The causes of IHD are many, involving social and psychological factors. For example, the death rate for men in 1990 in England and Wales was 33 per 10 000 compared to 25.6 for women (Chew, 1993), and, as Fig. 5.1 shows, there is a marked regional variation within the UK. The wealthier south of England has the lowest rates while the poorer north, together with Wales, Scotland and Ulster, have the highest rates. When deaths from all circulatory diseases are considered, only Sweden and Denmark amongst the advanced industrial countries have mortality rates 60–70% that of the UK, while in Japan it is well under half the UK figure (Chew, 1993). Clearly, therefore, social factors play a major role in the causation of this disease.

IHD is a disease of late middle age to old age. The death rate from IHD of men aged 25–44 was only 19 per 100 000 in 1990. Amongst men aged 45–64 this rose to 325 and in the age group 65–74 the rate was 1318 deaths per 100 000. (Figures for England and Wales only; Chew, 1993).

The majority of deaths from IHD occur soon after the onset of pain. Rawlins (1981) reported that 30.1% of those who died did so within 15 minutes after the onset of pain, and 56.3% had died by 2 hours after the onset. Thompson and Webster (1992) cite a typical figure of 60% of deaths occurring within one hour of infarct (see Fig. 5.2).

It is important to differentiate between angina and a myocardial infarction (MI). If the diseased coronary artery circulation is unable to meet an increased oxygen demand from the myocardium (usually

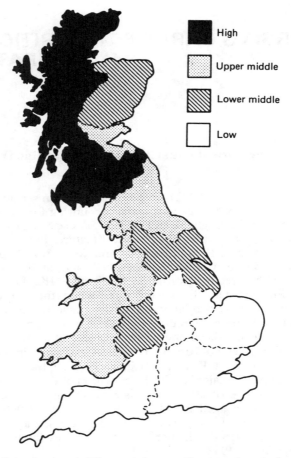

*Fig. 5.1   Regional differences in mortality rates from ischaemic
heart disease in men aged 45–54 years (Thompson and Webster,
1992)*

due to exercise), metabolic changes occur in the hypoxic myocardium
which produce the classic pain of angina pectoris—a diffuse, retro-
sternal pain which will often diminish with rest. The pain can be
easily confused with that of gastric disorders.

If, instead of an inadequate blood supply (angina), there is a

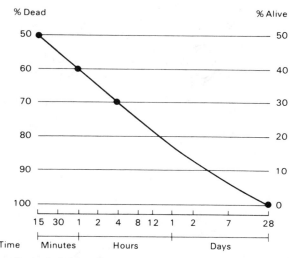

% Dead · % Alive

Time · Minutes · Hours · Days

Fig 5.2   Cumulative fatality against time in 348 coronary heart attacks where death occurred within 28 days (adapted from Tunstall Pedoe, 1978)

complete occlusion of the blood supply to a portion of the myocardium, that part will die, and a myocardial infarction will have occurred. The pain is localized in the centre of the chest. It is usually severe and crushing in nature, radiates into the left arm and possibly into the jaw, and it is not relieved by rest. The pain may be atypical, however, and in the elderly in particular, pain may be absent or at least not reported by the patient.

Assessment

The initial step is to let the patient describe the pain—its intensity, location, duration, what brought it on and whether there is any relevant previous history. A history of angina is common in patients presenting with an acute MI. Key observations are whether the pain has eased with rest or responded to GTN. If the answer is no, it is very likely to be an MI rather than an angina attack.

Mental state should be assessed as chest pain is a very frightening experience, and as fear and anxiety can make the condition worse.

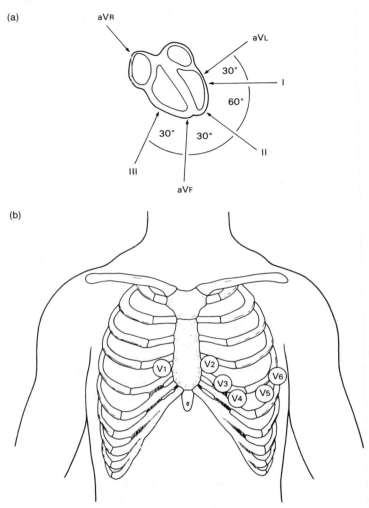

(a)

(b)

Once the general appearance of the patient has been noted—is it consistent with shock?—the vital signs need to be recorded. A rapid respiratory rate is usually seen in cardiac pain, associated with pulmonary congestion and/or the effects of anxiety. The pulse must be assessed for both rate and rhythm. A bradycardia carries a poor

(c)

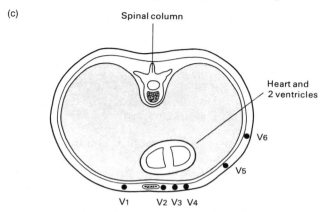

Fig 5.3 (a) *Front view of heart showing how the 6 standard or
limb leads relate in space*
(b) *View of chest showing correct position of 6 chest leads*
V1 4th intercostal space, right border sternum
V2 4th intercostal space, left border sternum
V3 midway V2 V4
V4 5th intercostal space, midline of clavicle
V5 5th intercostal space, tip of clavicle
V6 5th intercostal space, axilla
(c) *View of heart showing position of V leads*

prognosis in acute MI. A systolic BP below 90 mmHg usually
indicates shock, and if the patient is indeed suffering from an acute
MI, then the presence of cardiogenic shock also indicates a very
poor chance of survival. An accurate temperature reading is essential
to help to eliminate chest infection as an alternative possible cause of
the pain. Extensive research has shown that the thermometer needs
to be *in situ* at least 4 minutes for an accurate reading (Walsh and
Ford, 1989).

The next step in assessment is to carry out a 12-lead ECG in order
to discover any arrhythmia and evidence of MI or ischaemia. Before
performing an ECG, the nurse should explain *in language the patient
understands* exactly what is to be done and why—e.g. 'This machine
will take a recording of your pulse rate which will help us find out
what is causing your pain.' Explanations overheard by the author
vary from nothing at all (doctor) to 'This machine will do an
electrocardiographic recording of your heart' (medical student) to 'I

am just going to do a tracing of your heart' (nurse). The medical student's jargon frightened the patient, while the nurse's language conjured up images of pencils, tracing paper and a procedure akin to brass rubbing. None of the three approaches meant anything to the patient, increasing fear and anxiety as a result.

If nurses are to perform ECGs in A & E, they must understand what they are doing. In brief, they are recording the electrical activity of the heart with a delicate and sensitive machine. The machine should be handled with respect, and every effort should be made to obtain good electrical contact. A conducting medium is required for good contact (e.g. gel). The electrode should not be positioned on hairy parts of the body—the inside of the arms should be used and a razor for removing excess hair should always be on the ECG trolley. Alcohol swabs may also improve the quality of the ECG by removing excess body oil and sweat (Thompson and Webster, 1992). Patient movement, muscle tremor, and simple mains electric background hum will all cause interference.

Of the leads that are attached to the limbs, the right leg lead is an earth and plays no active part in the recording. There are, therefore, three limb leads which the machine uses to record the heart's electrical activity in six different combinations. Each of these leads gives a different view of the heart, together with the chest lead which is also used in six different positions. The result is 12 different views of the heart (see Fig. 5.3) which make it possible to localize the damaged part of the myocardium depending upon which leads show evidence of infarction. If, for example, leads II, III and aVf show the characteristic changes of an MI, it can be deduced that it is the inferior part of the heart that is damaged.

The basic components of an ECG are the:

P wave	Spread of electrical activity through the atria.
P-Q interval	Conduction of electrical impulse via the bundle of His to the ventricles.
QRS complex	Spread of electrical activity through the ventricles. The Q wave represents the first electrical activity away from the bundle of His in the intraventricular septum.
T wave	Repolarization of cells ready for next contraction.

Fig. 5.4 shows how the heart's conducting mechanism is related to the ECG. The machine is set to record a current towards the electrode as an upwards deflection.

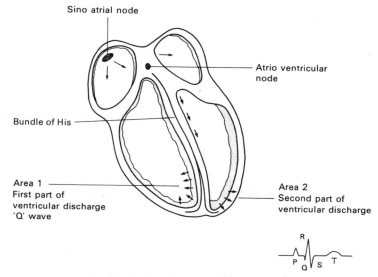

Sino atrial node

Atrio ventricular
node

Bundle of His

Area 1
First part of
ventricular discharge
'Q' wave

Area 2
Second part of
ventricular discharge

Fig 5.4   Conducting mechanism of the heart and the ECG

The A & E nurse should be able to recognize the following three ECG changes if correct triage of patients is to occur (see Fig. 5.5).

1. *Pathological Q wave.* An exaggerated Q wave indicates an area of dead myocardium, i.e. an MI has occurred at some time. However, as this is a permanent change in the ECG, it could relate to an episode that happened a year or more ago. Therefore, on its own, a pathologic Q wave does not indicate an acute MI. Consideration of Fig. 5.4 shows that the Q wave is normally lost in the electrical activity of area 2. However if area 2 is dead myocardium, there will be no electrical activity present and the whole of the normally activity in area I will be recorded, producing an exaggerated Q wave. The dead area of myocardium acts as an 'electrical window', allowing us to record activity normally swamped by healthy myocardium.

2. *Elevated ST segment.* This indicates acutely damaged myocardium and may be thought of as being due to the damaged cells leaking potassium ions (K^-) after each contraction. This leads to an excess of positive charges and hence the ST section is elevated above the normal baseline of the EGG (the isoelectric state).

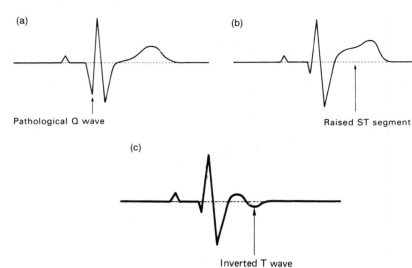

Fig 5.5   ECG changes associated with IHD
(a) Dead myocardium: pathological Q wave
(b) Damaged myocardium: raised ST section
(c) Ischaemic myocardium: inverted T wave

3. *T wave inversion.* This indicates myocardial ischaemia, but not an actual MI.

In addition to evidence of MI, the ECG will reveal if there is any serious arrhythmia present. Therefore, a 30 second rhythm strip from lead II should be obtained, and the patient should be continually attached to a cardiac monitor.

The need for explanation to the patient of what a cardiac monitor is cannot be understated.

The following are the major life-threatening arrhythmias which the nurse should be able to recognize on a monitor (see Fig. 5.6).

1. *Asystole.* No cardiac activity, cardiac arrest. It is essential to check the patient before instituting CPR as disconnected electrodes can produce a trace very similar to that of asystole.

2. *Ventricular fibrillation (VF).* Rapid quivering of the ventricles associated with a rapid, disorganized pattern of electrical activity. No output produced. Effectively VF is cardiac arrest. It requires

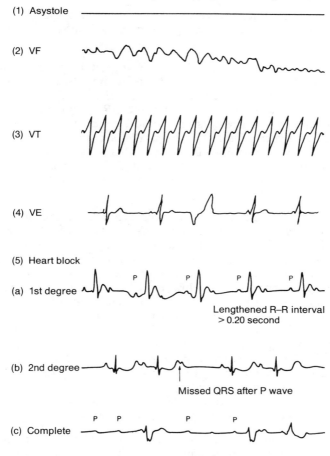

Fig 5.6   Serious arrhythmias

defibrillation and full CPR. Check first the patient's condition and responsiveness as electronic gremlins such as loose leads may be responsible!

3. *Ventricular tachycardia (VT)*. Caused by a ventricular pacemaker taking over pacing the heart and firing at a very rapid rate, 150–250 beats per minute. There are no P waves, only regular, bizarre ventricular complexes. Cardiac output falls to very low levels. There

is insufficient time for the ventricles to fill between each beat. The patient loses consciousness and proceeds to VF unless spontaneous remission occurs.

4. *Ventricular ectopics (VEs)*. If there is an irritable focus in one of the ventricles, it may begin firing off pacing impulses itself, leading to premature ventricular contractions or VEs. No P wave is seen, the beat comes early, and the shape of the QRS complex is different from normal as it represents an atypical conduction of electricity through the myocardium. Occasional VEs are not a cause for concern, but if they start to occur in runs, there is the possibility of a VT developing. Bigeminy is the coupling of a normal beat with a VE immediately afterwards. Trigeminy occurs when every third beat is a VE.

5. *Heart block*. First degree block involves a delay in the conduction of the electrical impulse through the AV node. The P–R interval is, therefore, lengthened and if it is greater than 0.2 seconds, first degree block exists. This condition may worsen until some of the impulses are not conducted at all. In this case, P waves may be seen with no QRS complexes to follow and a ventricular beat is dropped as a result. This is second degree block and may progress into a complete heart block (CHB) where the AV node fails to conduct any impulses at all. A ventricular pacemaker may take over to produce a slow rhythm (approximately 20–30 impulses per minute) which bears no linkage to the regular pattern of P waves which may still be seen. Such a slow rate leads to heart failure, and if the ventricular pacemaker fails to fire, the patient collapses with no cardiac output (Stokes–Adams attack) which will be a terminal event unless the ventricular pacemaker picks up again very quickly.

The key steps therefore in assessing the patient with chest pain are to obtain a description of the pain, assess the patient's appearance and mental state, record vital signs, and perform and interpret an ECG.

Intervention

In the case of patients with chest pain, prioritization of patients for the attention of A & E medical staff is the vital first step in nursing intervention. This is because of the close relationship between the time of death and the onset of symptoms (see p. 89). If the assessment described in the previous section is carried out accurately by the nurse, the patient may be assigned the correct priority and triage will have been correctly carried out.

One of the main thrusts of intervention is to limit the area of damage to the myocardium. To this end, high concentration oxygen should be administered at once. The patient should be cared for sitting upright to assist respiration. Unrelieved pain will contribute to higher levels of anxiety, stimulation of the sympathetic nervous system and hence increased cardiac activity, the result of which is that myocardial oxygenation is seriously compromised. Pain relief is, therefore, an urgent priority. Pain may be effectively relieved by the use of Entonox gas, which has the advantage of being 50% oxygen. Narcotic analgesia such as diamorphine should be administered IV immediately, usually in doses of 2.5 to 5.0 mg until pain relief is achieved. An anti-emetic drug such as prochlorperazine (12.5 mg) should also be given prophylactically and naloxone, the specific antidote to opioids should be immediately available in case of accidental overdose.

The relief of fear and anxiety will also assist in pain reduction. Psychological support is therefore essential. The patient should be cared for in a special 'cardiac cubicle' removed from the noise and bustle of the busy department, where monitoring can be carried out unobtrusively, i.e. with the monitor volume control on zero, and with the monitor invisible to the patient (but visible to staff). Explanations of what is happening together with the nurse's own attitude will reduce tension and fear, as will relief of pain, and the presence of family/friends.

The admission procedure to CCU should be expedited as much as possible, remembering the high risk of cardiac arrest in the immediate post-infarction period.

Medical interventions requiring nursing support will be limited to siting and heparinizing an IV cannula for venous access. Thrombolytic therapy aimed at dissolving the clot should be instituted at the earliest opportunity as necrosis of the ischaemic myocardium is almost complete within 6 hours of the occlusive event (Thompson and Webster, 1992). Agents used include streptokinase, urokinase and rtPA (recombinant tissue-type plasminogen activator). X-rays should not be obtained in A & E as this delays transfer to CCU; they should be taken later with a portable machine in CCU.

It should be the aim of an A & E unit to be able to transfer a patient with chest pain to CCU within 15–20 minutes of arrival. The transfer should always be undertaken with two porters and a qualified nurse and with necessary resuscitation equipment discreetly placed out of sight underneath the trolley. It is not a good idea to take relatives over to the CCU with the patient in case an emergency should develop in transit. It is better to take them over a few minutes later when the patient has been safely bedded down. It is important to prepare both patient and relatives so that they know what to expect in CCU; the array of monitors and other high-tech equipment can be very frightening and anxiety provoking.

Evaluation

Once a patient has been prioritized, they must not be forgotten. Their progress must be monitored and if necessary they should be afforded a higher priority if their condition changes. Effectiveness of pain relief must be assessed, and in the case of administration of narcotic analgesia, respiratory effort must be closely watched due to the depressant effect of opioids on respiration. Periodic checks on oxygen administration are required. The patient may remove the mask, especially to answer questions from the doctor, and leave it off.

It is very important to note how the patient's emotional state is progressing, as a modification in the environment (e.g. noise) or in the nursing personnel looking after the patient may be required to reduce anxiety.

Finally the nurse in charge of the patient must be continually checking progress against the target time of 20 minutes for transfer to CCU and not allow things to drift.

Care of the Patient with Respiratory Distress

Pathology

The principal causes of respiratory distress (other than trauma) are:

1. *Pulmonary oedema.* This in itself is not a disease but rather it is a symptom. The most usual causes are heart failure, MI and other cardiac conditions, but there are many other possible diseases that give rise to pulmonary oedema. The usual picture is one of back pressure from the left side of a diseased heart into the pulmonary circulation. The increased pressure in the pulmonary capillaries interferes with the normal osmotic pressure gradient. This causes fluid to move from the cells into the capillaries. The result is fluid oozing into the alveolar spaces and interfering with oxygen exchange.

Normally the amount of fluid in the lungs is equivalent to one-fifth of lung weight. In severe cases of pulmonary oedema, this may rise to the equivalent of ten times lung weight, a twenty-fold increase.

2. *Asthma.* The incidence of asthma appears to be increasing at a worrying rate with 2000 adult deaths per year, many of which are thought to be preventable. The effects of atmospheric pollution by motor vehicles may well help explain this increase. Whatever the cause, the result is obstruction of the bronchial tree due to bronchospasm. This is characterized by increasing mucosal oedema, constriction of the bronchial muscles leading to constriction of the bronchi, and plugs of mucus within the bronchi all of which obstruct the bronchi and lead to overdistension of the lungs (Corbin-West, 1992). This condition is associated with many other diseases such as bronchitis, pneumonia and emphysema. This leads to the characteristic asthmatic wheeze, hypoxia and understandable anxiety. Failure to respond to treatment leads to the severe condition of status asthmaticus.

3. *Acute on chronic bronchitis.* Chronic bronchitis is very strongly class-linked and in winter acute infections in already chronically diseased lungs lead to a very serious illness. The patient is often elderly.

4. *Spontaneous pneumothorax.* See p. 63.

5. *Pulmonary embolism (PE).* This occurs when a portion of thrombus in a systemic vein on the right side of the heart is dislodged into the circulation and lodges in either the main pulmonary artery (usually fatal) or a smaller artery. When a smaller artery is involved, a PE usually leads to an area of infarcted lung.

6. *Foreign body.* Small children are prone to inhaling all sorts of objects, some of which may lodge in the lower bronchial tree and cause serious chemical damage to lung tissue (e.g. a peanut) and/or areas of lung to collapse distally. Adults tend to come to A & E complaining of animal bones (e.g. fish or chicken bones) or other food being 'stuck in my throat'. Often they have swallowed the offending object but it has left a tear on the pharynx wall which produces a sensation of an object being stuck.

7. *Smoke inhalation.* Modern synthetic materials contain substances which, when burnt, release toxic fumes (e.g. synthetic materials in carpets may release hydrogen cyanide and ammonia). This means that in addition to possible burn injury, the patient may suffer

serious respiratory impairment due to chemical lung damage or asphyxia from increased levels of carboxyhaemoglobin caused by carbon monoxide inhalation.

8. *Drowning.* Sea water is a hypertonic solution and therefore it exerts an osmotic pull, drawing fluid into the alveoli. Fresh water, on the other hand, is hypotonic and will readily diffuse into the blood through the alveolar wall. In doing so, however, the contaminants invariably contained in the water will destroy lung surfactant and the fluid will seep back into the alveoli. The result in either case is pulmonary oedema.

Of great significance in immersion injury victims is the time spent in the water and the temperature of the water. Hypothermia develops quickly leading to circulatory collapse. Ironically if the victim is floating in an upright position in the water (e.g. wearing a life jacket), the hydrostatic pressure of the water on the lower limbs has a similar effect to MAST, which may preserve life for a considerable period. However, once the victim is rescued, that pressure is lost, the compromised circulation collapses and death occurs within minutes.

Immersion in cold water can produce serious cardiac arrhythmias, including bradycardia which makes the patient appear lifeless upon rescue as there is no immediately palpable pulse or obvious respiratory effort. However, recovery is still possible. This is well documented in cases of persons falling through ice on frozen lakes.

9. *Hysterical hyperventilation.* Hysterical overbreathing disturbs the blood chemistry by blowing off large amounts of CO_2. This leads to an alkalosis and upsets the normal levels of serum calcium. The result is muscle spasm (tetany) which typically causes hyperextension of the fingers and abdominal pain (see Fig. 5.7).

Assessment

The rate and type of respiration should be observed together with the other vital signs. If the patient is mouth breathing, the temperature may be recorded in the axilla for a minimum of 5 minutes. Wheezing indicates expiratory difficulty and is associated with asthma primarily, but may be found in other conditions, e.g. drowning and smoke inhalation. Stridor indicates difficulty on inspiration, often caused by a foreign body. The nurse should observe whether the breathing is easy or laboured and involving use of the accessory muscles of respiration (the shoulder girdle). A peak flow meter

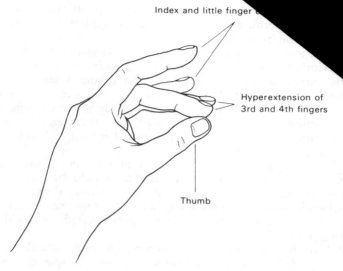

Index and little finger

Hyperextension of
3rd and 4th fingers

Thumb

Fig 5.7. Carpo-pedal spasm

should be available as peak flows form a good guide to progress in treating asthmatic patients.

The following key points should be noted in assessing respiration:

- The longer the period of expiration the greater the degree of obstruction.
- A grey, sweating, dyspnoeic patient sitting upright is in grave danger of respiratory arrest.
- Respiratory rate does not equate with the degree of dyspnoea, it slows down as the patient becomes more tired with the effort of breathing.
- Dyspneoa in the elderly patient may be the only presenting sign of acute myocardial infarction (Corbin-West, 1992).

If the patient is Caucasian, observation of skin colour is a key step in assessment. A cold, clammy pale skin is frequently found in heart failure. Cyanosis, on the other hand, is a late sign and indicates severe respiratory failure. Inhalation of carbon monoxide (CO) produces a deceptively healthy pink skin due to the formation of large amounts of carboxyhaemoglobin.

Mental state must be assessed as respiratory distress is a very ʒical support will be essential.

.gn of respiratory failure as it is

atient has any pain and to obtain
ɔain requires treatment as for a
be a pulmonary embolus that is
ɛralized pain over one side of the
back, made worse by coughing or
ɔ stabbing character, is caused by
will be associated with acute infec-

A histuɪ ɔ   cult to obtain due to the patient's
respiratory distress. ɪⅽ_   or friends should be closely questioned. In questioning the patient, it is useful to try to phrase
questions if possible in such a way that the patient has only to make
'yes' or 'no' answers that can be communicated by nodding or
shaking the head.

In examining the rest of the patient, the nurse should look for
certain clues. The hands may reveal carpo-pedal spasm, typical of
hysterical hyperventilation. Fingers may be nicotine-stained, indicating a heavy smoker who is prone to chronic chest infections. Alternatively, fingers may display the characteristic clubbing at the ends
associated with long-standing pulmonary disease. Chronic obstruc-
tive airway disease produces a typical barrel-shaped or 'pigeon'
chest. The legs should be examined for evidence of a deep vein
thrombosis (DVT) that could have led to a pulmonary embolism.
Are the calves the same size? Is there calf tenderness?

A specimen should be obtained of anything expectorated. Is it
blood stained or purulent?

The medical assessment will include a detailed chest examination,
X-rays and arterial blood gases.

Intervention

The patient should first be sat upright to help breathing and then
high concentration oxygen should be administered. The one exception to the use of high concentration oxygen is the patient with a
long-standing history of respiratory disease, hence the importance of
obtaining a history and checking for signs such as clubbing of the
fingers and barrel chest.

The respiratory drive is normally stimulated by rising levels of

CO_2 in the blood. However, in a patient with chronic respiratory disease, the body has adapted to high CO_2 levels and the respiratory drive, therefore, depends upon the secondary mechanism of low O_2 levels in the blood. Giving high concentration oxygen to such a patient will so increase arterial oxygen levels that the respiratory drive will cease to be effective and the patient may lapse into respiratory arrest. Consequently, if assessment indicates the existence of a chronic respiratory disease, oxygen should only be administered in low concentration—24% or 28%.

The patient who is confused because of cerebral hypoxia may not tolerate an oxygen mask. One solution is to use nasal oxygen cannulae or, as a temporary step, the nurse may hold the mask over the patient's face but without the mask touching the skin.

Psychological support is essential as the patient will be anxious and often very distressed. The nurse's own emotional behaviour will play a large part in determining the patient's (see p. 17). Particularly in conditions such as hyperventilation and to a lesser extent asthma, reducing anxiety will help to resolve the respiratory problem itself. The nurse being always visible and providing explanation of what is happening, and why, will help the patient. Nothing could be worse than the acutely distressed patient, abandoned in a dark corridor, awaiting a chest X-ray, alone with the feeling that there is no way they can summon help if they need it. The presence of members of the family may have a beneficial effect on the patient's psychological status, and hence on their breathing. But it can also work the other way, especially when large numbers of people are involved or when certain key individuals are present with whom there is a relationship problem.

Frequent monitoring of vital signs is required, with the respirations deserving maximum attention. Pulse oximetry is essential in the management of patients in serious respiratory distress.

If confusion is present, precautions should be taken to prevent the patient from coming to harm—cot sides, close observation, and reality orientation, carried out at every opportunity, may all be necessary.

Nursing support will be required for medical interventions which usually centre around establishing an IV line and administering drugs via that route. Examples of commonly used drug therapy in A & E for the patient with respiratory distress include IV frusemide 80 mg for pulmonary oedema (diuretic), IV aminophylline 250 mg and hydrocortisone 100 mg for asthma (bronchodilator and anti-inflammatory), IV heparin 5000–10 000 units for a pulmonary embolism (anticoagulant) and nebulized salbutamol 5 mg for asthma (bronchodilator).

In addition to trying to calm the hysterically hyperventilating patient (which often involves the removal of friends), a further useful step is to make the patient breathe in and out of a paper bag. The effect of this is to make them rebreathe their own CO_2 which will increase their CO_2 levels to normal, restore normal blood chemistry, and relieve the muscle spasm (tetany) that exacerbates the distressed state they are in. In many cases, it should be possible to have the patient breathing normally, without tetany, in 5–10 minutes.

Patients in respiratory distress should be afforded a high priority for medical attention. From the nursing point of view, the optimal care will be provided by the administration of the correct oxygen concentration, the positioning of the patient so as to facilitate breathing, the offering of psychological support to relieve anxiety, and continual observation.

Evaluation

Just because the patient is put in the correct position with the correct oxygen mask *in situ* does not mean that they are going to stay that way! They may remove the mask or slip down the trolley. Continual evaluation is essential to pick up these sort of problems and to correct them. Some of the drugs given during respiratory distress are very potent, which makes it essential to watch patient progress closely; for example, aminophylline and salbutamol can have cardiac side effects. ECG monitoring during the use of IV aminophylline is strongly recommended therefore. To take another example, if the patient has been given IV frusemide, the nurse should note whether they pass urine or not. If not, have they a bladder palpable? Are they in urinary retention as a result?

Due to the significant effect that anxiety can have on respiration, it is important to be continually evaluating the effectiveness of our psychological support for the patient and how the patient is relating to the friends/family that are present. (See Fig. 5.8 Critical pathway for patient with acute respiratory distress.)

Care of the Patient with Impaired Consciousness

Pathology

There are many reasons why a person's level of consciousness might

	0–5 min	6–15 min	16–60 min
Documentation	Registration as A & E patient	Notes ready for CO Hospital notes available	Admission forms complete
Assessment	Seen by triage nurse. RR, P general appearance, conscious level. Triage as top priority	BP, T, 12 lead ECG Pulse oximetry ABGs Chest XR continue RR, P ECG monitor CO exam patient	Continue vital signs, ECG and pulse oximetry Bloods for routine lab work
Medication	–	Bronchodilator by inhalation, IV frusemide as ordered	Continue as ordered
Treatment	Commence O_2	Continue O_2. Insert and heparinize IV cannula	O_2 therapy
Nursing care	Sit patient upright psychological support, close observation	Undress patient. Continue psychological support and explain procedures, ensure upright position and comfort, observe carefully	Continue as before, ensure bedpan/urinal available if IV frusemide given Inform receiving ward
Referrals	–	On call medical team	–
Family	Obtain relevant history, inform if not present	Inform of progress	Allow family member to see patient
Discharge	–	–	Transfer to ward when fit and bed available. Ensure all notes/XRs go with patient

Fig. 5.8   Example of critical pathway for patient with acute respiratory distress

be diminished. The following section concentrates on some of the more common causes of patients presenting at A & E with impaired consciousness with the exception of head injury and the effects of drugs and alcohol. Head injury has been dealt with already and drugs and alcohol will be discussed in Chapter 17.

1. *Cerebrovascular accident (CVA)*. The cause may be bleeding from a cerebral blood vessel leading to either a subarachnoid haemorrhage or intracerebral haemorrhage. The onset will be sudden in most cases. Alternatively, there may be occlusion of a blood vessel due to a thrombus (a more gradual onset) or an embolus (a sudden onset).

2. *Fits.* Fitting may be a sign of a range of pathological conditions although there may also be no apparent cause of the fitting behaviour (idiopathic epilepsy).

In grand mal epilepsy, the problem is an abnormal discharge of electricity within the brain which first produces a characteristic aura if it is located near one of the sensory centres (e.g. smell, visual disturbance) and then goes on to produce a tonic period of some 30 seconds or so when the patient's musculature goes into spasm and the patient is, as a result, unable to breathe. This is followed by the clonic stage of convulsions which passes into a deep coma from which the patient gradually wakes up. At this stage, often referred to as the 'post-ictal stage', confusion is likely.

3. *Diabetes.* In hyperglycaemic states, the metabolism of fats leads to the formation of ketones whose effects on the brain lead to unconsciousness and brain damage if the ketotic state is not reversed. The body's efforts to excrete the excess glucose in the urine lead to dehydration, hypovolaemic shock and electrolyte imbalance. Ketone formation leads to acidosis which the body seeks to correct by reducing CO_2 levels in the blood (CO_2 dissolves in water to form a weak acid). Hence the deep, sighing respirations characteristic of the hyperglycaemic state.

In hypoglycaemic states, the lack of blood glucose affects the brain to produce drowsiness, confusion and unconsciousness. As urine output has been normal, the patient will not be dehydrated or hypovolaemic.

4. *Acute infections and toxaemic states.* Any acute infection involving the brain, for example meningitis or encephalitis, will obviously affect the level of consciousness. Furthermore, any infection that

leads to hypoxia (e.g. chest infections) will diminish consciousness as will toxaemic states (e.g. uraemia).

Assessment

The first step must always be to assess airway, breathing and circulation, before moving on to assessing level of consciousness.

A history of the event together with any relevant medical history should be obtained. An epileptic fit may be described or the patient may be known as a diabetic. In undressing the patient, clues such as Medic-Alert bracelets, sugar lumps, out-patient cards and injection sites should be searched for. Identification of the patient is essential, not only so that next of kin can be informed, but also so that hospital notes can be obtained.

In assessing vital signs, the nurse will find further evidence of the cause of the patient's problem. The person in a hyperglycaemic diabetic condition will be dehydrated and hypovolaemic. The CVA patient will often be hypertensive. Rapid respiratory rate will indicate hypoxia and a pyrexia an infection. The patient may also be hypothermic if they have been in a cold environment for several hours with impaired consciousness. A rectal temperature below 35°C indicates hypothermia.

Blood sugar should always be tested, using a needle prick stix test.

Limb weakness should be assessed for evidence of hemiplegia (or monoplegia). Plantar reflexes should be tested by stroking the outer soles of the feet with a sharp object. An abnormal upward curling of the toes indicates an upper motor neurone lesion such as a CVA or a post-epileptic state. Extensor response to pain indicates a brain stem CVA.

A urine specimen should be tested, the hyperglycaemic patient's urine revealing glucose and probably ketones. A uraemic state will cause protein to appear in the urine. An unconscious diabetic patient may be catheterized to obtain a specimen as the presence of ketones in the urine is a very important medical sign.

The medical assessment will include a detailed neurological exam, radiography and blood samples for culture and biochemistry. Lumbar puncture is best performed on the wards and not in the A & E department.

Intervention

The immediate interventions with regard to airway, breathing, circulation and unconsciousness have already been discussed. However, if the patient is conscious but confused, steps must be taken to protect the patient from potential harm. Cot sides should be set up and carefully checked. There should be continual nursing observation and, if necessary, the patient can be nursed on a mattress on the floor. Reality orientation is required with the nurse telling the patient what has happened, what time it is and where the patient is, in order that the patient may make some sense out of the situation. The information should be kept simple as consciousness is impaired.

By providing reality orientation, nurses can help the patient hang on to reality. Try to imagine waking up in totally unfamiliar surroundings, with complete strangers standing around, a gap of maybe several hours in your consciousness and your mental processes impaired by illness. You will then appreciate the importance of reality orientation as a major nursing intervention.

Specific problems revealed by the assessment should be dealt with on their merits. Therefore, if the patient has had a fit, along with care of the patient in a confused post-ictal state, the possibility of the patient having a further fit should be considered. Observation is essential, with the aim of preventing accidental self-harm should a further fit occur. In such a situation, the patient is best left to get on with their fit, intervention being restricted to protecting the head if possible by using a blanket or pillow and by removing any objects that may harm the patient. The nurse should not attempt to restrain the patient or to force an airway into the mouth during either the tonic or clonic stages. This is dangerous and can lead to either the patient's teeth being knocked out or the nurse accidentally being bitten. Once the patient has stopped convulsing, he or she should be turned into the recovery position. The nurse should only then consider the use of an airway and then only if the patient tolerates it. Incontinence may occur due to relaxation of muscle sphincters at this stage. Therefore, the nurse must be prepared to clean the patient accordingly. If fitting is continuous and does not resolve after one attack, status epilepticus is said to be present. This serious condition requires medical intervention to control the fitting (to prevent anoxic brain damage). This intervention usually consists of intravenous diazepam or if needed a general anaesthetic and muscle relaxants to facilitate airway management and prevent further anoxic cerebral damage.

If assessment reveals that the patient is hypoglycaemic, and if the patient is able to drink, a glucose drink should be given immediately. A supply of Lucozade in the A & E drugs fridge is invaluable. If the patient cannot drink, IV dextrose 50% is given via a butterfly needle; 50 ml is usually sufficient to restore the patient to a normal level of consciousness.

In a hyperglycaemic state, the medical staff will need to correct the dehydration rapidly with an IV infusion. The first litre is usually given as quickly as possible, together with a stat dose of intravenous insulin (one of the rapid-acting varieties). Nursing assistance will be required, together with accurate fluid balance and vital signs monitoring, and usually catheterization to test for ketones and manage the urine output.

If a pyrexia of over 39°C is present, active steps, such as fanning and tepid sponging, must be taken to reduce the temperature. This is because if it rises to 40°C or above, fitting will often develop.

A space blanket should be used if the rectal temperature is below 35°C.

The possibility of an infection that could be transmitted to other patients in the department should be considered and the appropriate steps taken in line with hospital policy (e.g. disposal of waste and linen).

Pressure area care does not begin on the wards. It begins in A & E, and this fact is particularly important for patients with impaired consciousness. The trolleys in most A & E departments are very hard, and delays in moving patients to the wards are common, therefore patient care should include full pressure area care. Nurses should also check for incontinence which must be cleaned up at once to protect the skin and the patient's own self-image and pride. Nurses should make sure that the patient understands how to summon help if needed for the toilet or any other purpose. The phrase 'basic nursing care' is easily paid lip service to, but this should not be the case in A & E where with the help of Orem's model of nursing the patient's self-care demands should all be met.

Evaluation

Frequent checks should be made of level of consciousness and orientation to assess progress and the effectiveness of reality orientation. Temperature monitoring will reveal the effectiveness of measures such as tepid sponging and the use of a fan. Finger prick tests allow capillary blood sugar to be checked frequently so the effectiveness of care of the patient with a diabetic problem can be evaluated. Regular examination of the patient is needed, to ensure intervention as frequently as required, if there is a risk of incontinence and pressure sores. After a patient has had a fit, it is important to check that there is no evidence of a head injury and to monitor level of consciousness subsequently during the post-ictal period.

Care of the Patient with Abdominal Pain

Pathology

Detailed accounts of abdominal emergencies can be found in many surgical nursing textbooks. It is, however, useful to present a brief table of the most common emergencies seen in A & E (see Table 5.1). Many patients who present with abdominal pain are self-referred or sent in by a GP without the correct referral procedure to the 'on take' surgical team. The first person they meet is a nurse. Therefore, it is essential that the A & E nurse be able to prioritize such patients correctly.

Assessment

In order to decide upon the priority with which the patient will be seen, the nurse needs to determine the degree of pain the patient is in and the history of the illness and the associated pain. The vital signs are also essential in making this decision.

In assessing the pain felt by the patient, nurses are in a very subjective area for, as already discussed, different people from different backgrounds interpret pain and illness in different ways. It may help to ask the patient to rate the pain on a five point scale, and then try to obtain a description of the pain. Is it constant or intermittent? A steady pain or a gripping sharp pain? Is it localized to one area? Shooting into another part of the body (radiating)? Or generalized over the whole abdomen? Gripping pains of an intermittent nature are known as colic and indicate obstruction of the gut, ureter or bile duct (e.g. biliary or ureteric colic). The pain of appendicitis is localized to the right iliac fossa. The pain of peritonitis is generalized over the whole abdomen.

In taking a history of the illness, the nurse should be checking for

Table 5.1
Common causes of abdominal pain seen in A & E

System	Disease/Disorder	Typical Age	Comments
1. Gastro-intestinal	Indigestion	Young/middle age	Often presents as chest pain
	Alcoholic gastritis	Young/middle age	History of heavy alcohol intake
	Gastroenteritis	Young	Diarrhoea, risk of cross-infection
	Constipation	Any	Dietary advice and enema needed
	Appendicitis	Young	Nausea and low grade pyrexia
	Peptic ulcer	Middle/elderly	Haematemesis and melaena. Peritonitis – rigid abdomen; shock if perforated
	Obstruction	Elderly	Possible cause of obstruction – cancer, adhesions, strangulated hernia 'Drip and suck'
	Biliary colic	Young/middle age	Colic type of pain
2. Urinary	Renal/ureteric colic	Young/middle age	Colic type of pain, haematurea
	Cystitis	Young (female)	Need MSU and urinalysis
	Retention of urine	Elderly (male)	Palpable bladder, catheterize
3. Vascular	Aortic aneurysm	Elderly	Hypovolaemia, immediate surgery
	Saddle embolism	Elderly	Circulation to legs lost/impaired
	Mesenteric embolism	Any	Circulation to gut impaired

vomiting, the type of vomit—whether coffee grounds, fresh blood or bile—and any history of unusual bowel actions, such as diarrhoea, melaena or clay-coloured stools. Previous medical history should be noted as it may contain clues such as changing bowel habits and weight loss (carcinoma?), previous abdominal surgery (adhesions?), and episodes of similar pain relieved by eating (peptic ulceration?). Urine should be tested also.

The nurse should examine the patient's abdomen, palpating to see if it is soft or rigid. The bladder should be felt for. Is it full? An

Table 5.2
Nursing assessment of abdominal pain – important factors in prioritization

Medical Attention is Required

Urgently	*Soon*	*Can wait*
BP less than 80 mmHg systolic	Coffee grounds vomit	BP 110 mmHg or more systolic
Severe constant abdominal pain	Melaena	Soft abdomen
Pulsatile abdominal mass	Palpable bladder	Normal stools
Cold leg(s)	Temperature over 38°C	Constipation
No femoral pulse	Colicky pain	
Rigid abdomen	Haematurea	
No bowel sounds		
Haematemesis		

aneurysm will be readily felt as a pulsatile mass in the midline. Stethoscopic examination should be carried out to listen for bowel sounds, their absence indicating a paralytic ileus.

The mental state of the patient, together with any social problems, should be assessed as urgent intervention may be needed. Sudden illness, pain and vomiting constitute a very stressful event for most people. Table 5.2 is not a rigid set of rules but rather a set of general guidelines. Each patient must be assessed in their own right as an individual.

Intervention

Pain relief is a major priority. This can be achieved with Entonox in many cases. Whatever the patient's pain levels, psychological support for both patient and family is required. The patient should be allowed to assume whatever position is the most comfortable for them.

Surgical intervention is frequently needed. Patients, therefore, should all be kept nil by mouth and, as far as possible, the correct hospital pre-operative procedures with regard to matters such as consent, property and identification bands should be followed. Fear of surgery is to be expected and everything must be done to keep the patient and family informed of what is happening and why. This will help to reduce anxiety.

The traditional 'drip and suck' regime will often be asked for by the surgical team. This requires the passing of a nasogastric tube to aspirate stomach contents and the hydration of the patient by intravenous fluids. Accurate fluid balance together with careful recording of stools is needed.

Evaluation

The degree of relief from pain and anxiety should be noted; further intervention may be needed. Remember that it is the responsibility of the nurse in charge to check that theatre protocols have been correctly carried out by junior staff—for example, is the denture pot labelled with the patient's name? Continual monitoring of vital signs is needed to assess progress. It is important to check that the patient fully understands what has been said with regard to theatre, especially with elderly patients who will often nod in agreement to anything said by doctors without really understanding fully the implications. It is the responsibility of the nurse to check the degree of comprehension by the patient concerning future treatment plans.

References

Chew R. (1993). *Compendium of Health Statistics 1992*. London: Office of Health Economics.
Corbin-West A. (1992). The patient with bronchospasm: assessment, triage and teaching adjuncts. *Journal of Emergency Nursing*, **18**:6, 511–15.
Rawlins D. C. (1981). Study of the management of suspected cardiac infarction by British immediate care doctors. In *Immediate Prehospital Care* (Basket P., ed.). Chichester: John Wiley and Sons.
Silman A. J. (1981). Routinely collected data and IHD in the UK. *Health Trends*, **3**, 39–42.
Thompson D., Webster P. (1992). *Caring for the Coronary Patient*. Oxford: Butterworth-Heinemann.
Tunstall Pedoe, H. (1978). The Tower Hamlets study. *British Heart Journal*, **40**, 510.
Walsh M., Ford P. (1989). *Nursing: Rituals, Research and Rational Actions*. Oxford: Heinemann Medical Books.

SECTION III

Nursing Care of the Injured Patient

6 Fractures and Dislocations

7 Plaster of Paris Application

8 Soft Tissue Injury

9 The Burnt Patient in A & E

10 Eye Complaints and Emergencies

11 ENT and Dental Emergencies

12 Children in A & E

13 Elderly People in A & E

14 Women's Health Problems in A & E

15 Major Disaster Planning and Radiation Casualties

Chapter 6

FRACTURES AND DISLOCATIONS

Pathology—Causes of Fractures

Fractures are usually thought of as being due to trauma. This is not always the case, however, as repeated stress on a bone can lead to its fracture by a process similar to metal fatigue. Such a fracture is logically known as a stress fracture and is commonly seen in the foot (metatarsal) or the lower limb (fibula). Alternatively, bone can be so weakened by disease that it fails with little or no force involved. This is known as a pathological fracture and is seen, for example, where a tumour has led to secondary deposits in the bone (bony metastases).

Overall, however, the vast majority of fractures *are* due to trauma, and these are described as direct or indirect. In an indirect fracture, the break occurs at some point other than that where the force impacted against the bone; for example, a fall on an outstretched hand may lead to a fracture of the clavicle or wrist. Conversely, a direct fracture occurs when the bone breaks at the point of impact; thus, an over-the-ball-tackle in football leads to a fractured lower third of tibia and fibula.

Types of Fracture

One very important distinction in considering fractures is whether or not the fracture is open or closed. If the fracture site is in direct contact with the outside environment, no matter how small the wound, it is an open fracture. The importance of this consideration stems from the risk of infection which can involve the bone, leading to the very serious condition of osteomyelitis.

Fracture types may be described according to the diagram in Fig. 6.1. Such a classification is important as the orthopaedic

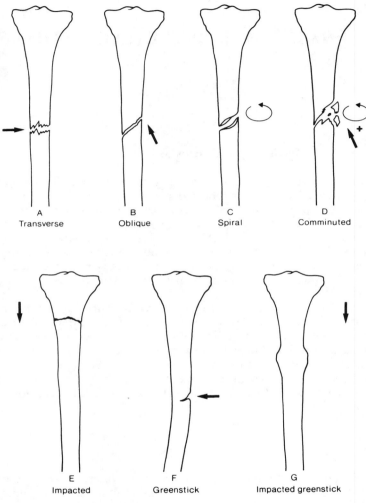

A	B	C	D
Transverse	Oblique	Spiral	Comminuted

E	F	G
Impacted	Greenstick	Impacted greenstick

Fig. 6.1   Common patterns of fracture and associated forces

surgeon needs to know the mechanism of injury if the fracture is to be successfully reduced. This is because the logical way of reducing a fracture is to reverse the forces involved in the original injury.

Fractures and Children

Children's bones have different properties that make fractures a special case when compared to fractures in adults. The much higher proportion of collagen fibres to calcium salts in children's bones means that the bones are less rigid. The result is the greenstick type of fracture where there is only an incomplete break and some cortical continuity remains. As bone growth is occurring at the epiphyseal cartilages located at either end of the bone, fractures involving this region are cause for special concern due to the risk of deformity from damage to the growing area. Such fractures are known as Salter's fractures and are graded I through V in order of seriousness.

Fracture Healing

Fracture healing is a complex process that requires an infection-free environment, fracture immobilization and a good blood supply. Where possible the aim of management is to provide such a situation so that healing can occur conservatively. However, if it is felt that the nature of the fracture is such that this will not occur or that the hazards of lengthy immobilization are too great (e.g. in the cases of a pathological fracture or a fracture of the femur in an elderly person), then the surgeon may opt to fix the fracture internally by an operation.

The first step in healing is the formation of a haematoma at the fracture site (Fig. 6.2). The haematoma takes little active part in the healing process and is quickly absorbed as cells from the deep surface of the periosteum divide and invade the haematoma. These cells are precursors of the osteoblasts, the cells that play an active part in the construction of new bone. The osteoblasts are responsible initially for the formation of callus which is an immature matrix of collagen and polysaccharides that becomes impregnated with calcium salts and as a result is visible on X-rays. As the callus matures into bone, the final stage of healing occurs with another type of cell, the osteoclasts, helping to remodel the bone by stripping off the surplus bulge from around the fracture site and reopening the medullary canal.

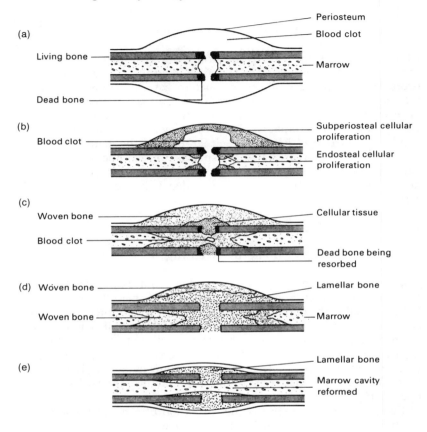

Modified from Crawford Adams J. (1983). *Outline of Fractures, including Joint Injuries*, 8th edn. Edinburgh: Churchill Livingstone.

Fig. 6.2   Pathology of fractures and the healing of fractures. (a) Haematoma, with necrosis of the bone next to the fracture. (b) Subperiosteal and endosteal cell growth. The haematoma is absorbed. (c) Callus formation. The cells, osteoblasts, lay down intercellular substance which calcifies to form bone. (d) Consolidation. Osteoblasts lay down lamellar bone. The woven bone diminishes. (e) Remodelling. Along the lines of stress, the bone is strengthened. Elsewhere it is reabsorbed.

Dislocations

When a joint is dislocated, by definition the two joint surfaces are so far displaced that there is no apposition between them. This dislocation also causes serious ligament and joint capsule damage. The term subluxation is used when there has been a partial dislocation so that there is still some apposition of joint surfaces.

Complications of Fractures and Dislocations

If the fracture is open, the most feared complication is osteomyelitis. Gas gangrene and tetanus are further major complications that are possible with a badly contaminated wound.

If there is pressure on a nerve or blood vessel due to the abnormal position of the bone or to tissue swelling, serious neurovascular complications can arise which in extreme cases can lead to the loss of the limb or to serious disability. Fracture above the humeral condyles can lead to the brachial artery being trapped, cutting off the blood supply to the forearm. This is most often seen in children and leads to Volkmann's ischaemic contracture, a flexion deformity of the hand and wrist. Arterial damage in leg fractures can lead to amputation.

Bleeding from a fractured bone can cause hypovolaemic shock. One litre of blood may be lost from a mid-shaft fracture of the femur and two litres may be lost from fractures of the pelvis (Paton, 1992). In joint injuries, bleeding into a joint is called a haemarthrosis; such is the limited space within a joint capsule that the result can be a very tense painful joint indeed. If a fracture enters a joint, it is essential for the surgeon to seek as anatomically perfect a reduction as possible as any irregularity left in the joint will lead to the rapid development of osteoarthritis.

Assessment

The triage nurse will have to carry out a rapid assessment of the injured patient and should be looking for the following key signs.

A cardinal sign to look for is localized bony tenderness, i.e. pain upon palpating the fracture site. This sign is best elicited by gently feeling along the bone and watching the patient for discomfort associated with pressing a discrete area over a bone. Deformity of the limb may not be present if the fracture is undisplaced, therefore localized bony tenderness is *the* key sign.

Once the probability of a fracture being present has been assessed, the next step is to assess the amount of pain that the injury is causing the patient and the patient's understanding of the possible injury. Patient compliance with treatment will only be fully forthcoming if the patient understands fully the nature of the injury.

The neurovascular state of the limb should be assessed distal to the injury by feeling for a pulse, the location of which should be marked on the skin. Serious damage can occur if a blood vessel or nerve is involved in the fracture. Dykes (1993) recommends nurses remember the 5 'p's of pain, pulses, paraesthesia, pallor and paralysis in assessing injured limbs. They should all be checked for distal to the fracture to ensure there are no signs of neurovascular damage. Any wound present should be examined with the possibility of an open fracture borne in mind.

Patient assessment should not be confined to the one limb where there may be an obvious fracture. If there has been sufficient force to break one bone, there may be other less obvious injuries as well, including fractures of other limbs. Taylor et al. (1994) showed, in a survey of 250 consecutive patients with fractured shafts of femur, that 85 had other serious injuries. Of this sample, 37 were motorcyclists and 92 were pedestrians; well over half of these patients had other significant injuries, yet in the 81 patients whose fractured shaft of femur stemmed from falls, only 7 had significant other injuries. The type of accident therefore has a major role in determining the risk of further injuries. Vital signs should be recorded to give a baseline from which any deviation indicative of hypovolaemic shock may be detected. The blood loss from fractures alone may cause this condition, in addition to which there is the possible loss of blood from soft tissue injury. As a rule of thumb, an open fracture has twice the blood loss of a closed one.

The psychological and social status of the patient should not be overlooked. This is of great importance in dealing with the elderly because very often it is these factors rather than physical problems that determine management.

Similar considerations apply if the patient has a dislocated joint. Lack of normal joint movement, pain and deformity are the key signs that the nurse will find present upon assessment.

Intervention

Provided that there is no other life-threatening problem immediately identified, the first goal of intervention should be pain relief. Immobilization of the fracture will make a contribution towards this goal. Home-made or ambulance splints should be removed to allow adequate assessment of the limb (using Entonox as required) and should be replaced with one of two kinds of splint.

If there is a femoral shaft fracture, traction will be required. The traditional method was the use of the Thomas splint with skin traction to overcome the very strong pull of the thigh muscles and to immobilize the fracture. A more modern approach involves the use of the telescopic Tracsplint system developed in the USA.

For fractures of the other long bones, traction is not required in A & E. The best method of immobilization for these fractures involves the use of a vacuum splint. This is a bag full of polystyrene beads that can be placed around the limb; when evacuated by use of the wall suction, it collapses under atmospheric pressure, forming a rigid splint and moulding to the shape of the limb. Such a system is far superior to old-fashioned methods involving bandaging the injured limb to a rigid splint. In the new system, the limb is not under pressure, the splint is radiotranslucent and the limb is fully visible all the time to allow continual observation of its vascular status. Furthermore, in application, the new vacuum splint is far less painful for the patient.

The next step in relieving pain is to try to minimize swelling by elevation. Hand and wrist fractures should be in a sling; fractures of the lower limb should be elevated by elevating the foot of the trolley. Rings and other constricting jewellery should be removed as soon as possible before swelling becomes a problem.

Movement of the injured limb should be minimized. The situation should not be allowed where successive doctors all want to look at the fracture, resulting in the splint being removed and reapplied several times. Entonox can be freely used for pain relief and in head injury cases this may still be used as the powerful opioids may be withheld for fear of depressing the level of consciousness.

Fear and anxiety will only increase the pain felt by the patient and tend to make for less cooperation. Clear explanation of what is happening and why, together with attention being paid to matters such as informing next of kin, will make a substantial contribution to pain control and the patient's well-being.

The pain of a dislocation may be partly relieved by supporting the limb, thereby removing any weight that the joint has to take. Psychological support and Entonox will also be useful for pain relief.

If the injury involves a wound, steps should be taken to wash out any gross contamination with a litre of normal saline immediately. A dressing should be applied, consisting of saline soaks and gauze pads soaked in iodine solution (e.g. Betadine). It may be assumed that the patient will be going to theatre soon; therefore, hospital protocols should be followed as for any patient going to theatre. Formal toilet and debridement in theatre is essential to prevent infection by washing out all traces of contamination and excising all dead or dubious tissue from the wound.

If a fracture is displaced or a joint dislocated, manipulation is required to restore the normal anatomical position of the bones involved. This is frequently undertaken in the A & E department. As nursing assistance will be required, the nurse needs to know something of the procedures which may be carried out.

Gross fracture dislocations of the ankle (the foot rotated at 90° relative to the tibia) require immediate reduction under Entonox by disimpacting the fracture and rotating the foot back to the normal position. If reduction is not immediate, serious neurovascular damage will result. This is a first priority *before* X-ray. Severe injuries of the lower part of the leg in particular may require amputation and, as Clarke and Mollon (1994) have shown, primary amputation results in discharge home in half the time compared to patients where amputation is delayed (mean time in hospital of 24.3 and 49.8 days respectively). Criteria for primary amputation are discussed by these authors and include complete disruption of the posterior tibial nerve, severe crush injury and serious associated multiple injuries.

The most commonly manipulated fracture in A & E is the Colles fracture using the Bier's block technique. A double cuff tourniquet is placed around the top of the arm which is then elevated to allow venous drainage before the cuff is pumped up to above arterial pressure as recorded by the attached pressure gauge. Local anaesthetic is then infiltrated into the arm via a butterfly, effectively anaesthetizing the whole forearm. The danger is that the anaesthetic drug may leak past the cuff if it deflates. If this occurs before the drug has been bound and rendered inert by plasma proteins, a serious and possibly fatal reaction may occur. For this reason lignocaine

	0–5 min	6–20/30 min	20/30–75 min
Documentation	Registration as A & E patient	A & E notes ready for CO	Admission referral form complete
Assessment	Triage nurse, check appearance and function, localized bony tenderness, pain, signs of neurovascular compromise	BP RR P CO exam patient Send to XR. Check for other injuries or medical conditions When did last eat or drink?	Is patient fit to be discharged? Check neuro-vascular status of limb distal to POP. Patient under-standing of POP care? Check XR if MUA
Medication	–	Opioid analgesia	Prn analgesia
Treatment	–	Consent for MUA if needed Set up IV if risk of hypovolaemia Dressing if open # Check Tet Tox status	MUA and/or POP or traction if # shaft femur
Nursing care	Remove splintage to allow exam. of limb. Psych support, NBM	Immobilize injury Monitor pain and neurovascular status of limb Remove constrictions such as rings. Cont. NBM, Psych support Explain procedures	Assist MUA/POP Teach POP/crutches care. Inform wd or make discharge arrangements. Role as patient advocate
Referrals	–	–	Orthopaedic-trauma team. Ward or follow up clinic, GP/Dist. Nurse?
Family	Inform if not present	Stay with patient in cubicle, keep informed	Keep informed Can they cope if discharged?
Discharge	–	–	Wd/OPD

NB. Times are variable depending upon severity of injury and whether patient is to be admitted or discharged.

MUA = Manipulation Under Anaesthetic; POP = Plaster of Paris

Fig 6.3   Example of critical pathway for patient with fracture or dislocation of limb

and Marcaine are no longer used, the safer prilocaine being preferred. Even with this safer drug, however, the cuff must remain inflated for at least 20 minutes. It is essential that a nurse stay with the patient throughout the manipulation and check X-ray stage, observing the cuff pressure gauge to ensure there is no leak, and observing the patient, who will be probably very grateful for somebody to talk to.

Another common manipulation carried out in A & E is for dislocated shoulders. This technique involves the administration of intravenous diazepam (muscle relaxant) and an opioid analgesic (e.g. pethidine) before manipulation. The patient is, therefore, not anaesthetized, but will be very drowsy. There is a signficant hazard of respiratory depression so close nursing observation is required in the post-manipulation period.

See summary boxes (pp. 130–136) for brief descriptions of some of the more common fracture and dislocation injuries seen in A & E.

After the fracture has been successfully manipulated (if necessary) and immobilized in plaster of Paris (see Chapter 7), the nurse must consider the problems associated with discharge. These include transportation to home, a follow-up appointment (usually the following day to check the plaster), whether the patient fully understands how to use crutches and/or what precautions need to be taken with the plaster, and finally, whether the patient can cope. In dealing with the elderly, especially those who live alone, it is often the case that the fall that brought about the current injury was the final episode in a steadily deteriorating situation. The A & E nurse must, therefore, carefully assess the patient's ability to cope at home and if there is any doubt, discuss the matter further with the medical staff, remembering the nurse's role as patient advocate, in order to mobilize fully community support or explore the possibility of admission to a care of the elderly ward. The final thought before discharging the patient should be—have they got any analgesia? A timely reminder to the medical staff can save a lot of unnecessary pain with a quick prescription.

If the patient is being admitted because of the fracture, preparation for theatre in accordance with hospital protocols is required. In addition, an intravenous infusion is mandatory for fractures of the femoral shaft to prevent hypovolaemic shock. Fractures of the neck of femur, however, bleed very little and do not require an IVI to prevent hypovolaemia, although one may be erected to ensure adequate hydration of the patient in the pre-operative phase.

Elderly patients with fractures of the femur have a very high risk of developing pressure sores (Versluysen, 1985). It seems that the causes are largely to be found outside trauma wards in the form of hard A & E, theatre or X-ray trolleys, where elderly patients lie immobile for hours on end. Turning such a patient in A & E is impractical. However, Spenco mattresses are available in sizes which fit trolleys and at least one such mattress should be available in A & E. Every effort should be made to transfer the patient to a ward bed where pressure area care may be instituted as rapidly as possible. Note that sheepskins will be of little use in A & E for such patients as they only prevent friction.

Evaluation

The effectiveness of pain-relieving intervention should be continually checked, together with the neurovascular status of the limb. Although a limb has been elevated to reduce swelling, it should not be assumed that it will stay that way. Slings can slip and pillows can mysteriously vanish from under legs. Similarly, splinting should be checked at periodic intervals to ensure that it is still functioning effectively.

In evaluating the effectiveness of instruction given to the patient about either plaster of Paris or the use of crutches, it is important that the patient be asked to demonstrate that they have learnt what has been taught. Therefore, the patient should be asked to repeat the plaster instructions to ensure they know what to look for and the patient should be observed walking with crutches. It is not what has been taught that is important, but what has been learnt, and the only way to evaluate patient instruction is to assess what has been learnt.

If the patient is experiencing a minimum amount of pain and anxiety, if their injured limb is safely immobilized, and if its neurovascular status is secure, then the nursing intervention can be evaluated as successful.

Summary Boxes for Common Injuries

Foot Injuries

1. Fractures or dislocations of toes
Cause: 'Stubbed toe'. Treatment: Ring block and reduce if needed, strap to neighbouring digit for support with gauze padding. Watch out for swelling.

2. Metatarsal fractures
Cause: Heavy weight falls on foot or motorbike RTA. Treatment: Elevate foot, crutches, non-weight bearing (NWB), rest. Watch out for swelling and neurovascular damage.

3. Fractured calcaneum
Cause: Fall on to heel. Treatment: Elevate, ice packs, NWB, rest. Watch out for swelling and neurovascular damage.

Lower Leg Injury

Fractured lower tibia/fibula
Cause: Lateral force. Treatment: If it is displaced, manipulation under anaesthetic (MUA), POP cylinder, NWB will be called for. If an open fracture, wound debridement will be necessary. If undisplaced, a full-leg NWB, POP backslab will be necessary. Prone to non-union, usual risks if open.

Ankle Injuries

1. Fractures of medial and/or lateral malleoli with or without ligament rupture with displacement of talus
Cause: Rotation and/or abduction or adduction, e.g. twisted foot while falling. Treatment: Simple fracture of malleolus requires a POP backslab, complete NWB for 24 hours, crutches. If ligaments are ruptured, internal fixation with screws will be necessary when swelling permits. Backslab and elevation meanwhile.

2. Trimalleolar fracture
Cause: Vertical compression, e.g. fall. Joint completely disrupted with posterior part of tibia fractured. Treatment: Internal fixation. Risk of osteoarthritis due to joint surface damage.

3. Fracture-dislocation of ankle (open)
Cause: Severe rotational force. Treatment: Immediate reduction under Entonox due to neurovascular compromise. Toilet/debridement, internal fixation. Risk of osteomyelitis, osteoarthritis, gas gangrene.

Wrist Injuries

1. Fractured scaphoid
Cause: Fall on to palm of hand, usually in young adult. Treatment: Fracture often does not show on first X-ray, but if there is localized bony tenderness in 'snuff box', treat as fracture with POP to include base of thumb. Untreated, risk of osteroarthritis.

2. Fractured base of thumb (Bennett's fracture)
Cause: Longitudinal force, e.g. boxing. Treatment: Involves the joint, therefore, needs perfect reduction (possible internal fixation) to avoid osteoarthritis. POP to include interphalangeal joint.

Forearm Fractures

1. Fractured distal radius with posterior displacement (Colles fracture, see Fig. 6.4)
Cause: Fall on outstretched hand, elderly. Displacement requires correction by disimpaction, anterior manipulation and placing hand in ulnar deviation. POP backslab and sling, complete POP applied at 24 hours.

2. As above with anterior displacement (Smith's fracture)
Cause: Fall on hand in flexed position. Treatment: Manipulate as above with posterior manipulation. However, a POP which includes the elbow is necessary due to high risk of fracture redisplacing. May need internal fixation.

3. Fractured mid-shaft radius and ulna (see Fig. 6.5)
Cause: High energy injury, often seen in children as a greenstick fracture. Treatment: Manipulation needed under GA for children, then POP. In adults, often internally fixed.

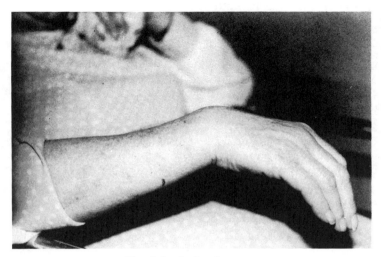

Fig. 6.4   Colles fracture

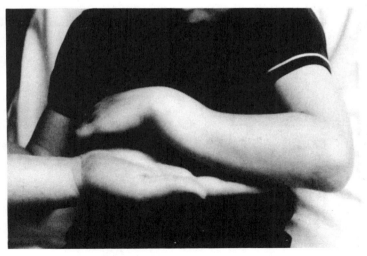

Fig. 6.5   Fracture of radius and ulna in 7-year-old boy

Elbow Injuries

1. Pulled elbow
Cause: Sudden arm jerk in young child age 2–3. Annular ligament slips over head of radius leading to painful elbow that the child will not move. Treatment: Reduce by pushing forearm upwards and rotating alternately into supination and pronation.

2. Dislocation of elbow
Cause: Heavy fall. Radius and ulna usually dislocated backwards relative to humerus. Treatment: Needs rapid reduction under GA due to neurovascular hazards.

3. Fracture of olecranon process
Cause: Fall on point of elbow. Treatment: Either treat by POP, by screw fixation internally or by excision of olecranon process.

4. Fracture of radial head
Cause: Fall on outstretched hand, young age group. Treatment: Often rest in a sling is all that is prescribed.

5. Supracondylar fracture of humerus
Cause: Fall in childhood. Treatment: Requires immediate reduction under GA due to risk to brachial artery. Long-term risk of deformity due to malunion—'Gun stock deformity'.

Injuries of the Upper Arm

1. Fractured shaft of humerus
Cause: Direct violence, usually in adults, or may be pathological. Treatment: Hanging U Slab POP, plus collar and cuff sling, or internal fixation. Complete POP later.

2. Fractured neck of humerus
Cause: Fall in the elderly, not usually displaced. Treatment: Sling or collar and cuff; emphasis is on mobility and exercise as the shoulder may become permanently stiff.

Injuries Involving the Shoulder

1. Dislocated shoulder
Cause: Fall on outstretched hand, usually anterior dislocation. Treatment: Reduce under IV diazepam and pethidine in A & E. Use Kocher method—apply traction along humerus with elbow bent at 90°, rotate arm laterally, carry elbow across body to midline, rotate arm so that hand falls to opposite side of chest. Alternatively pull along humerus with counter-traction in axilla.

2. Fractured clavicle
Cause: Fall on hand. Treatment: Conservative—with sling to support arm. Watch out for pressure on skin from bone ends.

Knee Injuries

1. Fracture of the tibial plateau
Cause: Blow from the side rotating femur on to lateral tibial condyle, e.g. car bumper hitting pedestrian. Treatment: After aspiration of haemarthrosis, POP, NWB. Osteoarthritis is long-term problem.

2. Fracture of patella
Cause: Direct blow. Treatment: If badly comminuted, patella is excised. If single fracture line, the two halves can be wired together.

3. Dislocation of patella
Cause: Flexion of knee. Patella always displaces laterally. The knee is held flexed. Treatment: Easily reduced under Entonox/IV diazepam. POP backslab.

Hand Injuries

1. Fracture or dislocation of digit
Cause: Direct blow. Treatment: Strap to neighbouring digit for support with gauze padding between. Encourage mobility. High arm sling for swelling.

2. Fractured metacarpal
Cause: Punching, usually fifth metacarpal. Treatment: If angulated, needs reduction and immobilization in volar slab in Edinburgh position, i.e. fingers extended and wrist cocked back. High arm sling.

Injuries to the Thigh and Hip

1. Fractured shaft of femur
Cause: High energy injury in young, pathological in elderly. Treatment: Traction to immobilize. IVI to prevent shock. Theatre for skeletal traction or internal fixation.

2. Fractured neck of femur (or trochanteric region)
Cause: Usually in elderly to very elderly a minor fall, or pathological due to osteoporosis. Leg shortened and externally rotated. Treatment: Requires internal fixation within 24 to 48 hours. Major social and psychological problems.

3. Dislocation of hip
Cause: High energy injury. Leg shortened and internally rotated. May be driven through acetabulum in central dislocation leading to long-term problems with osteoarthritis. Treatment: Reduction under GA in theatre.

4. Fracture of pelvis
Cause: In the elderly, usually due to a fall causing fracture of pubic rami; in young people, due to a high energy injury with fracture of pubic ring in two places. Blood loss up to 2 litres. Treatment: IVI urgent, risk of ruptured bladder or torn urethra. In the elderly, should be treated with bed rest. Major injury— requires pelvic sling or external fixation.

References

Adams J. C. (1983). *Outline of Fractures*, 8th edn. Edinburgh: Churchill Livingstone.

Clarke P., Mollon R. (1994). The criteria for amputation in severe lower limb injury. *Injury*, 25:3, 139–43.

Dykes P. (1993). Minding the 5ps of neurovascular assessment. *American Journal of Nursing*, June, 38–9.

Paton D. (1992). *Fractures and Orthopaedics*, 2nd edn. Edinburgh: Churchill Livingstone.

Taylor M., Bannerjee B., Algar E. (1994). Injuries associated with a fractured shaft of femur. *Injury*, 25:3, 185–7.

Versluysen M. (1985). Pressure sores in elderly patients: the epidemiology related to hip operations. *Journal of Bone and Joint Surgery*, 67(B), 10–13.

Chapter 7

PLASTER OF PARIS APPLICATION

Basic Principles

The plaster of Paris cast (POP) is an old, tried-and-trusted, effective and relatively cheap method of immobilizing a limb. It consists of hemihydrated calcium sulphate which is impregnated into bandage. Immersion in water causes an exothermic reaction to occur—heat is given off—as the hemihydrated calcium sulphate turns to hydrated calcium sulphate which sets to form the hard plaster cast.

There are, however, potential problems connected with plasters. If nurses are to avoid such problems, and to maximize the benefits for the patient, there are certain basic principles that must be observed.

Patient Understanding

The patient must understand what is happening and why. For the best results in applying the POP and in its subsequent after-care, a high degree of patient compliance and cooperation is required. This is unlikely to be forthcoming unless there is full comprehension by the patient concerning plaster care.

Adequate Padding of the Limb

A POP is very hard both on the inside and on the outside. Therefore, unless it is well padded, there are going to be problems with the skin, and the formation of broken areas leading to pressure sores is likely. There should be a layer of an elasticated tubular bandage (stockinet) next to the skin, overlaid by one of the proprietary padded bandages that are available for this purpose. Particular attention should be paid to padding bony prominences such as the ulnar styloid and the head of the fibula. The padding should extend above and below the plaster so that it may be turned back over the ends of the POP, preventing skin friction by the plaster edges.

Water Temperature

Water temperature determines setting time: the cooler the water, the longer the plaster takes to set initially. The nurse who is learning the techniques of plastering is, therefore, recommended to always use cold water, remembering to ensure that the bandage has been properly soaked through in the water, with some of the excess gently squeezed out before application.

Movement during Application

If there is any movement of a joint during the application or the initial setting phase, cracks will form within the POP which will seriously weaken the plaster and lead to its failure in the long term. Joints must be held perfectly still during the initial stage of setting.

Moulding

The plaster must be moulded to the shape of the limb in order to maximize comfort and support for the fracture. This means that speed is of the essence in applying the plaster. There must be time before it starts to harden for gentle moulding to be carried out.

Constriction

Tissue swelling accompanies most fractures and ligament injuries. If the limb is encased in a tight plaster, there will be no room for expansion to occur. This will cause compression of the soft tissues in the limb, leading to pain and a significant risk of neurovascular damage.

There are two main precautions that are taken to prevent this situation from occurring. First, in fresh injuries only a half plaster is applied, i.e. a backslab that covers only half the limb but that will still immobilize the injury while leaving room for tissue swelling to occur (Paton, 1992). Second, the limb must be elevated to encourage tissue fluid to move, under gravity, away from the injured region. Coupled with these two steps should be observation of the limb for

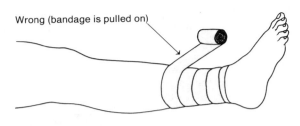

Wrong (bandage is pulled on)

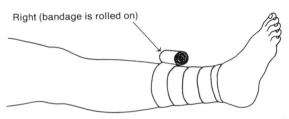

Right (bandage is rolled on)

Fig. 7.1   The incorrect and the correct method of application of plaster bandage

any changes in colour, warmth or sensation, in order to detect signs of neurovascular compromise as soon as possible (Morgan, 1989).

Many patients will be discharged home rather than kept in hospital. Therefore, it is essential that they fully understand what they are looking for and the need to get in touch with the A & E unit if they do observe or experience anything unusual.

Because of the hazards of tissue swelling, it is essential in applying plaster not to make the POP too tight. The plaster bandage should be rolled onto the limb rather than a length of bandage unwound and then wrapped around the limb as shown in Fig. 7.1. This latter technique will make for a plaster that is too tight. This should also be remembered in applying the outer bandage to a backslab.

There has been some controversy in the medical literature concerning the effectiveness of backslabs in preventing increases in tissue pressure surrounding a fracture. Younger et al. (1990) claimed that on the basis of their experimental work the use of backslabs should be discontinued in favour of applying a full cast which is then split and spread apart. This technique produced a cast which was capable of easier expansion than the backslab. This work was not however carried out on real limbs—artificial arms specially constructed for the purpose were used.

Research carried out on real patients does not support the views of Younger et al., however. Bowyer et al. (1993) reported upon a series of 15 patients with backslabs applied to the lower limb after operative fixation of ankle fracture. In all cases the increase in pressure within the slab was minimal (mean 3.4 mmHg), had peaked within 3 hours of application and fell steadily thereafter. There were no clinical signs of neurovascular compromise in these patients.

The dangers of applying insufficient pressure within a cast are discussed by Moir et al. (1991) who were critical of plaster casts applied to Colles fractures. Pressure measurements inside casts carried out by these workers were considered too low to stabilize the fracture effectively. It is necessary for a cast to apply pressure to the limb at three points, one of which will always be opposite to the other two, to function properly to immobilize the fracture. Moulding the cast to the shape of the limb in order to comply with Charnley's three-point principle did increase the pressures but Moir et al. still recommend the use of functional bracing long term.

Limb Positioning

Once plastered, joints will remain in the same position for up to several weeks. It is essential, therefore, that they be plastered in the correct position. In the lower limb, the ankle should be at a perfect right angle. There should always be some 10° of flexion in the knee. In the upper limb, the usual position for the elbow is at 90° with the palm of the hand facing the body if the whole arm is to be immobilized. If the hand is to be placed in plaster (usually for a fractured metacarpal that has been manipulated), the position that should be adopted is the one shown in Fig. 7.2.

Complete Setting Time

The plaster may seem very hard after some 5–10 minutes. However, it does take 48 hours to set fully and this must be explained to the patient. If it is a leg plaster, no weight must be allowed on the

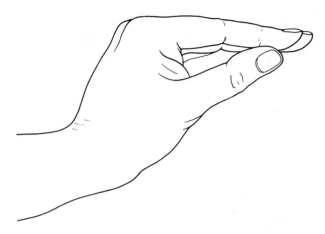

Fig. 7.2   Correct position for immobilization of the hand

plaster for at least 48 hours or else a crumbling disintegration of the nurse's best efforts will be the result. Crutches must be provided together with instruction and demonstration on how to use them. Clothes should not be worn over a freshly applied POP as this will delay setting by interfering with the drying process.

Plaster of Paris Backslabs

In a fresh injury, a backslab is usually applied to allow room for swelling and to facilitate easy removal, if required, of the plaster. It consists of a slab of several layers of plaster bandage, cut to the required length and shape, and applied over a well-padded limb. It is bandaged in place while still wet by an open-weave cotton conforming bandage. The end of the bandage is secured with a further piece of plaster sticking it down to the plaster underneath, but not to the open padding as this would effectively be completing the plaster. (See Figs 7.3, 7.4 and 7.5.)

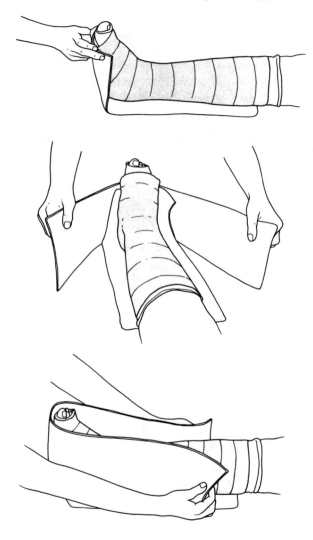

Fig. 7.3   Backslab for ankle/foot injuries

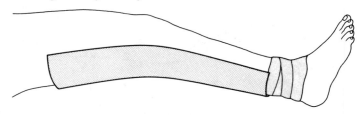

2 × 20 cm backslabs overlapping at the back of the leg.
Finish above the ankle which must be well padded.
Knee flexed at 10°.

Fig. 7.4   Backslab for knee injuries

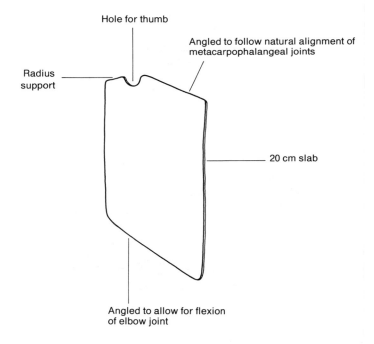

Hole for thumb

Angled to follow natural alignment of
metacarpophalangeal joints

Radius
support

20 cm slab

Angled to allow for flexion
of elbow joint

Fig. 7.5   Backslab for wrist injuries

Plaster Casts for Arm Injuries

Colles Cast

This type of cast will immobilize the wrist, but not the thumb. It is used for fractures of the distal radius. It should extend from just below the elbow to the metacarpophalangeal joints, leaving those joints free with a full range of movement. The thumb should be able to touch any of the fingers and the patient should have a reasonable grip. On the inner or palm-side of the wrist and hand (volar aspect), the plaster should extend no further than the proximal palmar crease. If the fracture has been manipulated, the position should be one of ulnar deviation and flexion. Plastering should commence with a 10 cm bandage turned twice around the proximal portion of the metacarpals and then passed twice between the thumb and index finger with a twisting motion before being continued up the arm in a spiral fashion. The plaster should be completed with a 15 cm bandage which should finish at the metacarpophalangeal joints.

Scaphoid Cast

Scaphoid fractures are exceptions to the rule about swelling, for there is usually very little associated with this injury. They can, therefore, go directly into a complete cast. Scaphoid fractures are notorious for not showing up on X-ray, but if the correct clinical finding of localized bony tenderness is noted over the scaphoid, the wrist should be plastered anyway. Very often the fracture will show on the second X-ray taken a week later, even though it did not show on the first.

The scaphoid cast is similar to the Colles cast, except that it immobilizes the base of the thumb (the first metacarpophalangeal joint—mcp) and should leave the interphalangeal joint of the digit free. If there is a fracture through the base of the thumb involving the mcp joint, it is called a Bennett's fracture and requires the interphalangeal joint to be included in the plaster.

Padding is, therefore, required around the thumb as well as the rest of the wrist and forearm. The plaster should be started with a 7.5 cm bandage turned twice around the proximal portion of the metacarpals before being taken twice around the base of the thumb, and completed with a 15 cm bandage. The patient should be able to touch finger tips with thumb when the scaphoid cast is complete.

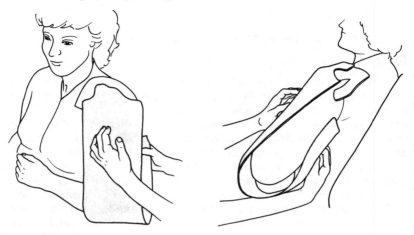

Fig. 7.6   Hanging U slab for humerus fracture

Full Arm Plasters

If the elbow is to be immobilized, the plaster will need to extend to the top of the upper arm. Particular attention should be paid to the area of the brachial artery to ensure there is no constriction in this region. Care should also be taken that the plaster is not causing discomfort under the axilla. It is usual to plaster the elbow at 90° with the palm of the hand facing the body. The wrist may be left out of the cast or included, depending on the injury. For example, if a Smith's fracture of the wrist is to be treated conservatively, it is typically done so in a plaster that will immobilize the elbow as well as the wrist due to the risk of the fracture slipping if the forearm is allowed to rotate, a movement that occurs at the elbow. Conversely, a supracondylar fracture of the humerus can be treated by leaving the wrist joint free, outside the plaster. (See Fig. 7.6.)

Plaster Casts for Leg Injuries

Below Knee Plasters

For a simple below knee plaster, a 20 cm bandage should be used, starting at the base of the toes and working up the leg to finish just below the head of the fibula. The ankle should be at a right angle. Two or three bandages will be required depending on the size of the leg. If a walking heel is to be added, scraps of plaster should be used to fill in the hollow that will be present on the sole of the plaster due to the arch of the foot. There must be a true, flat surface to attach the walking heel in the correct position. It should be secured using a 10 cm bandage woven in a figure of 8 fashion. The actual walking surfaces, however, should be left free of plaster. The walking heel needs to be centrally aligned if the patient is to be able to walk comfortably and safely.

Long Leg Cylinders

A long leg cylinder is usually applied for fractures of the tibia and fibula or injuries involving the knee. It should extend from just above the malleoli to the top of the thigh, and will benefit from having backslabs incorporated in it to give added strength. For fractures of the tibia and fibula, it is often easier if the plaster is applied in two stages. First, a below knee plaster should be applied to immobilize the fracture; then the cast should be completed by incorporating the knee and thigh in a second stage. For knee injuries, the idea of a two-stage plaster is also relevant, with the knee first being immobilized with a full leg backslab which, when set, can be plastered over to convert into a reinforced cylinder. The ankle should have plenty of padding to protect the malleoli and achilles tendon area; the knee must be in a slight flexion of about 5 to 10°.

Discharging the Patient with a Plaster of Paris Cast

When an individual is discharged with a POP, they are confronted with a series of real problems in self-care. Reference to Orem's model of nursing (see p. 34) shows that the patient has a series of universal self-care demands to fulfil. Now, with the handicap of a POP, there are specific problems which require self-care. In addition, the patient has health deviancy self-care demands in terms of caring for the effects of pathology (pain), the side effects of treatment (the cast) and adapting to a change in self-concept. A substantial amount of knowledge and understanding is required if the patient is to achieve self-care successfully in all these areas. It is the A & E nurse's responsibility to teach the patient what is required in order that self-care may be carried out effectively.

Firstly, the patient must not leave A & E without discussion of pain, the offer of analgesics and information about the possible significance of increasing pain, e.g. the POP is too tight. The nurse now needs to consider the cast itself. Plaster of Paris will crumble if it becomes wet. The patient should, therefore, be instructed to keep the plaster dry, and should be told why this is necessary. The problems of swelling within the cast and the neuro-vascular complications that can occur due to compression of blood vessels and nerves should be carefully explained to the patient. The patient should also be instructed about the possible signs of problems—swollen digits, discoloration and altered sensation— and about elevating the limb. A sling can be used for the arm; for the leg, the patient should sit with the foot higher than the level of the heart.

The final major problem concerning the plaster itself stems from the fact that it takes 48 hours to set properly. This is not much of a problem for arm plasters, but if it is a leg cast that the patient will eventually be allowed to walk on, it is important that the patient understand that no weight can be taken by the plaster for 48 hours. Crutches must be supplied together with instruction on how to use them. The patient should be asked to demonstrate their competence in using the crutches before being allowed to leave the department.

The loss of function and stiffness associated with having a limb in plaster will affect all the patient's universal self-care demands. The patient should, therefore, be encouraged to retain maximum move-ment in the limb by having various exercises demonstrated. For example, if a wrist plaster has been applied, finger exercises should be taught to the patient to maintain both extension and flexion; the importance of keeping the elbow and shoulder joints mobile should also be made clear. This is of special importance in elderly patients whose joints stiffen up very quickly.

The final area of health deviancy is that of adaptation. Lack of mobility may make some patients depressed or frustrated. This potential problem should be explored with the patient in advance in order that he or she be mentally prepared to cope with it.

Nurses need to consider that the plaster affects the whole person and not just the single limb. An example of this is the 75-year-old lady who has to use a Zimmer frame to get about. If this patient sustains a fracture of the arm, which is then placed in plaster, it may make it impossible for her to use the Zimmer frame. There will no longer be a balance between rest and activity. Social interaction will be severely limited, and if the patient tries to mobilize without a Zimmer, she will be exposed to a much more hazardous environment. There is, therefore, a major deficit in self-care which nurses must try to fill either by involving family or community services, or, if that fails, an admission to hospital may be required.

Before discharging a patient home in plaster, the A & E nurse must consider whether self-care can be achieved in terms of the universal requirements associated with everyday living, and in terms of specific problems relating directly to the plaster. Orem's model of nursing makes an elegant framework around which to plan for the patient's care after discharge. Initially the A & E nurse fills a partly compensatory role by immobilizing the injury for the patient (thereby meeting the patient's self-care deficit). Then the nurse moves on to the educative/advisory role in preparing the patient for self-care on discharge.

Synthetic Casting Materials

In recent years a variety of synthetic casting materials have become available as alternatives to POP. They are more expensive but have the great advantage of setting very quickly. Thus, an elderly person having a below knee cast for an ankle injury will find it very difficult to be non-weight-bearing on crutches for 48 hours while the POP sets. However, a synthetic cast will set hard for weight-bearing purposes in a fraction of that time, allowing patients to retain their independence and self-care ability. Plastics are also available which, when heated, become malleable, allowing splints to be moulded in A & E which can be bandaged in place to support joints such as the wrist.

References

Bowyer G., Iu M., Reynard M. (1993). Pressure in backslabs after surgery for ankle fractures. *Injury*, **24:**2, 121–2.
Moir J., Wytch R., Ashcroft P., Neil G., Ross N., Wardlaw D. (1991). Intracast measurements in Colles fractures. *Injury*, **22:**6, 446–50.

Morgan S. (1989). *Plaster Casting*. Oxford: Butterworth-Heinemann.

Paton D. (1992). *Fractures and Orthopaedics*. Edinburgh: Churchill-Livingstone.

Younger A., Curran P., McQueen M. (1990). Backslabs and plaster casts: which will best accommodate increasing intracompartmental pressures? *Injury*, **21**:3, 179–81.

Chapter 8

SOFT TISSUE INJURY

Wounds and other injuries to muscles and joints make up a large proportion of an A & E department's workload, some of which are old infected wounds rather than acute injuries. Research by Walsh found that 448 patients (22.4%) out of a sample of 2000 adult ambulatory patients required wound treatment. Of this group, one-third needed dressings only and two-thirds required suture or steristrip. The late night period was marked by the highest proportion of patients requiring suture, although in absolute numbers, the morning saw most attendances that required suture. The most frequent cause of wounds requiring suture was works accidents.

Many patients with wounds and minor injuries are suitable for treatment by nurses without lengthy delays to see busy casualty officers and Jones (1993) has described one such nurse-run clinic which operated very successfully over a 6-month trial period. The clinic saw 906 patients of whom 291 (32%) had problems relating to wounds and a further 183 (20%) had minor soft tissue injuries requiring support bandage/strapping. Walsh also found 20% of his A & E sample required support bandage/strapping of some sort. The nurse practitioner role in A & E clearly has a major part to play in the future treatment of patients with such injuries.

Pathology

Soft tissue injury can either be closed, as in bruising or a ligament sprain, or open, in which case some sort of wound will be present. The wounds seen in A & E are rather different from the surgical incisions that the nurse will have encountered elsewhere: A & E wounds can be in all shapes and sizes, and are all caused by non-sterile agents, with an accompanying high risk of infection. The following summary of wounds commonly seen in A & E will be of use as an introduction:

1. *Laceration.* A linear cut in the skin, usually superficial but may involve deep structures.

2. *Crush injury.* Fingers and toes are the most commonly involved. There may be a fracture of the bone underneath which will, therefore, be an open fracture. The force of the impact causes the soft tissue to burst open; a very painful injury with much swelling involved. Crush injuries carry a high risk of infection due to the damaged and devitalized tissue present (Fergusson, 1993).

3. *Penetrating wound.* A narrow but deeply penetrating track is involved. The cause can be anything from treading on a nail to a stabbing or gunshot wound.

4. *Abrasions.* A superficial but very painful injury. Dirt and grit is commonly ingrained or tattooed into the skin and has to be removed by scrubbing.

5. *Bites.* Ragged wounds are produced by bites and have a high risk of infection. Human bites carry a very high risk of infection as the mouth is heavily contaminated with bacteria, whilst the risk of hepatitis B or HIV transmission also exists (Wardrope and Smith, 1992). Such wounds should not be sutured due to the risk of infection.

6. *Degloving injury.* If a force is involved that is parallel to the skin, layers of tissue may be torn away, exposing a whole area of deeper structures.

7. *Burns.* See next chapter.

The normal healing process will produce fresh epithelial cover within 48 hours if the wound has been closed, although the healing process below the surface will take much longer (Westaby, 1985). An impaired blood supply, infection or the presence of foreign material will all delay or prevent healing. The aim in A & E, therefore, is to clean the wound thoroughly, removing foreign material and reducing the risk of infection, and then to close the wound so as to promote rapid healing with the minimum of scar formation and infection risk.

The most feared pathogens are the anaerobic Clostridium family. *Clostridium tetani* gives rise to tetanus, and *Clostridium welchii* and

Clostridium sporagenes are involved in gas gangrene. The spores of these organisms are found in the soil, and the fact that they are anaerobic means that they can live without free atmospheric oxygen. Therefore, if they are present in a wound that is closed over, they will thrive.

Tetanus is characterized by the toxins which are released by the *Clostridium tetani* attacking the nervous system. The result is severe muscle spasm which could be fatal once the muscles of respiration become involved. In established cases, therefore, the treatment involves long-term ventilatory support.

In gas gangrene, putrefactive changes occur within damaged or dead tissue. The clostridia are responsible for forming various hydrogen gases which escape into the tissue planes, giving the characteristic odour. The gas increases the pressure in the tissues surrounding the wound. This further impairs blood supply. Meanwhile, the toxins released by the bacteria cause a severe toxaemia. The condition is extremely painful and carries a high mortality rate.

A wide variety of other pathogens cause wound sepsis. As the patient in most cases is going home after treatment, it is important that the signs of infection be carefully explained. The patient should be given instructions to return should there be any signs of infection, such as pain, swelling, redness or inflammation tracking up the limb along the line of a vein.

The elderly have very fragile skin, and suturing is not necessarily the best means of closing wounds in this case as sutures may simply cut through the skin. The pre-tibial flap laceration is a common injury seen in elderly ladies and is best treated by the use of steristrips rather than sutures. If it is proximally based (see Fig. 8.1), there is a good chance of healing. The distally based flap, however, has a very poor blood supply and often necroses, and a skin grafting operation is needed.

In dealing with gunshot or shrapnel injuries, it is important to consider the velocity and hence energy of the projectile. If the velocity exceeds that of sound, the particle is supersonic and is defined as a high energy missile. It will behave in a very different way from a subsonic particle (a particle travelling below the speed of sound). For example, the muzzle velocity of the average handgun is some 550 feet per second. The velocity of sound is 1100 feet per second. A modern military rifle, on the other hand, has a muzzle velocity of about 2500 feet per second and the Colt Armalite exceeds 3000 feet per second. At these supersonic speeds, there is a high

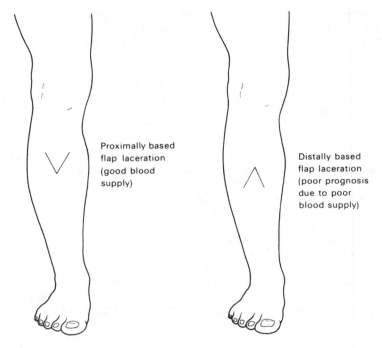

Proximally based
flap laceration
(good blood
supply)

Distally based
flap laceration
(poor prognosis
due to poor
blood supply)

Fig. 8.1   Pre-tibial flap laceration

pressure shock wave preceding the projectile and, in its wake, there
is a vacuum. The result on hitting the human body is an instantane-
ous pressure wave, causing catastrophic damage. This is followed by
the vacuum which sucks gross contamination deep into the wound.
A volume of tissue roughly equal to that of a football may be
destroyed by a single bullet, with only a tiny entrance and exit
wound to show for it. Bone is shattered, muscle and soft tissue
infarcted and blood vessels destroyed, simply due to the pressure
wave and without any physical contact with the projectile.

Of the closed soft tissue injuries, one of the most common categories are the sprains. These consist of ligament injury where the
ligament is grossly intact, but some individual fibres have been torn.
The result is painful and associated with a lot of swelling, but the
joint is stable. Bruising can have serious consequences because in

areas such as the foot and calf there may be little room for expansion to accommodate the extra tissue fluid. Pressure levels can rise to such a point that the microcirculation is impaired and serious neuro-vascular complications can develop.

Other commonly seen injuries include trauma to cartilage and bursae. In the knee, a tear of one of the semilunar cartilages is commonly associated with a twisting movement when the knee is flexed, resulting in the patient's knee locking in a flexed position. Repeated wear and tear on the bursae of the elbow or knee can lead to inflammation, swelling and pain, the so-called housemaid's knee or tennis elbow.

Although not traumatic in origin, the A & E department is commonly visited by patients with a wide variety of skin lesions. Table 8.1 makes a useful summary of the more common rashes and their origins.

Assessment

In order to assign the correct priority to the patient (triage) an accurate assessment of the wound and its effects on the whole patient is essential. The patient may be very distressed as the effect of the sight of blood can be very dramatic for some people. Therefore, the nurse needs a calm, reassuring manner in order to obtain a history. The nurse needs to find out what caused the injury, how and when and how much blood loss there has been. It is worth remembering, however, that the lay person is prone to exaggerate blood loss.

Taking a pad of gauze, the next thing the nurse should do is examine the wound itself, carefully removing the patient's own first aid dressing. The nurse should look for the depth and extent of the wound, see if any deep structures such as tendons are visible and if so whether they are damaged, note any contamination and, if bleeding occurs, note whether it is pulsatile and therefore arterial in nature. Finally the degree of pain felt by the patient should be assessed. Universal precautions against the transmission of blood-borne disease should be taken at all times.

The assessment should then move on to the area distal to the wound to see if there is any evidence of damage to structures such as tendons and nerves. The nurse should test sensation and movement with this consideration in mind and also note the colour and warmth of the skin.

Table 8.1   Common rashes seen in A & E

Disease	Chief Complaint	History
Herpes Simplex Type 1 (Cold Sore)	Usually around mouth or nose; group of vesicles rupture leaving painful ulcer with yellow crust.	Colds, fever, menstruation or overexposure to sunlight may precede outbreak.
Herpes Simplex Type 2 (Genital Herpes)	Small grouped vesicles around genitals and mouth.	Sexual contact with infected person.
Herpes Zoster (Shingles)	Grouped vesicles or crusted lesions along nerve root.	Chicken pox, reactivation of virus may cause attack.
Verucae (Warts)	Slightly raised papules.	Previous history of warts.
Rubeola (Measles)	Rash begins with macules on hairline, neck and cheeks, spreads downwards over rest of body. Appears 2–4 days after other symptoms, lasts 4–5 days.	Exposure to infected person 10–14 days previously. Cold, cough, fever before rash.
Rubella (German Measles)	Maculopapular rash begins on face, spreads to trunk.	Exposure to infected person 14–21 days previously. Adolescents have malaise, fever, anorexia and headaches before rash.
Varicella (Chicken Pox)	Appears first on trunk, spreads to face and scalp. Small red papules and clear vesicles on red base which break and dry leaving a crust. Itching.	Exposure to infected person 13–21 days ago. Malaise and anorexia before rash.
Tinea corporis (Ringworm)	Intense itching. Round red scaly lesions, central area heals while lesion continues outward.	Exposure to infected animals or persons. Most common in children.
Tinea capitis (Scalp Ringworm)	Mild itching, small spreading papules cause hair loss.	Exposure to infected persons.

Table derived from Holderman, M.C. (1984): *Nursing 84*, November, pp 22–23. Philadelphia, Pa.: Springhouse Corp.

The psychological state of the patient should be assessed as the sight of blood can be a very frightening experience; the possibility of either the patient or relative fainting as a result should always be kept in mind.

When there has been significant blood loss, or a penetrating injury, it is essential to record vital signs and then monitor them as necessary, as hypovolaemia can develop very quickly. Remember that a small entry wound in the case of a penetrating wound can conceal devastating injury within.

The patient's anti-tetanus status should also be ascertained, together with any other information relevant to wound healing, such as whether the patient is a diabetic or on steroid therapy.

In assessing closed soft tissue injuries, a history should first be obtained. Then the nurse should move on to look at the injury. It needs examining for localized bony tenderness, which would raise the possibility of a fracture, and for swelling, pain and degree of function. It is important to know how rapidly the existing amount of swelling occurred so that a reasonable estimate can be made of future swelling and, therefore, whether there is a significant risk of neurovascular compromise.

A common type of lesion that is presented at A & E is the wound that has become infected because the person did not seek treatment at the time. In addition, people present with a wide range of abscesses, some of which can be extremely painful. In assessing the patient, the nurse should obtain a history of how long the problem has existed and of any likely precipitating factor. The area should be examined for signs of the infection spreading such as a red prominent track along the line of a vein or the swelling of lymph nodes. Due to the association of infective lesions with diabetes, the patient should have a routine stix test performed for blood glucose. Temperature and pulse should also be recorded to assess the degree of systemic involvement.

Intervention

Control Bleeding

The first intervention is to stop any bleeding. This may be done by direct pressure over the wound with a firm dressing—initially this can be held by hand, remembering to use universal precautions, but a firm bandage will suffice once the bleeding has been stopped—and by elevating the injury, for example, by using a roller towel and a drip stand for a hand or arm injury. Injuries as extreme as traumatic amputations of limbs may be dealt with in this way. There is no indication for the use of a tourniquet in A & E other than to provide a temporary bloodless field for a brief examination of the wound.

Cleaning the Wound

Whether it is a major wound that will require repair in theatre or a minor wound that can be dealt with in A & E, it will need cleaning out thoroughly. If the wound is major, irrigation with a litre of normal saline in A & E is recommended. This can be followed by a dressing of saline soaks and iodine to keep the tissue in the best condition possible for theatre, where a formal toilet and debridement will take place. The aim is, in addition to a thorough toilet of the wound to wash out all contamination, to remove surgically any dead or dubious tissue which may act as a focus for infection (e.g. gas gangrene). The surgeon may leave badly contaminated wounds open for 3 days after surgery, covering them with only a light dressing. Only when absolutely sure that there is no evidence of sepsis, will the surgeon proceed to a delayed primary suture. This procedure is mandatory for all high velocity missile wounds.

In dealing with smaller wounds, research indicates that cleaning with antiseptics is of little value in preventing infection because the solution is not in contact with micro-organisms long enough and resistant strains are increasingly common (Walsh and Ford, 1989). A further major problem is that naturally occurring body fluids can make most antiseptics ineffective (Fergusson, 1993). A thorough cleansing with a sterile saline solution (e.g. Normasol) is therefore recommended and if the wound is very contaminated, hydrogen peroxide may be used as its effervescent effect may help loosen debris. It should be noted, though, that it has little if any antiseptic action, and there have been reports of tissue damage and near fatal air embolism associated with its use (Fergusson, 1993).

Abrasions demand special attention as grit may be tattooed into the wound. If left there, it will cause infection and possibly a permanent disfiguring mark. The use of a scrubbing brush or toothbrush may be the only effective way to remove such grit. Needless to say this is a very painful procedure and the patient should have the benefit of either a general anaesthetic, Entonox and local anaesthesia, or IV pethidine.

Wound Closure

The main techniques used in A & E for wound closure are suturing and steristripping, although the use of tissue glue is a recent development which may have much to commend it. The suture or steristrip should always be applied at right angles to the wound, skin edges should never be inverted (turned under) as this delays healing, and the tension in the skin around the wound should be evenly distributed. If there is too much tension in the skin the wound will break down. The nurse should therefore resist the temptation to pull skin edges together tightly. They should only be placed in opposition. Fig. 8.2 shows the correct technique for suturing.

If more than one stitch is required, the area should first be infiltrated with local anaesthetic which should be introduced via a needle inserted parallel to the wound and injected as the needle and syringe are gradually withdrawn. Lignocaine 2% is the agent of choice. However, in a very vascular area, such as the scalp, where bleeding often proves a problem, lignocaine with adrenaline may be used. Such a solution should never be used on a finger or toe as the vasoconstrictor effects of adrenaline are so great that peripheral gangrene may result.

The needle should be firmly gripped half-way to one-third along its length by the needle holders. When the needle is introduced into the skin, it is important that the wrist be rotated in alignment with the curvature of the needle, otherwise the needle will be bent. The needle should enter some 4 mm from the wound edge and exit the same distance from the opposite side of the wound. Dissecting forceps may be used to hold the wound edge to facilitate passing the needle through.

The knot is tied as shown in the diagram, some three turns being needed, each in the opposite direction from its predecessor. Each stitch needs to be about 3 mm from its neighbour. In cutting the stitch, the nurse should remember that a colleague will have to remove that stitch in a few days time—3 days for faces, 5 days for scalps, 7 days for elsewhere. For faces, 5–0 size suture material is usually used; 4–0 is used elsewhere although if considerable force is involved (e.g. over a knee), 3–0 may be used. Scalps are also often sutured with 3–0. For a more detailed discussion of suture technique the reader is referred to Wardrope and Smith (1992).

Steristrips are simply thin strips of adhesive paper (see Fig. 8.3). They are suitable for many wounds, do not require local anaesthetic

(a)

(b)

(c)

(d)

(e)

(f)

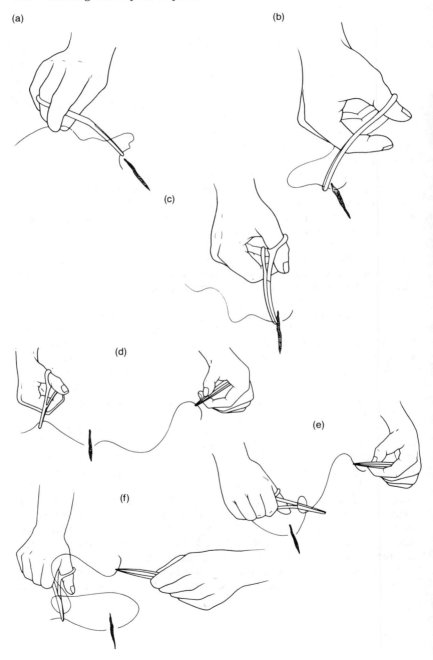

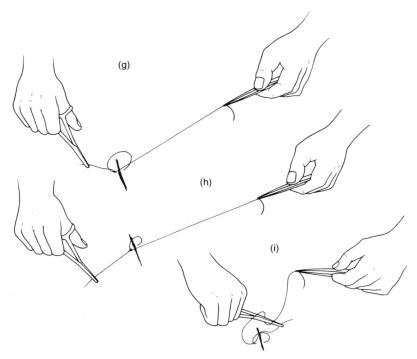

Fig. 8.2   Suturing technique
(a) Note that needle holders grasp the needle approximately one-
third along the needle and not at the end. The point of the needle is
perpendicular to the skin at point of entry. The point of entry should
be 3–4 mm from wound.
(b) By rotating the wrist, bring the needle through and out of the
wound.
(c) Re-enter on the opposite edge of the wound, rotating the wrist
to bring the needle out 3–4 mm from the opposite side of the
wound.
(d) Pull the suture through the wound, ready for tying the knot.
(e) Start tying the knot by making a loop with the needle holders.
(f) Grasp the end of the suture.
(g) Pull the end of the suture through the loop.
(h) Pull it firmly but not too tightly, laying the knot to one side of
the wound.
(i) Then repeat this twice, looping in the opposite direction on each
occasion.

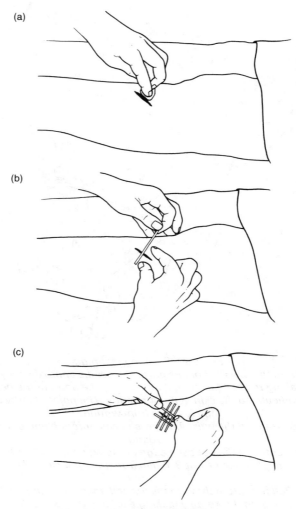

Fig. 8.3 Steristripping technique
(a) *After a thorough cleaning of the wound, wipe the skin on either side of the wound with tinct. benzene.*
(b) *Pinch the skin edges together and lay the strips across it.*
(c) *Leave gaps between the strips and finish by laying two anchor strips parallel to the wound.*

and leave less scar than sutures. They cannot, however, be applied to hairy areas such as the scalp, and if the wound is over a joint, they will probably be pulled apart by tension in the skin as movement occurs.

The skin on either side of a wound should be prepared by having tinct. benzene spray wiped over it to improve its adhesive properties. For most wounds 3 mm strips will suffice; 6 mm or 12 mm are available for bigger wounds. The strip should be attached first to one side of the wound. The wound is then pulled together and the strip stuck down onto the skin the other side. In large or ragged wounds, it may be necessary to perform a two-stage closure, using some strips initially to approximate the wound edges, and then proceeding to close the wound fully with further strips, removing the first strips in the process.

A gap should be left between strips to allow for drainage of any fluid from the wound. Finally, anchoring strips should be applied parallel to the wound to distribute skin tension evenly.

If tissue glue is used (Histoacryl) it should be remembered that it is only suitable for simple lacerations less than 3 cm long and should not be used around the eyes or mouth. Cockerill and Sweeting (1993) recommend the use of forceps to oppose the two skin edges and suggest one nurse should apply gentle lateral pressure to elongate the wound while the other brings the skin edges together with finger pressure which should be maintained for a minute or until the glue becomes opaque to ensure bonding has occurred. As with steristrips there is the advantage of not requiring infiltration with local anaesthesia. It is therefore very useful in treating children with minor lacerations (Pope, 1993).

Minor scalp lacerations can be effectively dealt with by simply tying together strands of hair from either side of the wound.

Dressing the Wound

The optimum dressing should produce a moist, sterile environment with minimum trauma to newly forming tissue (Westaby, 1985). Dressings which shed loose fibres into the wound will significantly delay healing. They should therefore be free from toxic or particulate material (James, 1994). Additionally, they should cause the minimum interference to the patient's normal activity, remain in place as long as required and be easily removed.

Plain dry gauze should not be in direct contact with the wound itself because it absorbs blood and exudate to form a hard, adherent mass that can be very difficult and painful to remove. One of the non-adherent proprietary dressings should be used in contact with the wound itself. Eyre (1993) has argued strongly against the use of the traditional paraffin impregnated gauze dressing for abrasions and other wounds, as there are many superior dressings now available which have far less of a problem with regard to adherence and 'strike through', i.e. the dressing soaking through to the outside with wound exudate. James (1993) is equally critical of these traditional dressings in A & E. Antibiotic impregnated gauze should never be used as it is expensive, ineffective and contributes to the development of resistant strains of bacteria.

The dressing may be secured to the skin with a hypoallergenic tape (e.g. Micropore) applied longitudinally as any swelling may give rise to circulatory impairment if there is a circumferential constriction around the limb or digit. Many modern dressings though are self-adhesive.

The use of an elasticated tube type of bandage (e.g. Tubigrip) is recommended, rather than the traditional crêpe bandage, to complete the dressing. It is cheaper, easier to apply, gives a more even pressure over the limb with no risk of the wrinkles that can cause skin problems, and will stay in place far more effectively than a crêpe bandage.

Finger dressings can be retained with a tubular bandage (e.g. Tubinette), the important point being to tie the bandage at the wrist, and not at the base of the digit, in order to avoid the risk of circulatory impairment. If swelling is anticipated, the hand should be placed in a high arm sling (see Fig. 8.4). The use of Flamazine cream or Granuflex for finger tip injuries is highly effective compared to traditional dressings (Eyre, 1993).

Head wounds may need a pressure bandage even after suture. A size F Tubigrip, 10 cm long, worn as a headband provides a very simple and effective solution to the problem, rather than the intricacies of head bandaging so beloved of the first aid manuals. Similarly the elasticated tube bandages (e.g. Netelast) provide a better means of securing dressings to the trunk than does the traditional body bandage.

Tetanus Vaccination

The effectiveness of the anti-tetanus immunization programme in the UK can be judged from the fact that there are no more than one

(a)

(b)

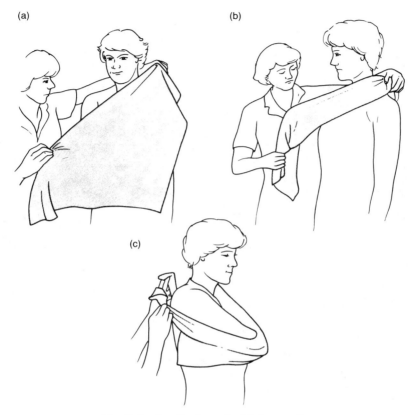

(c)

Fig. 8.4   Application of a high arm sling
(*a*) *This shows the position of the sling. Ensure that the hand that is
injured is placed on the opposite shoulder.*
(*b*) *Wrap the sling around the arm and hand. Pin to ensure that the
hand is enclosed.*
(*c*) *Tie the sling at the back.*

or two dozen cases per year compared to the death toll from tetanus of approximately a million per year in developing countries.

The adsorbed tetanus toxoid that is given to patients in A & E units is a form of active immunization in that it stimulates the patient to manufacture their own antibodies. Wardrope and Smith

Table 8.2   Characteristics of ideal dressings

Provide the optimum environment for wound healing (a moist environment) at the wound/dressing interface

Allow gaseous exchange of oxygen, carbon dioxide and water vapour

Provide thermal insulation (wound healing is temperature dependent)

Impermeable to microorganisms in both directions

Free from particulate contaminants

Non-adherent (many products are described as non-adherent but are low-adherent)

Safe to use (non-toxic, non-sensitizing, non-allergenic)

Acceptable to the patient

High absorption characteristics (for exuding wounds)

Cost-effective

Carrier for medicaments, e.g. antiseptics

Capable of standardization and evaluation

Allow monitoring of the wound (transparent)

Provide mechanical protection

Non-inflammable

Sterilizable

Conformable and mouldable (especially over sacrum, heels and elbows)

Available (in hospital and community) in a suitable range of forms and sizes

Require infrequent changing (products should be left in place for as long as possible)

NB. In practice, no single dressing will possess all these characteristics fully.
Table from Morgan, D. (1994) Establishing a dressings formulary, *British Journal of Nursing*, **3(8)**, 387–92.

(1992) recommend that a full course be completed by two subsequent injections at monthly intervals and that the average adult needs a booster at ten-yearly intervals thereafter. Anti-tetanus injections are a normal part of the childhood injections received in the UK. Therefore, any child that has had its triple injections as an infant will have received anti-tetanus cover.

If the patient states that they have never received any anti-tetanus immunization, it is possible to give passive immunity in the form of the appropriate human immunoglobulin if the medical staff assess the risk as being significant.

Closed Soft Tissue Injury

The usual aim is to treat closed soft tissue injury conservatively by rest and support. Swelling can be reduced by elevation and ice packs if necessary. Gradually the area can be mobilized as pain and swelling ease off. A tubular support bandage should be used to lend support to the injury in this stage. If a sprain of the ankle is so severe as to prevent full weight-bearing, consideration should be given to plaster of Paris to immobilize the injury. Crêpe bandage is of little effective use.

Abscesses and Infected Wounds

Abscesses are commonly treated by surgical incision and drainage, under general or local anaesthesia. The appropriate preparation of the patient is, therefore, required in line with hospital procedure, together with a full explanation of what is to happen and how long the procedure will take.

In dressing an old infected wound or a recently drained abscess, the principles of providing a sterile moist environment which can heal from the bottom up remain. In a review of the research, Walsh and Ford (1989) have shown that traditional solutions such as mercurichrome and the chlorine-based antiseptics (Eusol, Chloramine T) are ineffective and potentially very harmful. The authors conclude that they should be withdrawn from use and point out that there are many far superior new products on the market to debride and dress infected wounds (e.g. Iodosorb and Granuflex). Although more expensive per dressing, they are cheaper in the long run since they achieve healing much more quickly and safely, requiring far fewer dressings and much less nursing time. The characteristics of ideal dressings are summarized in Table 8.2.

	0–5 min	6–20 min	21–60 min
Documentation	Registration as A & E patient	A & E notes ready	Wound assessment chart started for follow-up A & E notes completed with sketch of wound
Assessment	Triage nurse, check wound for type size bleeding, patient for pain and anxiety	Obtain history from patient. Check wound for FB (?XR) and contamination, also damage to any underlying structures, check Tetanus status	Assess dressing when complete. Patient's understanding of care post discharge?
Medication	–	–	Anti-tetanus Antibiotics Analgesics as needed
Treatment	–	–	Debridement and thorough clean of wound, closure with suture steristrip or glue
Nursing care	Apply pressure dressing, limb elevation, psych support	Maintain as before	Lie patient down, explain procedures, close wound and dress. Give medication and wound care teaching
Referrals	–	–	Follow up in A & E or refer to health centre
Family	Inform if not present, psych support if needed	–	Include in patient teaching
Discharge	–	–	Ensure appropriate referral letter written

NB. FB = Foreign body

Fig. 8.5   Example of critical pathway for wounded patient

The patient will usually be discharged with a course of antibiotics and analgesics. The nurse should ensure that the patient understands the labels on the bottles and knows which are the analgesics and which the antibiotics. The patient also must understand the need to complete the full course of antibiotics even if the infection appears to clear up before completion. The nurse can remember that the patient's care from now on will be self-care until they return for their next appointment when the nurse will be able to check progress on the healing of the abscess. The use of a wound assessment chart to monitor progress is essential for professional nursing care, although the change involved in introducing such a chart needs careful management (Banfield and Shuttleworth, 1993). If necessary, patients may be given dressings to take home and may change the dressing themselves, provided that correct instruction is given in A & E first. The value of developing a self-care approach to nursing in the mode of Orem is evident from just this one common example of A & E care.

Self-care

It is important that the patient be instructed in self-care of the injury before discharge. Key points include the need for elevation, keeping the dressing dry and clean, the length of time until dressing or suture removal, and instructions about how to remove the dressings or where to go to get the sutures removed. The patient should be alerted about the signs of infection and instructed to return immediately if there is any suspicion of infection. If a full course of tetanus is required, the patient should be given a card with the dates of the next two injections and the nurse should emphasize the importance of the follow-up injections. In this case, the nurse is filling the educative/supportive role of Orem after the partly compensatory role which will have been filled at an earlier stage during treatment.

Evaluation

All dressings performed by junior staff should be checked before the patient is discharged, for if they are done incorrectly, they go home wrong and remain wrong.

In many respects, the only real evaluation of treatment is if the patient returns or not. If the patient does not return, the assumption is that the nursing interventions have been successful. If the patient does return with a problem, however, the nursing staff should try to see how nursing care could have been better carried out. This will benefit other patients in the future.

In order to evaluate the effectiveness of self-care instruction, it is essential to question the patient to see that they fully understand what has been taught.

References

Banfield K., Shuttleworth E. (1993). A systematic approach with lasting benefits. *Professional Nurse*, **8**, 234–8.

Cockerill J., Sweeting A. (1993). Nursing management of common accident wounds. *British Journal of Nursing*, **2**, 578–82.

Eyre G. (1993). Alternative wound dressings in A & E. *Nursing Standard*, **7**, 25–8.

Fergusson A. (1993). Wound infection—the role of antiseptics. *Accident and Emergency Nursing*, **1**, 79–86.

James H. (1994). Wound dressings in A & E departments. *Accident and Emergency Nursing*, **2**, 87–93.

Jones G. (1993). Minor injury care in the community. *Nursing Standard*, **7**, 35–6.

Pope S. (1993). The use of Histoacryl tissue adhesive in children's A & E. *Paediatric Nursing*, **5**, 20–21.

Walsh M., Ford P. (1989). *Nursing Rituals, Research and Rational Action*. Oxford: Butterworth-Heinemann.

Wardrope J., Smith J. (1992). *The Management of Wounds and Burns*. Oxford: Oxford University Press.

Westaby S. (1985). *Wound Care*. Oxford: Butterworth-Heinemann.

Chapter 9

THE BURNT PATIENT IN A & E

Pathology

The key factors in burn pathology are the area of the burn, the depth of the burn, and any special areas of the body, such as the respiratory tract, that are involved.

Area

The burnt area will almost immediately begin to lose fluid which is very similar to plasma in its composition. If sufficient fluid is lost from the burn, hypovolaemic shock will develop. The area of the burn is, therefore, crucial as it determines the volume of fluid lost. Area may be estimated using Wallace's Rule of 9 (see Fig. 9.1).

As a rule of thumb it may be assumed that in burns of 15% of surface area or greater in adults, and 10% or greater in children, hypovolaemia will develop. In these cases, therefore, the patient will need an IVI. If such an infusion is not commenced and the hypovolaemia not vigorously treated, the outcome may be fatal.

In reading about burns, the nurse may be confused by the different statements that are made about the type of fluid that should be used to correct hypovolaemia from burns. This is because there is a marked difference of opinion among the various specialists in the field. The basic requirements in the burn patient are protein, salt and water in such a form as will stay in the circulation. Sodium chloride is lost in great quantities in the burn exudate, along with protein, and therefore must be replaced. However, the hypovolaemic patient also needs fluids that will stay in the circulation rather than those which rapidly escape into the various other fluid compartments of the body. Thus, although normal saline contains the sodium chloride required, it will not effectively expand the circulation and, although Haemaccel is a plasma expander, it does not contain sodium

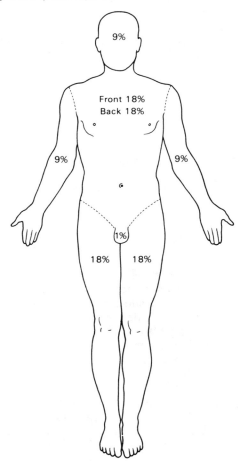

9%

Front 18%
Back 18%

9%   9%

1%

18%   18%

Fig. 9.1   Wallace's Rule of 9 for estimating area of burns

chloride. Solutions such as Dextran 70 and plasma protein faction (PPF), however, have both properties.

Fluid loss from a burn continues for over 24 hours after injury. This is of significance in planning dressings for patients who are to be discharged home with relatively minor burns. For the major burn requiring in-patient treatment, the continual fluid loss has to be

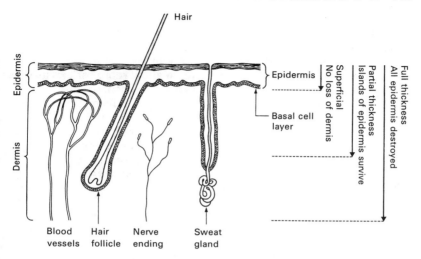

Fig. 9.2 Depth of burns.

taken into account in working out an IVI regime. Various formulae are used in this connection, one of the best known being the Mount Vernon formula (Wardrope and Smith, 1992), which calculates a unit volume of fluid from the patient's size and the area burnt.

Unit volume = Area burnt (%) × Patient's weight (kg) ÷ 2.
This unit volume of fluid is then administered in blocks of 4 hours, two blocks of 6 hours and one block of 12 hours, measured from the time of the burn and subject to adjustment in the light of the patient's condition.

Depth

The 1st, 2nd and 3rd degree burns classifications are to be avoided as they are imprecise terms that can mean different things to different people. It is more appropriate and precise to describe the depth of burns as either full thickness, partial thickness or superficial.

A full thickness burn is one in which the full thickness of the skin has been destroyed (see Fig. 9.2). The appearance is a typically dull grey area, or in flame burns, a dark brown or black. Because the nerve endings have been destroyed, there is usually a loss of sensation. The remaining tissue is hard and leathery. This poses a special problem in circumferential burns because the inelastic surface tissue will act as a tourniquet around the limb, within which there will be swelling due to the burn oedema. The result is occlusion of the circulation, gangrene and loss of the limb, unless the limb is excised longitudinally through the eschar tissue to allow room for expansion and for the release of pressure. This is known as escharotomy.

Healing of a full thickness burn occurs by the formation of scar tissue, which is both unsightly and inelastic. The inelasticity will give rise to loss of function and severe contractures. The need, therefore, is to treat full thickness burns by skin grafting in order to retain maximum function and avoid contracture formation.

If the burn is only partial thickness, then areas of epithelium survive around hair follicles and sweat glands. This permits the re-epithelialization of the burnt area, provided that it is kept free from infection. Skin grafting is, therefore, not usually required and healing should occur with a full range of movement. Partial thickness burns usually leave the nerve endings intact; therefore, they may be differentiated from full thickness burns by a pin prick sensation test. Scalds and flash burns are typically partial thickness.

Superficial burns involve a reddening only of the most superficial layers. This is known as erythema and is of minor importance compared to the other two types so far discussed. In estimating burn areas, erythema should be excluded.

One final type of burn that should be mentioned is the burn due to electricity. It is characterized by a small surface wound where the current entered the body, but within there may be major damage with burns extending down to the bone and involving structures such as tendons, muscles and nerves. The potential effect of the electric current on the heart should be the first focus of nursing and medical attention.

Special Areas Affected by Burns

Oedema of the face and neck can have serious implications for the airway. Inhalation of flames or hot gases will cause burn oedema in the respiratory tract itself. The threat of an occluded airway is very real in such cases and an early tracheotomy or intubation, if possible, is indicated.

Facial oedema will quickly make it impossible for the patient to open their eyes. This has two implications; first, if the eyes are to be examined properly, they must be examined immediately, and second,

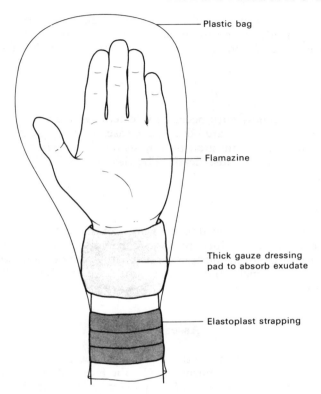

Plastic bag

Flamazine

Thick gauze dressing
pad to absorb exudate

Elastoplast strapping

Fig. 9.3   Flamazine bag treatment for hand burns

the patient may fear that their sight has been lost altogether, when the problem is simply that they cannot open their eyes.

Immobilization of hands in bulky dressings will lead to long-term problems of joint stiffness. For this reason, the 'Flamazine bag' dressing is recommended for burnt hands rather than more traditional methods (see Fig. 9.3). Flamazine is silver sulphadiazine, a very effective antibacterial agent.

Psychological Effects

The nurse should realize that there are profound psychological effects from a burn which affect not only the patient but also their relatives. There is the fear of disfigurement and altered body image on the one hand, and on the other, there are the inevitable feelings of guilt associated with the parent of a young child that has been burnt.

Infection

If a partial thickness burn becomes infected, healing will be delayed until the infection is cleared up. In the case of a full thickness burn, infection will make skin grafting impossible. In severe cases, infection from burns can cause death. The risk of tetanus should not be forgotten.

Other Later Effects

After the patient has moved to the ward, complications can develop. These include renal failure, toxaemia, anaemia, paralytic ileus, and in the case of children 'burn encephalopathy'. These complications can combine to make the burns victim an extremely challenging person to care for.

Assessment

Assessment of the burns victim starts with the airway. The nurse should note whether the burns involve the face and neck areas, and whether there is any evidence of the patient having inhaled flames or hot gas. Such evidence would include soot in the nasal passages or blistering around the mouth and lips.

It is important to obtain a history of the accident—what caused the burn, the time the burn occurred and what, if any, first aid has been applied. The next point to determine is how much pain the patient is feeling. Some burns cause remarkably little pain; ironically they are usually the more severe full thickness burns as the actual nerve endings have been destroyed, but other burns can be extremely painful.

The area of the burn should be estimated, using Wallace's Rule of 9 (see Fig. 9.1). This rule divides the body area up into multiples of 9%. For small areas, the area of the patient's hand can be taken as 1% of the body area. Areas of superficial erythema and redness should *not* be included in this calculation.

The last point to estimate is the depth of the burn. The appearance will give some clue: a full thickness burn is typically a dull grey colour with tough leathery eschar tissue; a partial thickness burn is usually red or pink in colour. Sensation is absent in the full thickness burn but present in a partial thickness burn. This may be tested for with the pin prick method.

A sketch of the burn is a useful means of recording its extent; areas of suspected full thickness burn can be shaded in and labelled as such.

Baseline observations are important to monitor the circulatory status of the patient and to detect any signs of hypovolaemic shock at the earliest stage. They should be repeated as frequently as the patient's condition indicates.

The psychological effects of the burn on the patient and on the family should be assessed, especially where young children are involved. Is the mother hostile and defensive, or anxious and expressing feelings of guilt? One important aspect that has to be assessed is whether the child's injuries match the story of the parent, as burns constitute a common form of child abuse.

In electrical burns, it is important to take an ECG and to monitor the patient's heart rhythm continually on a cardiac monitor. Function should be assessed together with sensation in view of the risk of damage to deep structures such as tendons and nerves.

Intervention

First Aid

The appropriate first aid for burns is irrigation with copious amounts of cold water. This will retard the process of tissue destruction due to heat and also afford the patient considerable pain relief.

Airway

The first priority for the burns patient is to safeguard the airway, and if assessment reveals problems due to oedema, tracheotomy or intubation will be considered. The A & E nursing team must be able to respond at once to the need for emergency tracheotomy or intubation in such a situation. Upper airway oedema peaks at 24–48 hours after injury. Treatment in less severe cases consists of administering humidified oxygen, maintaining close observation, an upright position and chest physiotherapy aimed at preventing atelectasis (Hudak and Gallo 1994).

Pain Relief

The application of cold soaks (gauze dressing pads and sterile water for irrigation) to the burnt area will usually reduce the pain felt by the patient though the risk of hypothermia should not be overlooked. The generous administration of Entonox gas will further relieve pain.

In major burns, the administration of intravenous morphine is recommended by many authorities. The best method is to dilute 10 mg of morphine in 10 ml of water for injection, and then to give, slowly, sufficient of the drug to achieve the desired degree of sedation and pain relief.

In dealing with young children, sedation is very important as it is impossible to dress properly limbs that are flailing in all directions at once. Furthermore, the more distressed the child, the more distressed will be the parents who are already probably feeling desperately guilty and blaming themselves for their young child's misfortune. A child may be sedated with oral trimeprazine syrup, but it must be remembered that the child can still feel the pain and that therefore some other analgesic agent is required in addition. Wherever possible, when dressing burns on young children, nurses should allow them to sit on their parent's lap as being held by a parent will be a source of comfort in what the child is currently experiencing as a very frightening experience.

Psychological Support

From the nurse's very first encounter with the patient, psychological support will be essential. Reference has already been made to the likely guilt feelings that parents of young children will be experiencing. In addition, adults will be fearing disfigurement as a result of their injuries.

It is very difficult at this early stage in A & E to deal with a straight 'Will I be scarred for life?' question. But this is precisely what is in the mind of the burn victim, and may even be on their lips. If asked, the nurse should try to answer the question fairly and frankly, pointing out that at this early stage it is very difficult to say with any degree of certainty what the outcome will be. Such an answer is better than bland reassurances about the wonders of modern plastic surgery. On the other hand, the question may remain unasked; if this is the case, the nurse should try to get the patient to verbalize their fears and to get the matter out in the open for realistic discussion.

The degree of distress displayed by the patient may be markedly reduced by simply talking about the problem and offering support as appropriate.

The IVI and Fluid Balance

If the burn is over 15% of the body surface area, an IVI will be required to prevent hypovolaemia. Apart from nursing assistance in siting the infusion, it will be a key part of the resuscitation effort that an accurate fluid balance be kept. Catheterization, with hourly urine measurements, is essential due to the risk of renal failure. The kidneys should be able to produce a minimum of 0.5 ml of urine per kg body weight per hour; failure to do so indicates that they are being underperfused and that, therefore, inadequate IV fluids are being given to deal with the burn shock. For an average adult, the hourly urine output should not drop below about 35 ml (Hudak and Gallo, 1994).

Burns Dressings

The aim of the dressing is to provide an aseptic environment in which, depending on the depth of the burn, either healing can occur or the wound can be readied for successful grafting.

The first step is to debride the wound. Contaminants such as charred clothing and soot should be washed away using copious amounts of sterile water for irrigation. After cleansing, a pair of non-toothed McIndoe's dissecting forceps should be used to remove all dead tissue and blisters. Alternatively, clean blister tissue may be left and the blister fluid aspirated with a needle and syringe. Little pain should be felt by the patient as the tissue is dead; once pain is felt, it is a signal to stop as that tissue is obviously alive!

The wound dressing should be occlusive and secure, in order to preserve the aimed-for aseptic environment, yet at the same time it should be easy to remove for redressing. These criteria are best met with the Flamazine and Melolin dressing technique which consists of spreading Flamazine cream over an appropriate sized sheet of

Melolin with a sterile spatula to a thickness of 3–4 mm and then applying this to the burn. The Flamazine will act as a powerful prophylactic agent in preventing infection of the burn, and yet it can also be used for treating infected burns as well; the Melolin will ensure that the dressing is easily removed without sticking.

Because burns will ooze exudate for at least 24 hours, there is a need for a considerable thickness of gauze backing up the Melolin, possibly two large dressing pads thick. The whole dressing should be secured with tape and then by an elasticated tubular bandage rather than crêpe.

Elevation of the burnt limb is essential because of the volume of oedema that is to be expected. If the patient is going home, this must be one of the key points made in discharge instructions.

The problems associated with finger stiffness after prolonged immobilization necessitate the special technique used for burns involving the hands—the 'Flamazine bag dressing' (see Fig. 9.3, p. 175). Debridement and cleaning are carried out as normal. Then the hand is smeared generously with Flamazine and inserted in a plastic bag which is securely taped to the wrist. A large dressing pad should be taped around the wrist inside the bag to soak up the oedema and the whole arm should be placed in a high arm sling. The key point about this dressing is that the fingers are unrestricted and therefore, provided that the patient remembers to exercise them, stiffness will not be a problem. Instruction about finger exercises is essential prior to discharge, in addition to warning the patient that the appearance of the hand may be alarming due to maceration of the skin. Daily bag change may be necessary initially due to the volume of tissue exudate produced.

The same technique may be used for burns to the foot and toes. The nurse will find it a great deal quicker than the traditional burns dressings which would involve separate dressings for each finger in addition to dressings for the rest of the hand.

If the patient has suffered a major burn, he or she is best treated in a regional centre and an immediate transfer should be arranged. The failure of A & E units to treat burns patients correctly has been alarmingly described by Palmer and Sutherland (1987) in a study of 152 patients transferred to their regional burns centre (see Table 9.1).

These figures include nine children with burns of over 10% who had no IVI, two of whom had already developed shock, and the fact that, of the 28 adults who had IVIs, in six cases they were not working. This disturbing study indicates that A & E units were not

Table 9.1
Problems encountered in treatment of burns patients on arrival at a
regional burns centre

Problem	Children	Adults
Total number of patients	54	98
No first aid applied after accident	17	64
Salt, flour etc. applied as first aid	3	8
No documented estimate of burn area	21	36
Not receiving IV fluids	46	70
Receiving inappropriate IV fluids	5	2
No written record of IVI	3	4
Suffering pain	27	26
Only given oral analgesia	8	5
Given no analgesia at all	11	7

managing burns patients correctly and emphasizes the need for a
major in-service training initiative for both nursing and medical
staff in this area. Recent experience with disasters only underlines
the need for A & E units to be proficient in managing patients who
have suffered burns and inhalation injury (Walsh, 1989).

Self-care of Burns Dressings

The majority of burns patients seen in an A & E department are
usually discharged home and followed up on an out-patient basis.
Therefore, the patient must fully understand how to look after the
dressing if best results are to be obtained and complications such as
infection are to be avoided. Key points are the need to keep the limb
elevated in fresh burns, the importance of exercising the fingers in
hand burns, and for any burn, the need to keep the dressing clean
and dry. The patient needs to know when he or she has to return
to hospital—i.e. at an arranged time such as a burns clinic held in
A & E, or if the dressing has soaked through, started to disintegrate
or emit an unpleasant smell, or if there is another indication
of infection.

The ability of the patient or the patient's family to care for the
dressing, and the effect that dressing will have on the patient's
universal self-care demands should be carefully thought about by
the nurse before discharge. Failure to do so can have serious implica-

	0–5 min	6–15 min	16–60 min
Documentation	Registration as A & E patient Burn chart available	A & E notes ready Fill in burn chart	Complete notes and burn chart
Assessment	Triage nurse, check breathing, area depth of burn, pain level. Top priority if serious burn	History from patient Vital signs Careful survey of burn depth and area. Check special areas e.g. mouth, eyes	Monitor vital signs, urine output, pain, limb colour distal to burn
Medication	Entonox	IV analgesia if needed, Entonox	Analgesia ATT
Treatment	Intubate if needed	Set up IV with wide bore cannula. O_2. Temporary dressing to protect burn	Debride and dress minor burns Catheterize major burns, continue resuscitation until stable
Nursing care	Psych support Cold compresses/ irrigation of burn	Continue. Assist with resuscitation	Burn dressing Psych support Fluid balance give medication Patient teaching if minor burn which will be managed as out-patient
Referrals	–	Regional burns unit if serious	Arrange transfer to regional unit
Family	Psych support Inform if not present	Continue. Keep informed	Cont. allow to be with patient, answer questions honestly
Discharge	–	–	Transfer only when stable. If minor burn, arrange follow-up and give teaching session

Fig. 9.4   Example of critical pathway for burnt patient

tions for the patient and make for a much more prolonged and painful period of ill health because of the problems that may arise if the burn becomes infected.

Evaluation

The psychological state of the patient, together with the degree of pain being felt, should be closely watched in order to determine the effectiveness of intervention in these two areas. It is also important to check that an elevated limb remains elevated as it may easily slip.

The effectiveness of the other main area of nursing intervention, the dressing, is usually measured at the patient's next attendance. It is important that senior nursing staff check the state dressings are in upon return to ensure that staff within the unit are carrying out effective burns dressings—i.e. dressings that will last, with a minimum infection rate and which can be easily removed without causing the patient undue distress. It is only by monitoring dressing standards that steps, such as teaching, can be taken to improve dressings to the standard required should there be a shortfall. (See Fig. 9.4 for Critical Pathway for Burns.)

Finally, it remains to check that the information that has been taught has been learnt, i.e. does the patient understand the self-care instructions that have been given? Only questioning of the patient will allow nurses to discover whether he or she has truly learnt what has been taught.

References

Hudak C., Gallo B. (1994). *Critical Care Nursing*, 6th edn. Philadelphia: J. B. Lippincott.
Palmer J., Sutherland A. (1987). Problems associated with transfer of patients to a regional burns unit. *Injury*, **18**:4, 250–7.
Walsh M. (1989). *Disaster, Current Planning and Recent Experience*. London: Edward Arnold.
Wardrope J., Smith J. (1992). *The Management of Wounds and Burns*. Oxford: Oxford University Press.

Chapter 10

EYE COMPLAINTS AND EMERGENCIES

Pathology

The human eye has been well-endowed by nature with defences such as the bony orbit and a very fast blink reflex. Despite these defences, however, eye injuries are common. In addition, the A & E nurse will see many patients who bring themselves to the department with a wide variety of eye complaints of a non-traumatic origin, although eye trauma remains the single most likely reason for attendance (Elkington and Shaw, 1988).

Non-penetrating Eye Injury

Trauma to Structures Surrounding the Eye

The bony orbit that surrounds the eye may be fractured as a result of facial or head injury. The injury may be an isolated fracture which is called a 'blow out' fracture or it may be a component of either a facio-maxillary injury or a fractured base of the skull. In a blow out fracture, the cause is a blow to the front of the orbit; the force from the blow is conducted as shock waves by the orbital floor and causes a sudden rise in intra-orbital pressure, the result being that an isolated piece of bone is blown into the adjacent sinus. The problem that this injury causes is that tissue, including muscle, herniates through the hole and becomes trapped; the mobility of the eye is restricted and double vision or diplopia develops.

In the more serious cases, where the orbital fracture is part of other fractures, the eye can be impaired by damage to the optic nerve, or one of the other facial nerves, leading to the development of a nerve palsy.

Soft tissue injury to the eyelids is a common situation; it usually causes bruising which resolves with the passage of time. Most lacerations are easily stitched or closed with tissue glue; however, Wardrope and Smith (1992) recommend that lacerations which go through both surfaces of the lid or involved structures such as the lacrymal duct should be referred to a specialist. Due to the speed with which swelling of the lids can develop, it is essential to examine the damaged eye promptly, as soon afterwards examination may be rendered virtually impossible by the swollen and bruised lids. In burns cases, it may be impossible to close the lids due to the burn damage. As the cornea must not be left exposed, this requires that antibiotic ointment be applied to the cornea and that urgent arrangements be made for a plastic surgery procedure to replace the destroyed tissue.

Foreign Body (Non-penetrating)

This is probably the most common ophthalmic complaint seen in A & E, the cause being any small particle such as dust, grit, woodsplinters or metal fragments. Foreign bodies which have failed to penetrate the eye will either be found lodged on the surface of the cornea or on the under-surface of the eyelid, the conjuctiva. In this latter case, it is known as a sub-tarsal foreign body.

Corneal foreign bodies, such as vegetable material, can produce severe irritation and infection and, in the case of metallic objects, can very quickly stain the cornea with a deposit of rust. Sub-tarsal foreign bodies produce the sensation of 'something in my eye' and, therefore, the eyelids should always be everted when a patient presents complaining of a foreign body.

Corneal Abrasion

This is an extremely painful condition in which the epithelium of the cornea is removed from the damaged part. It is usually caused by a glancing blow to the eye from any number of objects such as a finger nail, towel or newspaper.

Chemical Injury

The extent of the injury is related to the nature and concentration of the agent involved. Alkalis are the most damaging (e.g. substances containing lime such as wet cement) as they can rapidly penetrate the cornea and produce severe damage to the iris, ciliary body and lens while also causing ischaemia. Acids of equivalent strength are less damaging than alkalis as they combine with tissue components to precipitate deposits of protein which form a barrier against further penetration (Tannen and Marsden, 1991). Nevertheless, whether the injury is caused by an acid or alkali chemical, the effects can be devastating.

Radiation Injury

Ultra-violet light is the usual culprit, producing damage to the superficial layers of the epithelium of the cornea. Pain, photophobia and watering are the usual symptoms the patient presents with a few hours after exposure. Sun lamps and welding without proper goggles are the usual causes, the latter giving rise to the name of 'arc eye' by which this condition is informally known.

Keratitis or inflammation of the cornea is the usual result of exposure to other forms of radiation. Cataract formation is a long-term complication of ionizing radiation exposure. This is well-documented in survivors of the Japanese atom bombs, the cataracts tending to develop some 5 years after the bombing.

Contusion and Concussion Injury

Contusion refers to injury from the direct impact of the force involved. Damage to the eyelids has already been mentioned; the cornea can also be affected by contusion. The result can vary from corneal oedema through to rupture of the whole globe, depending on the force involved.

Concussion refers to the conduction of shock waves from the point of impact to other parts of the eye. The blow out fracture has already been discussed as an example of this type of injury. Within the globe itself, various very severe injuries are possible, including detachment of the retina or the ciliary body, vitreous or retinal haemorrhages, and/or the development of a hyphaemia. A hyphaemia is bleeding into the anterior chamber and can have devastating effects on sight due to the development of secondary glaucoma and corneal staining. Cataract of the lens or the dislocation of the lens may result from a concussion injury; the iris sphincter may be ruptured in concussion, leading again to the long-term risk of glaucoma.

Penetrating Eye Injury

Penetrating eye injuries may be classified into two groups: those in which the object responsible is withdrawn after penetration and those in which the object is retained in the eye, forming an intra-ocular foreign body. The prognosis for vision depends upon the size of the laceration in the cornea or sclera, and upon which part of the eye is involved. Penetration to the posterior chamber carries the worst prognosis.

In order that a foreign body may penetrate the eye, it must possess a large amount of energy. Typical objects are glass from a car windscreen (see Fig.10.1), flying debris from industrial processes such as drilling, and material propelled by a blast after an explosion. The most common form of retained foreign body within the eye is metallic—iron and steel account for between 85 and 98% of intra-ocular foreign bodies caused by industrial accidents, a similar proportion to that found in war casualties.

A much feared complication of penetrating eye injury is sympathetic ophthalmitis, where after injury to one eye, the uninjured eye

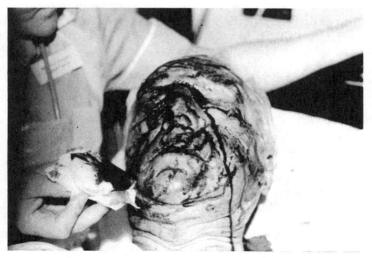

Fig. 10.1   Typical car windscreen injury. Serious damage to both eyes plus multiple lacerations to face

develops a severe inflammation some time after (from 3 weeks to 4 months has been reported). If untreated, this inflammation may lead to loss of useful vision in the uninjured eye. Prompt post-traumatic surgery and early enucleation of the injured eye, together with the use of steroid therapy, have greatly reduced the incidence of this complication which can lead to complete blindness.

In addition to the obviously disastrous effects that the foreign body may have on the delicate structures of the eye, there is a further risk of siderosis bulbi if the foreign body contains iron. This condition stems from the chemical reactions which occur within the eye due to the iron, its effects being seen some time after the injury. As the iron dissolves, it becomes incorporated into the cells of the eye, leading to chronic damage and eventually blindness. For this reason, it is mandatory that all ferrous intra-ocular foreign bodies be removed. An electromagnet is commonly used to do this.

Inflammation of the Eye

There are many varied eye conditions that bring patients to A & E other than trauma. There is not space to describe all of them, but it is worth noting some of the conditions that give rise to inflammation of the eye, for this is the most common eye problem after trauma (see Table 10.1).

Assessment

The first step is to obtain a history of the complaint from the patient. Important symptoms that may be mentioned and which should alert the nurse to give a patient high priority in the queue include: haloes around lights (classically indicative of an early attack of glaucoma), 'floaters' described by the patient as visible wisps or strands (indicating inflammation or debris from trauma), flashing lights (retinal damage) and, of course, sudden blindness. Other less helpful symptoms (less helpful because they are so non-specific) include photophobia, which may be associated with inflammation of the eye but can be associated with many other illnesses such as migraine and pain in the eye. Pain may be of ocular origin (e.g. inflammation of the cornea), but it may also be caused by many

Table 10.1
Common causes of inflammation of the eye

Condition	Pathology
Stye	Boil on lid margin.
Chalazion	Cyst within tarsal plate (eyelid).
Allergy	Reaction affecting both eyelid and conjunctiva.
Conjunctivitis	Redness of conjunctiva. There is discharge but no pain. Bacteria are the usual cause.
Keratitis	Painful inflammation of cornea. Common causes are an extension of existing conjunctivitis, corneal exposure, or the herpes simplex virus which leads to the formation of a dendritic ulcer.
Iritis	Acute inflammation of the iris.
Glaucoma	Raised intra-ocular pressure. Common cause is blockage of the aqueous circulation from the ciliary body via the pupils to the drainage angle in the anterior chamber. It can be either acute, chronic or secondary to some other condition such as iritis or hyphaemia. This is a potentially blinding condition.

other conditions such as sinusitis, where the patient attributes the pain to the eyeball. Furthermore, the pain of acute glaucoma can be described by some patients as being in the forehead and nowhere near the eyes.

It is also possible that the patient may present as an emergency complaining of sudden visual disturbances and loss of visual acuity which turn out to be associated with AIDS. Plona and Schremp (1992) report that in the USA 75% of AIDS patients develop ocular conditions and comment that the person may be totally unaware that they are HIV positive when they present. Typical pathological findings include cytomegalovirus (CMV) infections, Kaposi's sarcoma of the conjunctiva, retinal haemorrhages and vasculitis. There are many other systemic diseases which can affect vision of course, such as diabetes, but none perhaps so devastating as AIDS.

If the patient is presenting with a foreign body, it is essential to find out if it was a high energy or low energy accident due to the risk of penetration and if possible what the foreign body might be composed of. Similarly, if it is a chemical injury to the eye that the patient has sustained, then nurses need to know what chemical, how long ago and what first aid measures have been taken (hopefully copious irrigation with cold water).

After obtaining a history, the next step is to assess vision. Simple finger counting will assess whether there is any double vision present. The use of the standard Snellen Visual Acuity Test is strongly recommended for all patients with eye complaints. The chart consists of lines of letters of differing sizes which the average eye should be able to read at varying distances, depending on the size of the letters.

The patient is asked to read the chart from a distance of 6 metres, one eye at a time, the other eye being occluded. The results of each eye are carefully recorded, noting the last line to be read correctly. If the patient wears spectacles, this test should be carried out both with and without the spectacles. Each line has a number which refers to the distance at which the average eye should be able to read that line. The result is, therefore, recorded as a fraction, the top number referring to the distance at which the patient stood from the chart, the bottom number being the line number that was correctly read (i.e. the distance at which an average eye would be able to read that line). Thus vision recorded as 6/6 means that at a range of 6 metres the patient can read the same size letters that the average eye can read at 6 metres.

If the patient is illiterate or very young, an E chart is used, consisting of rows of the capital letter E pointing in different directions. The patient is asked to indicate using three fingers the position of the E.

After assessing visual acuity, the nurse should move on to the eye itself, working inwards in a regular sequence which the A & E nurse will find helpful to have as a standard pattern for assessing eyes. Both eyes should always be examined.

The eyelids should first be examined for evidence of disease or damage. This should include eversion to examine the under-surface of the lid (the conjunctiva). This is best done by asking the patient to look downwards, grasping the eyelashes, then gently pulling down, round and up while depressing the upper margin of the tarsal plate with a cotton applicator or similar implement. The under-surface of the eyelid should be readily visualized by this technique.

For assessment of the eye itself, a bright pen torch is essential. First the pupil responses and the shape of the pupil should be tested to check they are brisk to respond and equal and regular in size and shape. A pear-shaped pupil indicates significant eye trauma and disruption of internal ocular structures (Hartland, 1993). The cornea should be examined for evidence of a foreign body, a corneal wound or redness indicative of inflammation. Damage to the corneal epithelium is difficult to visualize under normal conditions, but the addition of a drop of sodium fluorescein will show the damaged area in bright green which is easily visible. Ocular position and movement should also be checked; a blow out fracture of the orbit is often associated with an apparently recessed eye, for example (Hartland, 1993).

Finally, the person as a whole must be assessed. Eye injuries produce great fear of blindness in many patients. Patients are, therefore, likely to be very frightened and anxious. Thus an assessment of the psychological state of the patient is needed as nursing intervention is required in this area as much as for the actual eye injury.

Amongst those patients who do lose their sight, the greatest psychological trauma has been shown to occur at the actual time of sight loss rather than later (Vader, 1992), which underlines the importance of the A & E nurse approaching such patients holistically rather that just focusing on the immediate physical problem. Vader (1992) reports that amongst those who lose their sight as a result of trauma there is profound remorse and recrimination together with anger, denial and self-pity. Plona and Schremp (1992) point out that in AIDS patients, the fear of blindness acts to increase the already high suicide risk as there is no greater fear than the fear of blindness.

The medical assessment will include a test of the field of vision, a detailed examination using both an ophthalmoscope and a slit lamp. A slit lamp is a binocular microscope with a strong light source that provides a well-illuminated and highly magnified view of the area in question. X-rays will be required if there is a risk of penetrating injury or fractures.

Intervention

The victim of an accident who has suffered serious eye injury will need considerable and immediate psychological support due to the fear of blindness which will probably be uppermost in his or her mind. It will be the lot of the nurse to deal with difficult questions such as 'Will my sight be alright?' and 'Am I going to be blind?' from a patient whose face will probably be swathed in bloody bandages. The approach described in the chapter on burns is recommended—i.e. sympathetic, honest and realistic.

If chemicals have been spilt into the eye, copious irrigation with water is the correct first aid procedure, and removal of contact lenses if worn. Irrigation will then be continued in A & E, with a sterile solution of water or saline. Tannen and Marsden (1991) recommend the use of an ordinary IV giving set, first accustoming the patient to the temperature of the solution by running it onto the cheek. The procedure is best carried out with the patient lying flat and the nurse standing at the patient's head. For effective irrigation to occur, the eyelids must be opened. This will require a great deal of tact and gentleness on the part of the nurse, for most people with an already irritable and possibly painful eye are understandably reluctant to have that eye held open while somebody pours fluid into it. Local anaesthetic such as amethocaine 1% applied in advance may facilitate this procedure. Nurses would do well to try to imagine themselves in the patient's position when deciding how to handle the victim of eye trauma. A kidney dish should be held against the face in order to catch the irrigation fluid and the fluid should not be allowed to soak into the patient's clothes. The nurse should work from the inner, nasal part of the eye outwards when irrigating and ensure that there is a constant flow of fluid over the eye, but that it is not under pressure—a gentle trickle provides sufficient force.

A subtarsal foreign body can be readily removed with a cotton applicator or a glass rod after eversion of the eyelid. Gentleness and reassurance are required in carrying out the procedure as the patient may find it frightening. Corneal foreign bodies are removed frequently with nothing more than a sterile hypodermic needle; however, the cornea first needs anaesthetizing.

Nurses are frequently required to instil various drops and ointments into the patients' eyes. These include antibiotic ointment, mydriatics to dilate the pupil and local anaesthetic agents for pain relief. Table 10.2 provides information on their uses.

After treatment, consideration should be given to padding the eye. However, eye pads do cause great inconvenience due to the monocular vision they produce (e.g. for drivers) which has significant implications for the patient's self-care demand. They should be used, therefore, only after careful consideration of how the patient will manage with monocular vision. The indication for padding an eye is if there is a defect in the corneal epithelium which will heal more quickly under a closed lid. Instillation of antibiotic ointment

Table 10.2
Eye drops and ointments commonly used in A & E

Type	Examples	Reasons for Use
Local Anaesthetic	Amethocaine	To relieve pain and allow examination. To allow procedures which involve contact with cornea.
Miotic drops (pupil constricting)	Pilocarpine	To open the drainage angle thereby restoring the aqueous circulation in glaucoma.
Mydriatic drops (pupil dilating)	Tropicamide Homatropine	To obtain a clear view of the posterior segment of the eye. Prevent adhesions between the iris and the lens in chemical burns. Patient should not be allowed to drive after use as the focusing mechanism of the eye will be disturbed.
Antibiotics	Chloramphenicol Drops 0.5% Ointment 1%	To prevent infection. If both eyes are being treated, two separate tubes should be used and labelled left and right, in order to prevent cross-infection. Drops are rapidly diluted and therefore need frequent application (hourly). Ointment will last longer.
Anti-viral	Idoxuridine 0.1% Drops	To treat dendritic ulcers caused by the herpes simplex virus. Requires frequent application.
Stain	Fluorescein	To obtain visualization of areas of missing corneal epithelium. Green indicates affected areas.
Steroids	Betamethasone	To suppress inflammation. Must never be used unless the corneal epithelium is shown to be intact as steroids' suppression of the natural defence mechanisms can have disastrous consequences in the presence of herpes simplex.

and padding may be carried out on a daily basis until healing is complete. The pad is best secured with tape (e.g. Micropore) and a short piece of elasticated tubular bandage.

In serious conditions such as a hyphaemia or detached retina, rest is essential as further sudden movements can exacerbate the situation. It is as well, therefore, to have a general rule in A & E that movement should be minimized for patients suffering from any eye injury. Effective channels of communication must exist between A & E and the nearest ophthalmic unit to ensure prompt specialist treatment for serious eye conditions.

Finally, before discharging a patient home from A & E, nurses must be sure that the patient understands what is required in terms of self-care of their eyes and that they are aware of the correct way to apply the ointment or cream that has been prescribed.

Evaluation

Continual assessment of the patient's psychological status is needed to assess how they are coping with the mental stress caused by the fear of blindness.

After irrigation, the nurse should carefully check the eye to ensure that there is no obvious material present, including by everting the eyelid. The degree of understanding of the patient of self-care requirements should be ascertained before discharge, for it is not what is taught, but what is learnt that counts.

References

Elkington A., Shaw P. (1988). *ABC of Eyes*. London: BMJ.

Hartland G. (1993). Nurse-aid management of ocular emergencies. *British Journal of Nursing*, 2, 823–6.

Plona R., Schremp P. (1992). Care of patients with ocular manifestations of HIV infection. *Nursing Clinics of North America*, 27, 793–805.

Tannen M., Marsden J. (1991). Chemical burns of the eye. *Nursing Standard*, 6, 24–6.

Vader L. (1992). Vision and vision loss. *Nursing Clinics of North America*, 27, 705–13.

Wardrope J., Smith J. (1992). *The Management of Wounds and Burns*. Oxford. Oxford University Press.

Chapter 11

ENT AND DENTAL EMERGENCIES

The Ear

Trauma

The external part of the ear, the pinna, is composed of cartilage and is commonly involved in injury. It may be lacerated, in which case it may be sutured and treated as any other wound, or it can suffer blunt trauma leading to the formation of a haematoma. Left untreated this will lead to deformity and the formation of a 'cauliflower ear'. Wardrope and Smith (1992) are pessimistic about the prospects for successful aspiration of such a haematoma and recommend referral to a specialist ENT surgeon for surgical drainage.

In severe injuries the whole of the pinna may be cut or torn off, e.g. in a knife fight. In such cases reattachment may be possible; therefore the wound site should be covered with a saline soak and the missing part retained, preferably dry and in a refrigerator though not frozen.

Foreign bodies in the external auditory meatus are common problems with small children. They vary from beads to live insects in which latter case they should be drowned with olive oil before removal is attempted, as the insects are easier to remove dead than alive. Great skill is required on the part of the nursing staff to gain the cooperation and confidence of the parents and the child. The best approach after explaining to the parents what is going to happen is to sit the child on the parent's lap, wrapped tightly in a blanket so as to keep little hands and arms safely out of the way, and then attempt once to remove the object. If the casualty officer cannot remove it immediately, it is best left and the case referred to an ENT specialist. Further attempts with a struggling child may well lead to the object being pushed further into the ear, risking perforation of the eardrum.

The eardrum is most frequently damaged as a result of a sudden pressure change, e.g. after an explosion or in landing or take-off when flying. A blow to the ear with the hand flat or slightly cupped can produce the same effect. Small perforations will usually heal themselves but large tears may require surgical repair. The usual result of a perforated eardrum is deafness on the affected side.

A common reaction is for people to hit themselves on the side of the head affected or to try to poke something down their ear. Both should be discouraged as they may lead to further damage to the delicate structures of the middle ear. In making disaster plans, it should be taken into account that if an explosion has occurred there may be large numbers of people with perforated eardrums and deafness as a result. It is important to attempt to convey the likely temporary nature of such deafness to people in order to allay anxiety.

Diseases of the Ear

It is probably true to say that in an ideal world people with diseases of the ear would not often be seen in A & E as they should have seen their GP who would have arranged the appropriate ENT specialist referral if needed.

A & E staff should not, however, be too dismissive of people with earache for two reasons. First, the ear may be very painful and the patient may be in considerable distress, especially if they cannot get an appointment to see their GP for two days, and second, ear pain may indicate a disease process which could have serious consequences for the patient if untreated.

The usual cause of a painful ear is infection: otitis externa, otitis media (which can be acute or chronic), or mastoiditis. Chronic disease of the middle ear (chronic suppurative otitis media) can lead to complications such as meningitis, brain abscess, and erosion and destruction of bone.

Chronic otitis media requires a careful toilet of the ear, a swab should be taken for culture of fungi and bacteria, and topical antibiotics applied, typically gentamicin and neomycin with a steroid. The nurse should enquire tactfully about personal hygiene as health education could significantly reduce the incidence of future episodes. Ludman (1993) states that cleaning the ear with a dirty towel, particularly after swimming, is the best way to produce otitis media.

Infections of the pinna of the ear include herpes (which may be accompanied by involvement of the inner ear leading to deafness, giddiness and vomiting) and the inflamed crusts of a staphylococcal infection seen in children with impetigo. If herpes is suspected it is essential the patient is given a triage category which ensures they see a doctor (Butler and Malem, 1993). A swollen painful earlobe may be associated with a recently pierced ear which has become infected. The earring should be removed and the person advised about hygiene.

One disease involving the ear that can lead patients to attend A & E in a very distressed emergency condition is vertigo. This condition gives rise to an illusion of movement, either that the person is moving, or that the environment is in motion. The cause is a conflict of information from the vestibular sources within the inner ear with information from other sensory systems, or alternatively, when the information supplied by the vestibular system about body movement cannot be coherently assessed by the central nervous system.

Vertigo always produces imbalance, although imbalance is not always caused by vertigo. The person suffering from an attack of vertigo will often fall to the ground and vomiting and nausea are common. The patient will present at A & E collapsed with vomiting. The patient should be laid flat on a trolley with cot sides in place and a vomit bowl available. Acute episodes of vertigo can be very frightening for the patient, therefore considerable psychological support is necessary. An intramuscular injection of prochlorperazine (Stemetil) 12.5 mg is often prescribed to help relieve the symptoms.

A common cause of vertigo is Menière's disease, affecting one ear only and most common in onset in people between 30 and 60 years of age. The result is a violent paroxysmal attack, rotary in nature, associated with tinnitus and deafness, which may be one of several attacks clustered together. Migraine is another common cause of vertigo, particularly in adolescent girls.

The Nose

Trauma

Fracture of the nasal bones is the most common facial fracture and is usually due to blunt trauma, e.g. a fall on the face or assault. Deformity which may be obvious at first will quickly be obscured by soft tissue swelling. Reduction should occur before 3 weeks, as fractured nasal bones will set within 3 weeks, but after one week in order to allow the swelling to go down. The need is, therefore, to make an ENT appointment for 7 to 10 days' time in order that the ENT specialists can manage the problem thereafter.

Nose Bleeds

There are many reasons for nose bleeds, ranging from trauma or simply blowing the nose too hard in young people through to hypertension and degenerative arterial disease in the elderly. In young people bleeding is usually venous, while in the elderly an area of multiple arterial anastomosis located on the septum, Little's area, is usually the culprit, giving rise to arterial bleeding.

Nose bleeds are potentially very serious, especially in the elderly, and should be carefully assessed by the nurse in the same way that any other serious bleed would be assessed. Blood loss should be assessed by interviewing the patient to find out how long the bleed has been going on, by examining any evidence such as a towel used to try to stop the bleeding, and by asking if the patient has been swallowing any blood as well as spitting it out. Blood pressure and pulse must be measured as hypotension and hypovolaemic shock are possible; an alternative finding is that the patient is hypertensive, and the hypertension has given rise to the nose bleed.

If the patient is hypovolaemic, then the full resuscitation procedure should be activated and should take priority over controlling bleeding in the first stages. Ludman (1993) states that 'An elderly patient who has lost a lot of blood is more likely to die during the next few hours from the effect of loss already sustained than from the results of continued bleeding.'

To try to arrest bleeding, the best procedure is to show the patient how to squeeze the *soft* lower part of the nose tightly. This will control bleeding by compression. Compression should be applied *continuously* for 20 to 30 minutes. The application of ice packs to the bridge of the nose may also be beneficial due to their vasoconstrictor effect. The patient should be sat upright if possible with their head tilted slightly forward and they should be supplied with a bowl and instructed to expectorate any blood that drips into their mouth. The patient should be instructed not to swallow the blood because it will lead to vomiting and also prevent measurement of the blood loss. If direct pressure is controlling bleeding, however, there should be little or no blood dripping down into the mouth.

If the patient is shocked from the bleed, their position should be modified to promote venous return and perfusion of the vital centres by elevating the legs and lying the patient as flat as possible.

We see in nose bleeds a good example of Orem's self-care model of nursing at work, as under nursing guidance the patient meets their own self-care demand in stopping the bleeding.

A spray of cocaine solution (2.5–10%), a head light and mirror, silver nitrate cauterization sticks, and a nasal packing set will be required by the medical staff to control the bleeding if direct pressure fails. The medical techniques used in A & E are either cauterization or nasal packing. The nursing staff must ensure that they know where this essential equipment is kept.

The sight of blood can have a very distressing effect on some people and, young or old, the patient suffering from a nose bleed may need considerable psychological support and encouragement from the nursing staff who should be aware that this is a potentially fatal condition. This is especially true of the situation where the patient is required to compress their own nose for 30 minutes. The temptation to let go soon becomes very great and all the good work done by 10 minutes of compression can be undone by 10 seconds' curiosity in wanting to see if the bleeding really has stopped.

The Throat

Trauma

Reference has already been made to the need to deal urgently with neck injuries due to the twin threats posed by spinal injury and damage to the soft tissues of the throat which may lead to swelling and airway obstruction.

A common problem encountered in A & E is that of adults who feel they have 'something stuck in their throat', usually a fish or chicken bone. Such objects are usually found at the level of the tonsils or in the upper part of the oesophagus.

In assessing the patient, the nurse should be alerted by the patient describing a sensation of sharp pain on swallowing, especially if it radiates to the ear, difficulty in swallowing saliva, and tenderness over the trachea. Any of these symptoms indicate a real risk of an object being lodged in the throat or upper oesophagus. Unfortunately many such objects are radiotranslucent, e.g. fish bones and many dental plates, but radiography is standard procedure still. If a perforation has occurred, even though the causative object may not show on X-ray, air in the soft tissues will allow the medical staff to make a diagnosis.

The picture is complicated by the fact that a sharp object that is swallowed may well scratch soft tissue, leaving behind a sensation of something sticking in the throat, even though the object has long gone on its way down the alimentary canal. Despite reassurance that there is not a problem and that nothing is stuck, the patient can still feel the sensation of something sticking there, and may not be convinced of the diagnosis. Considerable tact and diplomacy are required sometimes in this situation.

Perforation of the oesophagus or the development of an abscess in the upper respiratory tract due to impaction of a foreign body can have very serious consequences. It is advisable, therefore, to err on the side of caution and most A & E departments refer their patients on to ENT specialists if there is any chance of an impacted foreign body. If the patient is discharged, the nurse should reinforce patient instructions to return if symptoms do not improve or if any feeling of being unwell and feverish or if pain in the upper chest and neck region should develop. Mediastinitis developing from a perforation of the oesophagus will make the patient seriously ill, while if a pharyngeal abscess were to develop, there is a risk of occluding the airway.

Hoarseness and Stridor in Children

Stridor in a child with a previously adequate airway is usually caused by infection, but inhaled foreign bodies, trauma from ingesting corrosive agents and allergic oedema are other possible causes.

Croup is caused by acute laryngitis and can be a very frightening experience for both parent and child, a fact that should be remembered by the nurse. Dyspnoea is usually associated with more serious infections of the respiratory tract from the epiglottis downwards, rarely but most seriously epiglottitis. The throat and larynx of such young children in respiratory distress should only be examined by medical staff with considerable experience due to the risk of provoking laryngeal spasm which will lead to a total airway obstruction and cardiac arrest. Tracheotomy in a situation such as this is extremely difficult and the only way of providing an airway may well be by inserting needles into the trachea.

Facial and Dental Emergencies

Facial Trauma

Trauma in the form of a direct blow to the face tends to produce one of several characteristic fracture patterns, which may also involve the base of the skull, leading to CSF leakage (rhinorrhoea from the nose and otorrhoea from the ear).

Blunt trauma to the side of the face is most likely to fracture the cheek or zygoma characteristically in three places, the zygomatic arch, the posterior half of the infra-orbital rim and the frontal zygomatic suture, giving rise to what is known as a tripod or trimalleolar fracture.

High energy trauma affecting the front of the face can lead to fractures of the maxilla. Maxillary fractures tend to follow one of three characteristic patterns, first described by the French pathologist Le Fort (Fig.11.1). A Le Fort II fracture produces very heavy nasal and pharyngeal bleeding which endangers the airway. A Le Fort III fracture commonly involves a CSF leak as there is usually an associated fracture of the cribiform plate. The airway is also at risk in a Le Fort III fracture because, as can be seen, the whole of the front of the face is effectively separated from the rest of the skull.

Fractures involving the mandible are associated with injury to the jaw. A midline fracture will usually be associated with a fracture of the condyles as well. Fractures of the nose have been discussed elsewhere (see p. 197).

Assessment of Facial Injuries

The first priority in assessing the patient who has sustained facial trauma, as in all cases, is to assess the patency of the airway. Noisy, laboured breathing almost certainly indicates obstruction of the airway. The mouth should be examined for the cause of obstruction, e.g. bleeding, vomit, dentures and the tongue. The contours of the face should be assessed, as in a Le Fort III fracture the front of the face is separated from the skull and gives a characteristic 'shoved in' or dish-like appearance. This indicates a serious hazard to the airway due to the abnormal anatomy.

Bleeding should be assessed and its source identified if possible as

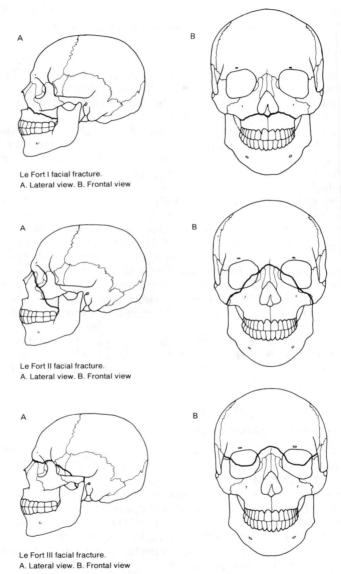

Le Fort I facial fracture.
A. Lateral view. B. Frontal view

Le Fort II facial fracture.
A. Lateral view. B. Frontal view

Le Fort III facial fracture.
A. Lateral view. B. Frontal view

Fig. 11.1 Patterns of fracture, Le Fort Types I–III

clots of blood constitute a major airway threat. CSF should be looked for, indicating a fracture of the base of skull if found.

Facial trauma inevitably means that the brain absorbs a substantial amount of the energy involved, leading to the possibility of brain damage. A thorough neurological assessment, with particular attention being paid to level of consciousness, is therefore required.

If the patient is able to cooperate, the ability to oppose upper and lower sets of teeth correctly should be assessed. Failure to do so indicates facial bone fracture such as a Le Fort or mandibular fracture. Gentle palpation of the face may well allow the nurse to feel the step associated with a fracture. A complaint by the patient of double vision should alert the nurses to the possibility of a blow out fracture causing tethering of the rectus muscle that controls eye movement (see p. 184).

Intervention

The first intervention priority is to clear and maintain the airway which is at hazard from bleeding, clots, dentures, fractured teeth, the tongue, vomit and the abnormal anatomy associated with certain fracture patterns such as a Le Fort III fracture.

The standard measures of mechanically clearing the oropharynx with suction and forceps (or gloved fingers), inserting an oral airway to lift the tongue forward (if tolerated), and positioning the patient on their side with the head down to aid drainage of blood, etc., should be followed immediately. Consideration should also be given to the possibility of cervical injury. In severe cases, intubation or tracheotomy may be required immediately in the A & E resuscitation room. The nurse should therefore know where the necessary equipment is located and be able to give whatever assistance is required by the medical team.

Due to the grave hazard posed to the airway by facial injuries, patients should never be left unattended or lying on their backs. Oxygen may be administered via a high concentration mask. Careful monitoring of the patient's neurological status is required due to the risk of deterioration in consciousness associated with brain trauma. A cervical collar is a wise precaution due to the risk of spinal injury.

Severe facial injuries can be very distressing to the patient, distress that can be compounded by fear of disfigurement. Psychological support from the nursing staff is therefore very important. Communication with the patient may be impeded as the injuries may interfere with normal speech. Nurses should, therefore, try to phrase questions so that the patient may answer simply yes or no.

Patients with facial fractures will usually have their fractures dealt with by wiring. They therefore need preparing for theatre in the usual way, according to hospital policy.

The effectiveness of nursing intervention needs to be continuously monitored. Evaluation should concentrate on the patency of the patient's airway and also on how much bleeding is occurring, particularly from the nose and mouth where blood can be caught in a bowl and the volume measured.

Dental Problems

A & E departments are commonly confronted with patients in severe pain due to toothache for whom there is little we can do apart from give them a bottle of paracetamol.

Bleeding from a tooth socket following an extraction earlier in the day is a familiar complaint seen in the evening at A & E. The presence of blood in the mouth which the patient continually has to expectorate leads to distress and anxiety, while swallowing it will cause nausea and vomiting.

The correct procedure is direct pressure to the bleeding socket applied by having the patient bite on a gauze swab. 'Intraoral bleeders can rarely be clamped and tied and electrocoagulation is of little value' is the verdict of Anderson and Cosgriff (1975), recommending that time and effort should not be wasted on these two techniques.

Usually 20 to 30 minutes of continual pressure will control the bleeding. If this is not successful, the use of an oxidized cellulose dressing should be considered.

It is helpful to ask the patient if there have been any other bleeding-related problems, as this may indicate a significant blood disorder that requires investigation.

Pain associated with facial swelling and an elevated temperature is indicative of a dental abscess, usually related to non-vital or degenerative pulp, the result of advanced dental caries. The patient will often complain of having been unable to eat, drink or sleep because of the condition.

While the medical staff will probably prescribe analgesics and antibiotics (penicillin), the nursing staff should ensure that the patient understands the need for complete rest, which tablets are for pain and which are the antibiotics. This last information should be written on the tablet bottle label as patients who have been suffering from a dental abscess are often tired and distressed and may not absorb fully information given verbally. Dehydration may be present; therefore advice should be given about the need to drink plenty of fluids. General dietary information concerning liquid nutrition may be of assistance in some cases. Such nursing interventions fit well into an Orem self-care model.

In severe cases, cellulitis may develop involving the soft tissue of the whole jaw. Admission for in-patient management is required in such cases.

References

Anderson D. L., Cosgriff J. H. (1975). *The Practice of Emergency Nursing.* Philadelphia: J. B. Lippincott Co.

Butler K., Malem F. (1993). Nurse and management of ear, nose and throat emergencies. *British Journal of Nursing*, **2**, 875–8.

Ludman H. (1993). *Otolaryngology*, 3rd edn. London: BMJ.

Wardrope J., Smith J. (1992). *The Management of Wounds and Burns.* Oxford: Oxford University Press.

Chapter 12

CHILDREN IN A & E

● Children are a major group of patients in A & E with problems unique to themselves. Powell (1991) for example stated that a quarter of A & E attendances are accounted for by the under sixteens while Wilson (1985) estimated that the average A & E unit will see 11 000 children aged fourteen and under in a year, admit 650, and witness the death of five of them.

● Children should not be treated as small-scale adults. Their needs are totally different and this is reflected in DoH guidelines concerning the provision of registered children's nurses in all areas of a hospital where children are cared for. Lancaster (1993) strongly argues the case for the provision of children's nurses and specialist children's facilities in A & E. Evans (1988) has shown that it is possible to create such a children's unit within the main A & E department for as little as £2000. The staffing of such units is critical and a careful study should always be undertaken to identify those periods when children are most likely to present in order that registered children's nurses can be most effectively deployed. Lancaster (1993) for example studied a large hospital A & E unit and found that the peak period for children's attendances fell between 1600 and 2000 hours which contrasts with Walsh's findings that the busiest period for adults was between 1000 and 1400 hours (Walsh, 1990).

Accident prevention in children has been targeted by the DoH in Health of the Nation (1992). The aim is a 35% reduction in childhood mortality from accidents by the year 2005. Many agencies will be involved if this target is to be attained and nursing staff have a major role to play with parents in working towards this goal (Levene, 1992).

However laudable this aim may be, there are those who are critical of the government's approach. George (1992) summarizes these criticisms by asking why the government makes no mention of non-fatal injuries and the subsequent disability and suffering that are associated with such trauma. This is particularly relevant to children who have a whole lifetime ahead of them. No new money is available to help implement these goals and even more telling is the strong association between poverty, social deprivation and childhood accidents which the government also ignores in their Health of the Nation targets.

Levene (1992) cites evidence that death from burns and scalds for example is six times more likely amongst children from a Social Class V home compared to Social Class I. Golding (1983) points out that the evidence of the 1970 Child Cohort Study showed that 65% of the children who died accidentally before the age of 5 had mothers who were in Social Class IV or V or were unemployed. Urban children were more likely to have accidents than those living in a rural area, a finding confirmed by Kay (1989). Further evidence of the effects of poverty comes from Whitehead (1987) who showed that the mortality rate amongst infants under one year of age in Social Class V is double that in Social Class I.

When national statistics are examined the major influence exerted by poverty and other social factors on childhood accidents and mortality rates is apparent. The Public Health Common Data Set (DoH, 1993) released to accompany the Health of the Nation shows mortality rates in England for accidents in the under fifteens almost twice as high in the Northern RHA (8.96 per 100000) compared to the South Western RHA (4.65 per 100000).

It is not surprising to see the North Western RHA with the second worst record (8.15) while at the other extreme, the SW Thames RHA is next to the SWRHA (4.93). The regions referred to are the English NHS Regions pre-1994 and this data refers to the period 1989–91. These figures also reveal that gender plays a key role, as the overall mortality rate for boys in England and Wales was 8.96 compared to 6.64 per 100000 for girls.

Given this linkage with poverty, it is worrying that the proportion of families with lone mothers as their head has risen from 7% in 1971 to 18% in 1991 (General Household Survey, OPCS, 1991). Of these women, 55% had no work and are totally dependent upon state benefit while only 18% had full-time employment. Figures such as these indicate that while nurses have a key role to play in reducing childhood accidents, so too does government in terms of tackling the fundamental evil of child poverty.

In order that a strategy may be developed to reduce childhood accidents, Cody and Waine (1992) have shown that the starting place is an analysis of A & E statistics in order that key problems may be identified and targeted. These workers demonstrated that in their study in North Wales, the two main causes of childhood accidents were environmental hazards and inadequate supervision. The most common presenting condition in children aged under 5 was head injury, accounting for 40% of attendances in the age group 1–4 alone. Findings such as these have major implications for health education and accident prevention programmes as well as for training of A & E staff to ensure they are well prepared to deal with the most common presenting childhood conditions.

Parents' perception of danger around the home was studied in an interesting piece of work by Cliff and Li (1983). They found that the three areas rated most dangerous by parents were the kitchen, stairs and bathroom in that order. However, when Cliff and Li looked at where accidents actually do happen, the most dangerous area is the living room, followed by the bedroom and finally the garden. The kitchen, stairs and bathroom were the least dangerous areas in their survey. Of the children involved, 72% of their parents stated that they had had no advice about home safety from a health professional. Based on this study, there is obviously a major role for A & E staff in health education.

The busy A & E department will see many children, both ill and injured, in the course of a day. It is important that the nursing staff are aware of some of the ways in which children differ from adults, starting with the way that children think.

The Way Children Think and How it Varies with Age

A child's way of thinking and of perceiving the world is very different from that of an adult. It develops through stages, each of which is very different one from the others. In order that the nurse may communicate effectively with the young child, due recognition of the child's cognitive development has to be made. It is to the work of Jean Piaget (1952) and his co-workers that nurses should look for guidance in describing the thought or cognitive processes of a child.

According to Atkinson et al. (1987), Piaget's ideas may be summarized by saying that children pass through the following stages.

1. *The sensori-motor stage, age 0–2.* At this age, the child is said to be egocentric, gradually learning that the world around is not just an extension of self. For the first 7 months of life, the child is without the concept of object permanence; therefore, if something cannot be seen it does not exist to the child. That something includes both mother and nurse! It is 18 months before the child's actions can be described as purposeful, i.e. the child can work out how to do something before doing it.

2. *Pre-conceptual thought, age 2–4.* Egocentricity is still very pronounced; the child believes that others, including the nurse, think and see the world in the same way that the child does. There is no idea of groups or classes, therefore the child is unlikely to realize that the nurse who has just appeared is the same sort of person as the nurse who was looking after him or her but who has now gone to lunch. The child cannot deduce as adults can, with the result that if X and Y are alike in some respects, the child may claim that they are alike in all respects. Thus if one medicine tastes nasty, the child may decide that all medicines taste nasty.

3. *Intuitive thought, age 4–7.* According to Piaget, it is at this age that the child begins to see things from other people's point of view. But the child is still unable to reverse mental processes with the result that understanding quantity is beyond the child of this age. If liquid is poured from one container into another of different shape, the child will claim that there is more in the container with a higher liquid level and will not be able to see that the volume remains the same. Thus in giving medicine to a reluctant 5 year old, a more successful approach may be to pour the medicine onto a spoon from the measuring pot as the child may think of this as a smaller volume.

4. *Concrete operational thought, age 7–11.* The child develops thought that is defined as logical by adult standards. Reversability and the ability to group and classify are now developed. However, the child cannot deal with abstract concepts, only with those that can be derived from first-hand reality. Thus when a 9-year-old Tarzan falls out of a tree and fractures his arm, the instructions to the boy upon discharge should centre upon care of the POP which he can see and understand rather than the healing process of the broken bones which he cannot see and which involves abstract concepts that will not be understood.

5. *Formal operational thought, age 12–14.* It is only in this age range

that the child learns to handle the abstract thought patterns and concepts that are taken for granted by adults.

In summarizing the debate around Piaget's ideas, Atkinson et al. (1987) point out that recent work suggests factors such as intelligence and environment play a big part in determining the rate at which children progress. It also appears that Piaget may have seriously underestimated children's developmental rates. A & E nurses must however consider that children of different ages tend to think in different ways and utilize Piaget's ideas as a guide.

In describing the child's physical development, there are the well-researched milestones which can be summarized by charts such as the Denver Developmental Screening Test. (For this test, see Helberg, 1983.) The use of such detailed screening tests is the role of the health visitor rather than the A & E nurse. However, in assessing young children in A & E, especially in cases of suspected child abuse, it is essential to know what the child should be able to achieve, as underachievement indicates possible under-stimulation and neglect. Furthermore, in planning A & E facilities for young children, their developmental level is essential knowledge if sensible plans are to be made.

Child Abuse

Abused children present to A & E every day of the week. Therefore, it is important for nurses to understand something of the background and the tell-tale signs that should make the nurse suspicious of child abuse—be it physical, mental or sexual. Child abuse is a large-scale problem and the situation is not helped by the subjective nature of the term and a lack of clarity of definition. Wheeler (1992) points out that different agencies make different definitions of child abuse and also reminds us that communication failures are a depressingly common theme that runs throughout all the enquiries that have been held into child deaths from abuse.

Dingwall (1983) is critical of the way many professional workers identify non-accidental injury cases by stereotyping parents such as single mothers as likely abusers yet excluding others from any possibility of abusing their children by virtue of social class. In his research, Dingwall did find that nursing staff in A & E units were more alert to and more effective in detecting child abuse than doctors who he criticizes for not looking beyond the physical evidence. There is another dimension to this debate, however, for as Niven (1992) points out there is a strong statistical association between sociodemographic factors such as financial deprivation, single mothers, young parental age, marital disruption and lack of social support with child abuse. However, the vast majority of children from such backgrounds, as Niven reminds us, are not abused, hence the importance of avoiding stereotyping.

In assessing any child in A & E for the risk of abuse the following factors should be noted as warning signs:

1. A delay in seeking treatment.
2. If there is an inadequate explanation of the injury.
3. If the explanation is inappropriate for the extent or type of injury.
4. Signs of previous injury, such as fading bruises.
5. Defensiveness and hostility, or alternatively apathy and disinterest towards the child by the parent.
6. Silence and withdrawal on the part of the child.
7. Evidence of failure to thrive; if the child has not reached appropriate milestones both for physical or mental development.
8. Frequent parental attendances at A & E (often for non-specific reasons) with the child.
9. Signs of physical neglect.

If any of the above factors are present, the child should be completely undressed to allow a thorough examination. The behaviour of the child and the parent or parents should be carefully watched as this may reveal clues to abuse that may not be noted if just the physical signs are searched for (Helberg, 1983). Mental cruelty, isolation and neglect of the child's developing mind does not leave physical evidence. Sexual abuse may not either, although the genitalia and rectum should be included in the physical examination. The incidence of sexual abuse of children is difficult to estimate because the better known the person is to the child, the less likely the case is to be reported to the police. Gillespie (1993) cites work estimating a likely figure in England and Wales of 6000 children a year who suffer abuse. It is likely that the abuser will be a member of the family or well known to the child, probably male, and the abuse will be a long-term process spread over years which has devastating long-term psychological implications for the victim.

At some stage in the proceedings, the child should be carefully questioned in private, out of earshot of the parents if this is possible. The stage of cognitive development of the child should be considered in phrasing questions. A doll may be helpful in the case of a young child who can demonstrate which parts of their body were interfered with more readily than they can describe with words where sexual abuse is suspected. The important role of A & E nurses in helping to select cases of child sex abuse cannot be underestimated (Saines, 1992).

Local authorities maintain a register of suspected and at risk children, a copy of which should be in the A & E department, updated frequently, and accessible to qualified staff. Information that is not accessible is not information. This register should be checked at even the slightest suspicion. Clearly laid down procedures which are followed, teamwork and close links with health visitors are essential as the Cleveland sex abuse controversy and other recent individual tragedies have shown. Later agency liaison is channelled through the Area Child Protection Committee which should have A & E representation, while there should be a hospital-wide protection network to raise the issue of child abuse wherever children are in hospital (Crow, 1993).

If there is a possibility of child abuse, it is usual procedure to contact the paediatric services who will involve Social Services. Meticulous attention to detail is necessary in recording injuries and marks on the child together with the child's general appearance as the case may well end up in court.

Dimond (1993) lists the following key sections from the 1989 Children Act which are relevant:

Section 43: Child Assessment Order; this gives legal authority for a detailed assessment to be carried out.

Section 44: Emergency Protection Order; this allows a local authority to take a child into care for protection.

Section 46: Police Powers; this permits a constable to remove a child to a place of safety or prevent anyone removing a child from a hospital or other accommodation.

Cases of child abuse can be very distressing for the staff involved. Feelings of anger and outrage at the sight of a pathetic rag doll of a child covered in bruises and burns are understandable human emotions. The suspicion of sexual abuse may also fill the nurse with revulsion and anger. However, anger is not a constructive force that will help the child. The child is, after all, the victim of anger and may have mixed emotions of guilt and anger as a result of the abuse (Saines, 1992). The nurse must be in control of him or herself if he or she is to be in control of the situation and to act for the child in the child's best interests. Remember we are not employed as judges; it is for others to pass judgement on the parents. It is worth noting the findings of Ward et al. (1993) that the mothers of assaulted children are more likely than other women to become the victims of assault themselves.

Some Common Childhood Emergencies

1. *Accidental poisoning.* A major recent study by Burton (1993) gives a good description of this problem. He found that in a study of 319 children presenting at a major A & E department, the most common age was 2–3 years old. Tablets were the most common substance taken (31%) followed by liquid medications (15%), household cleaners and paint thinners (10% each). He comments that taste and smell are no deterrent to young children and also that many parents stated they thought substances were safe because they were in high cupboards. This ignores the climbing ability of even young toddlers.

In the assessment of the child, nurses need to discover exactly what was taken, how much, when, and if there has been any vomiting since ingestion. Questioning should be tailored to the child's level of cognitive development and also to the parent or guardian's level of anxiety which can be very high and as a result interfere with their ability to think clearly.

There are few specific antidotes to ingested poisons; the approach is therefore to attempt to eliminate the substance before further absorption can occur. Gastric lavage is to be avoided if possible in children, and instead emesis is induced by giving 15 ml of syrup of ipecacuanha followed by about 200 ml of water which should be flavoured according to the child's taste with squash. If this does not work, the dose may be repeated. Vomiting is usual within 20–30 minutes and in the majority of cases admission is not needed. Gastric lavage is only considered if ipecacuanha has failed or if the child's level of consciousness makes vomiting hazardous. If this is the case, for lavage to be safely performed, the airway needs securing by intubation.

If a corrosive substance (e.g. bleach or a hydrocarbon-based chemical such as turpentine) has been swallowed, emesis is to be avoided and drinks of milk given instead. One of the most common and serious poisonings is that due to iron capsules prescribed for the mother's anaemia; they present a very attractive sight to the young toddler. The result is necrosis of the gastrointestinal wall and poisoning by the iron as it is so rapidly absorbed. Desferrioxamine IV should always be available to deal with this serious emergency.

In dealing with the accidentally poisoned child, we should be acutely aware of the mother's distress and guilt feelings. Awareness about safety might be raised tactfully if it is appropriate, as in Burton's study almost 20% of parents said they had never received any advice about the safe storage of drugs in the home.

2. *Febrile convulsion.* Children react to illness very quickly, and an acute infection can produce a rapid climb in temperature to over 39°C. It is during this phase of rising temperature that a convulsion is most likely with children aged 6 months to 5 years (Rogers, 1992). Such a convulsion can be a very alarming experience for the parents, who usually wrap their child up in a blanket, increasing the risk of further convulsions by raising the temperature even further, and then rush off to the nearest A & E department in a state of great anxiety.

Great reassurance is necessary, together with an accurate temperature reading (with the thermometer at least 5 minutes in situ, under the axilla). The use of the rectum is unsafe and unreliable and this traditional method should no longer be used with children (Rogers, 1992). If the child is indeed pyrexial, then cooling should commence by removal of clothing, blankets etc. but extreme measures such as tepid sponging are not recommended (Rogers, 1991). The nurse should be explaining to the parents all the time what is being done and why. Medication to reduce the child's temperature such as Calpol should be commenced as soon as the child is able to cooperate.

Epilepsy still has a major stigma attached to it in the minds of many parents, and this thought will be paramount in their minds in many cases. It is best to avoid the word 'fit' and handle the parents with great tact. It has been found, however, that about 2.5% of children who have a febrile convulsion subsequently develop epilepsy (Royal College of Physicians, 1991).

3. *Acute respiratory distress.* Pathology: the most common causes of acute respiratory distress in children are:

a. Foreign body: commonly nuts or beans cause an inflammatory response in addition to obstruction; can be anywhere between the nasopharynx and bronchus.

b. Infectious disease causing obstruction of the airway: a common problem is tonsillitis or a tonsillar abscess. Epiglottitis is a serious emergency as the swollen epiglottis can easily occlude the airway; the child is pyrexial, dysphagic, drooling, hypoventilating but not coughing. No attempt must be made to examine the epiglottis as this can cause spasm and respiratory arrest.

c. Croup: a bacterial infection of the larynx, trachea and bronchi leading to inflammation of the lining of the trachea and larynx. The child is very distressed, exhibits respiratory stridor and has great difficulty breathing.

d. Asthma: the bronchioles are in spasm leading to expiratory wheeze (see p. 101).

e. Bronchiolitis/pneumonia: the young child can be acutely ill as a result of infection of the lower respiratory tract. Parents may not always contact their GP and can bring such an ill child to A & E at any time of the day or night.

Nursing Interventions

Chapters 4 and 5 have already dealt with the care of adults with serious respiratory problems. The following key points are essential to remember in A & E because children are different in significant ways not least of which is the obvious fact that a child's airway is smaller than an adult's. Airway blockage is therefore easier in children whether the cause is a foreign body or oedema. The immature anatomy of an infant means that the normal process of clearing the airway by extending the neck has the opposite effect as this will compress the larynx; therefore, the jaw thrust manoeuvre should always be used (Soud, 1992). A much narrower endotracheal tube will be used with small children which means the risk of occlusion is always greater and therefore greater attention should be paid to suctioning the tube. If the child is conscious he or she should be allowed to find the most comfortable position, which may be sitting upright on a parent's lap. Children are much less likely than adults to tolerate an oxygen mask although the presence of a parent may help, especially if combined with the use of nasal cannula. In a child with serious respiratory distress, pulse oximetry and close observation of respiratory rate and effort, along with pulse, are essential throughout. The nurse should always remember the extreme anxiety of the parents involved, as well as the fear of the child, in such a situation.

Children with acute asthmatic attacks may be seen frequently in A & E. Some 10% of children are estimated to have asthma (Warner, 1989). The normal adult inhaler is not suitable for young children and the A & E nurse must be familiar with paediatric equipment such as the large volume spacers (Hurrell, 1993). Every effort should be made to encourage parents to try and allow their child to have as normal a lifestyle as possible (Wooler, 1993) and the A & E nurse should reinforce this message, although with sensitivity, and the parents may well be very anxious after their child has had an acute attack.

4. *Children with burns*. Although Chapter 9 considered burns in detail, it is worth raising the subject here to remind nurses that children are different to adults. This is particularly relevant in view of the findings of Irwin et al. (1993) who surveyed 100 children with burns referred to a regional burns unit. Of these children, 53 were injured by hot liquids, the next most common causes being flame burns (12 cases), domestic irons (8) and radiators (6). Irwin et al. found that the standard assessment and treatment protocols were frequently not followed in A & E units. In 60% of cases for example no estimate of burn area was made and in 51% of cases, no estimate of burn depth. When these estimates were made, they were frequently wrong. They urge the prompt introduction in A & E units of education policies concerning burn injury in children.

Pearce (1992) paints a similar picture of inappropriate treatment when it comes to burns dressings. She surveyed six A & E units to investigate their dressing policies for children with burns. Despite the recommendations on p. 163 she found the widespread use of traditional dressings involving bactigras, paraffin tulle and gauze, which research has demonstrated to be inferior products.

A final reminder of how A & E units can let down children with burn injury comes from Cox (1992) who developed a written information pack to be given to parents of children with burns upon leaving A & E. She found that, in a follow-up study of twenty-three children seen and discharged with burns, the A & E nursing staff only remembered to give the leaflet to five parents. The lessons to be learnt are clear from these examples: nurses in A & E must take children with burn injury more seriously, as should our medical colleagues.

5. *Sudden infant death syndrome (SIDS)*. Perhaps one of the most tragic scenes of all in A & E is played out several times each day in the UK as an ambulance rushes to hospital with the lifeless body of a young baby and a totally distraught mother who found her apparently healthy baby dead in the cot where she had laid him to rest not long before.

Despite the dramatic reduction in infant mortality in the last 100 years, the rate of SIDS has remained constant and therefore is now the commonest cause of post-perinatal mortality in infancy, accounting for 2000 deaths in 1991 (Henderson, 1992).

The age most at risk is 2–4 months and, according to some authorities, in this age range SIDS accounts for more deaths than all other diseases put together. The evidence is that most deaths occur in the early hours of the morning when infant and family are all asleep.

In reviewing the evidence to date, Henderson (1992) comments that although there are several factors involved, there is a strong consensus that if babies are not placed face down to sleep, then the risk of SIDS will be substantially reduced.

Returning to A & E and the nurse confronted with this situation, it has to be said that usually there is nothing that can be done for the infant, who is usually beyond resuscitation.

The nurse's attention has to focus on the parents. The nurse will readily appreciate the guilt feelings associated with this situation, especially if the baby has been left with a baby-sitter. It is imperative to try to dissipate this guilt by pointing out that there is no blame to attach and that there is nothing that could have been done. Accidental suffocation is a common idea that springs to the parents' mind in this situation. It is an idea that can be safely dispelled as this is not the cause of SIDS.

The grieving process begins in the resuscitation room and the parents should be encouraged to hold the baby. It is the first step in coming to terms with the reality of death, of accepting rather than denying death, of letting go.

It is essential to arrange support for the family; assistance should be given to contact other members of the family and friends. The health visitor, GP and Coroner's Office should be contacted. A post-mortem will be required. Support for the parents may be obtained from the Foundation for the Study of Infant Deaths. Their address is given at the end of the chapter. They are a world famous organization offering counselling and support through a network of local self-help groups, among their many other activities.

It remains to say that, in addition to the grief of the family, there is also the grief of the staff. Such grief is to be expected as a normal human response to any death, particularly a child's death, and staff should therefore be encouraged to verbalize their feelings and emotions. Students in particular find this situation very difficult to handle. In this day and age, there is no place for tears in the sluice and a brusque 'Pull yourself together, girl' from Sister, but rather there should be discussion of the event and support for staff. The dangerous myth of being 'too soft for nursing' should be laid firmly to rest. It is the senior nurses' responsibility to see that such discussion takes place and that staff feelings are thoroughly explored.

References

Atkinson R., Atkinson R., Smith R., Hilgard E. (1987). *Introduction to Psychology*. San Diego: Harcourt Brace Jovanovich.

Burton R. (1993). Eat, drink and be dead. *Accident and Emergency Nursing*, 1, 14–19.

Cliff K., Li H. (1983). Children in danger. Community Forum, *Nursing Mirror*, 156, i–viii.

Cody A., Waine N. (1992). Preventing childhood accidents: an intervention exercise in Clwyd. *British Journal of Nursing*, 2, 1059–64.

Cox B. (1992). Research into practice. *Paediatric Nursing*, 4, 24–6.

Crow J. (1993). Safety net. *Nursing Times*, 89, 42–4.

Department of Health (1992). *Health of the Nation*. London: HMSO.

Department of Health (1993). *Public Health Common Data Set*, vol. 1. London: HMSO.

Dimond B. (1993). Non-accidental injury and the A & E nurse. *Accident and Emergency Nursing*, 1, 225–8.

Dingwall R. (1983). Defining child mistreatment. *Health Visitor*, 56, 293–4.

Evans R. (1988). Somewhere for the children. *Nursing Times*, 84, 26–9.

George M. (1992). A piecemeal approach to accident prevention. *Nursing Standard*, 6, 22–3.

Gillespie F. (1993). Child sexual abuse: definitions, incidence and consequence. *British Journal of Nursing*, 2, 267–72.

Golding J. (1983). Accidents in the under fives. *Health Visitor*, 56, 293–4.

Helberg J. (1983). Documentation in child abuse. *American Journal of Nursing*, 83, 236–9.

Henderson M. (1992). Sleeping position and sudden infant death syndrome. *Paediatric Nursing*, 4, 12–16.

Hurrell F. (1993). Choosing inhaler devices for children with asthma. *Paediatric Nursing*, 5, 22–4.

Irwin I., Reid C., McLean N. (1993). Burns in children: do casualty officers get it right? *Injury*, 24, 187–8.

Kay E. (1989). Accidents will happen. *Nursing Times*, 85, 26–9.

Lancaster N. (1993). The right staff. *Paediatric Nursing*, 5, 22–4.

Levene S. (1992). Preventing accidental injuries to children. *Paediatric Nursing*, 4, 12–14.

Niven C. (1992). *Psychological Care for Families*. Oxford: Butterworth-Heinemann.

OPCS (1991). *General Household Survey*. London: OPCS.

Pearce S. (1992). Treatment and care of minor burns and scalds. *Paediatric Nursing*, May.

Piaget J. (1952). *The Origins of Intelligence in Children*. New York: International Universities Press.

Powell C. (1991). A better service. *Paediatric Nursing*, 3, 18–20.

Rogers M. (1991). Temperature recording in infants and children. *Paediatric Nursing*, April, 23–6.

Rogers M. (1992). Febrile convulsions. *Paediatric Nursing*, 5, 24–7.

Royal College of Physicians Working Group (1991). Guidelines for the management of convulsions with fever. *BMJ*, 303, 1345–6.

Saines J. (1992). A considered response to an emotional crisis. *Professional Nurse*, 8, 148–52.

Soud T. (1992). Airway, breathing, circulation and disability: what is different about kids? *Journal of Emergency Nursing*, 18, 107–16.

Walsh M. (1990). Why do people go to A & E? *Nursing Standard*, 5, 24–8.

Ward L., Shepherd J., Emond A. (1993). Relationship between adult victims of assault and children at risk of abuse. *BMJ*, 306, 1101–2.

Warner J. (1989). Management of asthma: a consensus statement. *Archives of Disease in Childhood*, 64, 1065–79.

Wheeler S. (1992). Perceptions of child abuse. *Health Visitor*, 65, 317–19.

Whitehead M. (1987). *The Health Divide: Inequalities in Health in the 1980s*. London: The Health Education Authority.

Wilson D. (1985). *The Epidemiology of Childhood Accidents*, London: CAPT Publications.

Wooler E. (1993). Asthma in children. *Paediatric Nursing*, 5, 22–4.

Note: The address of the Foundation for the Study of Infant Deaths is 35 Belgrave Square, London SW1X 8QB.

Chapter 13

ELDERLY PEOPLE IN A & E

Just as it is inappropriate to think of children as adults only smaller, so it is wrong to think of the elderly as the same as everyone else only older. The profound physiological, psychological and sociological changes associated with ageing mean that nurses must consider the elderly as having a unique field of problems that is deserving of special consideration.

The proportion of the population in the elderly age group has grown steadily in the last few decades, especially the very elderly. In 1971 for example 2.3% of the UK population were 80 or over; by 1991 that had reached 3.7% (CSO, 1993). In absolute numbers this translates into 2.2 million people in 1991 with a further 6.9 million aged 65 to 79. By the year 2001 it is predicted that the very elderly (80 or over) will have risen to 2.5 million while the 65–79 age group will have fallen slightly to 6.7 million (CSO, 1993). This elderly population is predominantly female as shown by the fact that 62% of those aged 75 or over were women in 1991 (*General Household Survey*, 1991).

As a person ages, he or she becomes more likely to be affected by various degenerative disease processes which will make that person more likely to attend A & E as an emergency (e.g. after a stroke or myocardial infarction). However, ageing also makes a person much more likely to have accidents and falls and brings with it increasing social problems for many elderly people. The social circumstances of the elderly patient must receive careful consideration by the nurse before discharge from A & E, and there are times when the patient advocate role of the nurse must be strongly to the fore.

Physiological Changes with Age

There will be a general deterioration of bodily function with age. This is only to be expected, but there are certain key areas which are worth focusing on in some detail, starting with the musculoskeletal system.

There is a loss of muscle bulk and osteoarthritis of various joints leading to pain and stiffness. Such changes seem to affect most old people. In addition there is also thinning of the bone, osteoporosis, which affects females more than males. Loss of bone mass increases fracture risk but the relationship between these two variables is complicated by other factors such as the effects of bone density decrease being more pronounced on cancellous rather than cortical bone (Downton, 1993). Other pathological processes affecting bone become more common in the elderly such as osteomalacia, Paget's disease and bony mestastases from malignancy.

It is a mistake to think that the elderly do not experience pain as much as younger people because of degeneration of the nervous system. It has already been stated that pain is an individual experience and the nurse must assess pain for each individual. Many of today's elderly population grew up in hard times and were firmly taught that pain was something to bear and stoicism a virtue. An elderly person is, therefore, more likely to bear pain with less complaint than might be expected.

A major problem area is that of temperature regulation which deteriorates with age in some people. Consequently, the elderly are prone to hypothermia. A range of social factors such as poverty and poor housing act with other physical factors such as lack of mobility and side effects of drugs to make hypothermia the problem it is today. A minimum estimate of the annual death rate from hypothermia in the UK would be 500 deaths per year.

The elderly experience many problems with the special senses. Vision deteriorates with age due to changes in the cornea and lens shape that affect focusing, leading most commonly to long-sightedness. Diminishing pupillary size and opacification of the lens with old age reduces the amount of light entering the eye to such an extent that a person of 85 needs eight times as much light to see objects as brightly as a younger person. Problems such as cataracts, chronic glaucoma and retinal detachment all threaten the sight of the elderly. If an elderly person is brought to A & E without a pair of spectacles, the nurse's assumption should not be that their sight is so good that they do not need spectacles, but rather that they may have left them behind somewhere in the process of being brought to hospital. The simple solution is to ask the patient or relative if the person normally wear glasses.

Hearing impairment increases sharply with age. Degenerative changes in the auditory nerve and cochlea cause a preferential loss of hearing for high frequency sounds, i.e. consonants, which are essential for understanding speech. Problems in sound conduction contribute further to deafness and many old people therefore rely on lip reading to understand what is being said. However, staff should be wary of the stereotypical assumption that all elderly people are deaf and should certainly refrain from shouting at a person who is hard of hearing. Slower, carefully enunciated speech, ensuring that the patient can see the speaker's lips, and a careful check on any hearing aid (is it switched on?) will be more productive.

The A & E nurse must care for the elderly person as an individual, not a collection of stereotypes. Respect and dignity must be afforded the patient, not childish sobriquets such as 'dearie'. The nurse who assumes that a woman patient will be incontinent, deaf, confused and probably will not feel much pain simply because she is 82 years old has no place in A & E or any other form of nursing.

The Psychology of Ageing

Confusion is often the first psychological problem to spring to mind in considering the psychological changes of ageing. It can either be a progressive chronic state, for example dementia, or it can be an acute episode brought on by physical factors and known as acute brain failure (Donovan, 1991). The nurse therefore needs to know the patient's normal level of mental functioning before making a judgement about any confusional state. Cerebral hypoxia may induce an acute confusional state secondary to a chest infection or heart failure, while other metabolic disturbances (e.g. electrolyte imbalance) can have the same effect.

However, confusion in the elderly may not have a simple physical cause, but may be situational in nature, i.e. it may be the environment and situation that the patient is in that is causing the confusion. It is important to recognize this possibility as simple environmental manipulation by the nurse may control and diminish the patient's confusion.

Mitchell (1973) looked at sensory deprivation in relation to nursing and described three situations which make the old particularly prone to suffer from this effect. Mitchell's three types of sensory/perceptual deprivation apply particularly to A & E.

She first talked of a 'therapeutically restricted environment' which corresponds to a typical A & E cubicle: bare walls, no indication of day or night or time of day—an environment totally lacking in stimuli. (Nurses can try lying flat on one of their own trolleys in a cubicle to see how long it takes to get bored.) Mitchell then talks of a 'socially restricted environment' typical of many old people living alone and isolated and also typical of many A & E cubicles where the old person lies for hours, while busy A & E staff go about their work elsewhere. Finally she describes 'sensory-perceptual deficits' associated with the deterioration of the special senses described already and which will be made worse if the patient's spectacles or hearing aid are not available.

If a patient who cannot hear or see properly is put in an environment with little or no sensory input, the patient will experience severe sensory/perceptual restriction. Experiments on sensory deprivation have produced mood changes, thought disorder and hallucinations in a matter of a few hours in young volunteers (Atkinson et al., 1987). Therefore nurses may considerably reduce confusion in elderly patients by providing them with an environment rich in stimuli and interaction with other people. A & E nurses should encourage friends/relatives to be with elderly patients at all times. Nurses should try to find time to talk to elderly patients, should arrange cubicles so that there are clues to time and date, should repeatedly tell patients where they are and why they are there (for short-term memory characteristically fails with age) and should make every effort to compensate for the elderly patient's failing eyesight and hearing. In short, nurses must provide an informative and stimulating sensory environment for elderly people in A & E.

Finally nurses ought to consider the ageing patient as a whole and how he or she views the current situation they are in. Physical limitations on activity can produce frustration; for some people retirement brings hours of empty time and a feeling of worthlessness which results in a fall in self-esteem. Death becomes all too familiar as lifelong friends and relatives succumb to the inevitable passing of the years and this leads to isolation. Anxiety and depression are commonly encountered in old age. The presenting symptoms of depression in the elderly can be confused with early dementia; these include memory impairment, poor communication, apathy and muddled thought processes (Donovan, 1991). This only underlines the importance of not stereotyping elderly patients.

The Sociology of Ageing

A & E departments are regularly confronted with elderly patients who cannot look after themselves but who are not suffering from an injury or medical condition that alone requires admission. As a result, A & E staff may question how caring and responsible the patient's family are being.

The traditional view of the extended, pre-industrial family caring for its elderly members in a way not seen today has little or no evidence to support it. However, there are three times as many frail elderly people cared for at home than in institutions and more women are now caring for elderly dependants than they are under 16 year olds. Many families actually perform heroics at great cost to themselves to care for elderly relatives and it is usually as a result of intolerable stresses and strains that they might leave an elderly relative in A & E with the statement that 'We just can't cope anymore'.

The evidence therefore suggests that the elderly person brought to A & E in a state of neglect will be unlikely to have a family to look after them, while if a family states that they cannot look after granny and she will have to stay in hospital, there are usually good reasons for the family to say so. It is certainly in the patient's best interest not to have conflict between family and hospital, which may easily arise if the A & E staff try to force the issue. After all, there are currently close to three million people aged 75 or over in the UK, the vast majority of whom are not in hospital. Who is looking after them? The answer is that families are.

Elderly People Who Fall Over

Having briefly considered some of the physiological, psychological and sociological problems that are relevant to the care of the elderly in A & E, this chapter concludes by looking at what is probably the most common reason for the elderly to attend A & E apart from illness, and that is a fall. Much of what is said, however, applies equally well to old people who attend A & E for other reasons.

Problems in mobility caused by joint stiffness, muscle wasting and bone disease are compounded by decay in neuromuscular coordination, cardiovascular function, environmental factors and drugs. Elderly people are therefore more likely to lose their balance than younger persons, and once they have done so, are less able to correct their posture, leading to a fall. Falls may be seen, therefore, in terms of intrinsic factors such as postural hypotension and extrinsic factors such as loose carpets or poorly fitting slippers. The frequency of falls in the elderly has been found to lie in the 28–35% per annum range in most studies which have looked at the elderly living at home (Downton, 1993). The rate amongst those in institutions is probably much higher. The Consumer Accident Unit (1988) found that most falls happened in the home (67%) and that the kitchen/bedroom/lounge area was the most common site, not the stairs as might be expected.

Terms used by the elderly tend to be very vague such as giddiness, blackout, and light-headedness, which makes retrospective medical diagnosis imprecise. The nurse in A & E is more concerned with the effects of the fall which can vary from the obvious immediate injury to a loss of confidence, which leads to the person becoming housebound, chair- and then bedbound, becoming increasingly more immobile and dependent (Redfern, 1986).

Common injuries suffered by the elderly in falls include fractures to the upper end of the femur, wrist (Colles fracture) and upper humerus, dislocation of the shoulder, and lacerations of the shin, scalp and face. Great care has to be exercised with the case of the confused elderly person with a head injury. Is the confusion due to the head injury? The sudden move to hospital in the middle of the night after falling out of bed? Or was the person already confused?

A fracture of the upper end of the femur is a serious injury that most A & E departments see in an elderly person every day on average. The classic clinical sign is shortening and external rotation of the injured leg. Two recent large-scale studies both reported mortality rates of 12% for such patients (Fox et al., 1994; Holt et al., 1994) and a female to male ratio of over 6:1. The study by Fox et al. showed the mean hospital stay was 31 days but those patients with dementia averaged 56 days and those with pressure sores 53 days. The Holt study found the best predictor of discharge mobility and post-operative complications were age and mobility pre-injury. The most common complication was chest infection, although the incidence of pressure sores is not referred to.

Every effort should be made to ward such patients as quickly as possible to prevent problems such as pressure sore formation. Surgery is performed to fix the fracture internally as soon as possible as the alternative conservative treatment requires a lengthy period of traction and bed rest. The complications of immobility are such that the elderly person would be unlikely to survive the period of time involved. Fractures of the wrist are usually reduced and plastered in A & E under regional anaesthesia and followed up on an out-patient basis; similarly dislocations of the shoulder are relocated using IV sedation and analgesia. Fractures of the neck of humerus require pain relief and a sling, but can be managed with minimal interference on an out-patient basis. Lacerations in elderly people are better steristripped rather than sutured in many cases due to the fragile nature of the skin. This is especially true of flap lacerations over the shins where careful application of steristrips, a non-adherent dressing and an elasticated tubular bandage (never crêpe as it always falls down) will produce the best results. On occasions, however, skin grafting is necessary.

Assessing the Elderly Patient in A & E

Assessment should include the psychological and social setting of the patient. Vital information about the state of the person's home can be obtained from the ambulance crew who bring the person to hospital: is it clean, warm and looked after or dirty, cold and neglected? What is the situation with regard to neighbours and family? This and much more key social information is to be gained from the ambulance crew. In undressing the patient, further information may be gleaned about social background by looking at the state of the clothes, skin and general hygiene. Bennett and Ebrahim (1992) rightly stress that the assessment of the patient's social networks in A & E is just as important as the physical state.

Talking to the patient will enable further information to be gleaned. A first assessment should be made of how oriented the patient is, and of any disabilities due to visual or hearing impairment. Short-term memory should be checked by asking the patient to remember some item and then repeating the question five minutes later. Some elderly people suffer from pathological short-term memory loss yet are able to keep a remarkably good facade of normalcy in conversation, so short-term memory should always be checked. Does the patient know where they are and why? This may seem an obvious question, but nurses will be surprised about how many elderly patients do not—small wonder they are then labelled confused!

In assessing the patient for physical injuries, the principle of multiple pathology should always be borne in mind. Just because there is an obvious fracture of the upper femur, nurses should not forget to look at the wrists and shoulders for possible fractures there also. A full set of vital signs is needed as there may be a whole range of cardiovascular, respiratory, urinary tract, gastrointestinal and endocrine pathologies present as well. Careful temperature recording is essential to eliminate the possibility of hypothermia. An ECG is fairly standard procedure to eliminate cardiac arrhythmias or a silent MI. Blood sugar should be tested by pin prick and a 'stix' method while urine should also be tested and an MSU obtained if possible.

Intervention—Care for the Elderly in A & E

The dangers of sensory/perceptual deprivation have already been discussed. Every effort must be made to keep the patient oriented in time and space using reality orientation techniques. Provision must be made for the poor memory if present by repeating vital information. Spectacles and hearing aid should be obtained if at all possible and great care exercised to secure effective communication. Consideration should be given to having a reality orientation board which includes a large clock, the date and a notice of where the patient is. The nurse should remember to use language that the patient will understand.

A & E trolleys are notoriously hard, and pressure sores can have their origins in a long wait in A & E. Pressure area care is therefore essential if patients are to be in A & E for over 2 hours. Turning is difficult but not impossible on narrow trolleys. If the patient has a fracture of the femur turning, will be impossible since the fracture will not be stabilized. The Spenco mattress offers a solution, as it is available in widths that fit trolleys. Sheepskins may be of value in relieving friction, but rubber rings should be discontinued as a pressure-relieving aid as they are of little value and are of positive harm (Walsh and Ford, 1989).

The availability of a commode in the department will help many patients for whom perching on a bedpan is very difficult. Small points make a big difference in caring for the elderly. Have they a call button available? The urge to micturate can come suddenly in many elderly patients, leading to the humiliation of apparent incontinence, which could have been avoided.

Hypothermia needs to be treated with a space blanket which by virtue of its high reflectivity warms the patient by reflecting their own body heat. The blanket should cover the scalp, from which a very high proportion of heat loss occurs and it should be next to the body. ECG monitoring may be required.

Old people are more likely to accept their lot uncomplainingly; they should not be forgotten therefore in the hustle of a busy A & E department. The offer of a cup of tea while waiting (if they are not waiting for a general anaesthetic) and a few kind words can mean a great deal, and can also obtain for the nurse information that might not have been otherwise volunteered. Elderly people often see real problems as 'something that you just have to put up with', rather than an important symptom.

The problems associated with discharging patients have been discussed elsewhere; however, they are never more pressing than in the case of the elderly. A clear picture of the social background to which we are discharging our elderly patient is necessary before such a step is taken. Given the communication difficulties that arise from declining vision, hearing and short-term memory, it is obviously important to be sure that what has been taught has been learnt with regard to points such as plaster instructions, medication, and follow-up appointments. Simple instruction cards in bold type and medicine bottles that can be opened by the elderly, whose manual dexterity may have declined, are simple examples of planning for the special needs of the elderly.

If care is planned around Orem's self-care model, nurses are more likely to appreciate potential problems from the patient's point of view and, therefore, to make more realistic plans for the patient on discharge. At the end of the day the nurse should not forget her or his role as patient advocate, and if you are unhappy about a medical decision that since the old lady did not break anything when she fell over she must go home, then you must say so. Busy but junior and inexperienced medical staff often overlook the social element of how the patient will cope at home. At the very least, you should ask the doctor to see if the patient can walk unaided, the basic requirement for going home. Many intended discharge decisions have been reversed by such a simple step. Most casualty officers are willing to listen to advice from nursing staff about the care of elderly people and their suitability for discharge or about how to get the community services involved, provided that the nursing staff go about it in a constructive way.

Evaluation

Evaluation of nurses' attempts to maintain an old person's orientation in time and space is achieved by talking to the patient, and always in language that they will understand. How effective instructions about care of an arm in plaster or about taking medication have been will be seen when the patient next returns—so to some extent we are shutting the stable door after the horse has bolted.

While the patient is in A & E, evaluation can be carried out by checking the condition of the patient at regular intervals to make sure that the trolley is not wet and that pressure points are being relieved.

References

Atkinson R., Atkinson R. Smith E., Hilgard E. (1987). *Psychology*. San Diego: Harcourt Brace Jovanovitch.
Bennett C., Ebrahim S. (1992). *Health Care for the Elderly*. London: Edward Arnold.
Consumer Accident Unit (1988). *Home and Leisure Accidents*. London: Consumer Accident Unit.
CSO (1993). Key Data. London: Government Statistical Service
Donovan L. (1991). Mental health problems in old age. In Garrett G. (ed.) *Healthy Ageing: Some Nursing Perspectives*. London: Professional Nurse.
Downton J. (1993). *Falls in the Elderly*. London: Edward Arnold.
Fox H., Pooler J., Prothero D., Bannister G. (1994). Factors affecting the outcome after proximal femoral fractures. *Injury*, **25**, 297–300.
General Household Survey (1991). London: OPCS.
Holt E., Evans R., Hindley C., Metcalfe J. (1994). 1000 femoral neck fractures: the effect of pre-injury mobility and surgical experience on outcome. *Injury*, **25**, 91–5.
Mitchell P. (1973). Sensory status, *Concepts to Basic Nursing*, New York: McGraw-Hill.
Redfern S. (1986). *Nursing Elderly People*. Edinburgh: Churchill Livingstone.
Walsh M., Ford P. (1989). *Nursing Rituals: Research and Rational Action*. Oxford: Butterworth-Heinemann.

Chapter 14

WOMEN'S HEALTH PROBLEMS
IN A & E

A significant number of women who attend A & E do so with complaints that are unique to women. It is essential therefore to explore the background of these conditions in order that the nurse may gain some insight into the psychosocial background involved in bringing women to A & E.

To understand the present we often have to look at the past, and to understand the origins of many women's health problems, such an approach is essential.

During the early 19th century women continued to make the transition from a rural or domestic working life into the factories of the established industrial revolution (Hall, 1989a). Whilst low wages are factors of rural and urban living, the towns and cities included atmospheric pollution and a diet controlled by what was available in the shops at greater cost. Hall (1989b) continues by discussing the impact of higher wages upon single women which encouraged men to protect their earning potential through the unions and government policies.

Women were forced into a dependency upon men, being expected to uphold the family structure, which the moralist implied was in imminent danger of collapse. At this time, women undertook piece-work to supplement the household income. However the outbreak of two world wars saw women being temporarily drafted into the industrial workforce and women became equated with a disposable workforce.

In parallel with the feminist movement has been a rise in the vision of education for daughters. Nevertheless, *Social Trends* (1994) indicates that currently a quarter of women between 16 and 59 years of age have no qualifications. Educational attainment is still dependent upon the social class of the parent.

Recent economic trends have resulted in changing employment patterns. Significantly more women are in part-time employment, and have more second jobs (OPCS, 1990). In 1994, *Social Trends* indicated that a third of women were classed as economically viable with 1 in 6 recorded as unemployed. The impact of employment needs to be considered in the context of other social patterns occurring simultaneously such as changes to the family unit. Many women still perform the dual role of wage earner and homemaker; the conflict of this balancing act may result in stress which in turn contributes to women attending the A & E department.

Stress and Women

Many women are now unsure of their place in society as a result of the changes described above. Stress amongst women results from a diversity of internal and external factors. Society, encouraged by the media, expects certain stereotypical behaviours from 'normal' women, e.g. the housewife, mother or working woman. Rarely in these images are women seen in combined roles. Guilt and disharmony occurs as women perceive that they have failed to achieve these images. Richardson (1993) urges us to remember that women are more than biological reproducers and providers, but sexual, feminine individuals.

Factors which induce stress include any significant life change, e.g. divorce, separation and single parenting. Statistics provide us with the occurrence of each of these events; however, the sociopsychological impact cannot be measured although 'risk scores' of stress provide some indicators to susceptibility.

There is a strong feeling of guilt when a single mother looks at her children and sees them totally as her responsibility. There is no one to share decisions or control of the children, no one to help to decide which bills should be paid now and which can wait. It is a great burden to fall on one pair of shoulders.

In 1991 there were 3 million single parents, only 1% of whom were lone fathers. Childcare facilities are poor: the General Household Survey of 1991 indicated that two-fifths of women use unpaid families or friends for childcare support.

In order to give good and appropriate care, A & E nurses should reflect upon the great stress that women have to live with, be they married or single, working or not, as a result of the tensions created by this dual role in society of woman the worker and woman the homemaker.

Stress may manifest itself differently but amongst women self-poisoning (parasuicide), alcohol abuse and smoking are well-recognized signs of stress.

Alcohol abuse is associated with social problems leading to mental and physical ill health. *Social Trends* (1994) indicates a regional variation from 6 to 14% of the population which consumes alcohol to excess (over 15 units per week). Research indicates a close association between alcohol abuse and suicide attempts (Merrill et al., 1992; Platt and Robinson, 1991).

Smoking continues to feature significantly on the health promotion agendas. Whilst smoking has decreased to 29% of women, the highest usage remains amongst those of lower social groups. It is significant that deaths from lung cancer amongst women have risen by 75% in twenty years (General Household Survey, 1990).

WHO (1993) figures indicate that the incidence of parasuicide amongst women is three times greater than men. The reasons for this discrepancy may not always be clear, although it may be the culmination of a period of stress which may have been treated with antidepressants. Hawton and Fagg (1992) indicated in their study that the incidence of self-poisoning declined in the early 1980s but increased to a rate of 711/100000 among 15–25 year olds by 1990. Of particular interest to the A & E nurse is the rise of paracetamol use from 14.3% in 1976 to 42% in 1990.

Stress may manifest itself in physical or psychological symptoms. Graham (1993) described how women fail to report illness in the normal way either because they are unaware of a deterioration in their own health or by being ill they will be unable to maintain current roles within the family. Women are less able to relieve the causes of stress by walking out or going to the pub.

Whether she turns up at the GP's surgery or at the A & E department, this woman is not a malingerer nor a time waster, she has a real problem that must be recognized. The nurse should be supportive and sympathetic, not dismissive with a 'Pull yourself together, of course you can cope' attitude. Physical complaints must be accepted and investigated at their face value, even if there is a suspicion that they may be conscious or unconscious rationalizations of the woman's desire for help. Nurses do not have the right to adopt a judgemental attitude in such cases.

The Battered Woman

'One night he came back at 2 am. We had an argument and he started hitting me. He jumped on top of me. He laid into me with his fists, with his knees, with his feet. I was bruised all over. My child woke up and came to sit with me. He carried on hitting me and split her lip too. Afterwards I started passing blood in my urine.'

This account of the violence that women suffer at the hands of men was given by an Englishwoman at the International Tribunal of Crimes Against Women, 1976. What makes even worse reading, however, is this woman's account of what happened to her when she sought help the following day:

> The GP? He gave me a lecture saying that I was breaking my marriage vows if I wanted a divorce.
>
> The hospital doctor? He patted me on the shoulder and said that such things occasionally happened.
>
> The social worker? Your husband is such a nice man and he is ever so sorry.

Why then do women put up with such treatment? First, they are afraid of even worse violence if their husband finds out that they have been talking about it to someone else. Second, there is the defence mechanism of denial—ignore it and it will go away. Then there is the guilt of failure. A woman must be a failure as a wife if her husband beats her, and then she feels guilty at being unable to do anything about the situation for each of the reasons described above. Pictures of the happy family are promoted every-day by the mass media. Not surprisingly, when her own family life fails in a welter of blows and kicks, the woman tries to preserve appearances and live up to the happy family image shown in the media.

Historically violence against women in the home was endorsed by society as acceptable; however, it is now seen as a socio-cultural problem. Smith (1989) provided an overall perspective of the nature and public responses to domestic violence against women. More recently research by Mooney (1994) is more specific, suggesting that as many as one in ten women in Inner London experience violence by a man known to them. Domestic violence can occur within any social group, particularly skilled. Pahl (1985) indicated that those with restricted financial independence were less likely to leave the relationship. The abuse will be physical and or psychological towards women and may include threats of harm to any children. Women typically live in fear and have low self-esteem; the abuser has power and control (Hadley, 1992).

The age at which battering most frequently occurs is more easily determined. The National Women's Aid Federation report the most frequently battered age group is from 27 to 32 years of age. An NSPCC study of matrimonial violence found the average age of the children involved in such families was 6.33 years. We therefore see a picture where most violence tends to occur in established marriages with young children.

Women attending A & E departments may present with a variety of injuries in unusual places: injuries to face, genitals, chest and breasts are common, in addition to spinal fractures and other injuries at various stages of healing. Psychological trauma may be manifested through panic attacks, self-mutilation, parasuicide and non-specific physical symptoms, i.e. abdominal pains, miscarriage, chest pains. If the history does not tally with the injury, the nurse should be aware that the woman may be a victim of violent abuse. It is important to remember that pregnant women are not immune. Indeed Bewley and Gibb (1991) discussed evidence that demonstrates abuse may begin or increase during pregnancy.

Once the nurse's assessment has suggested battering as the possible cause of a woman's injuries, it is more important than ever to give the patient an opportunity to talk. Privacy is essential and, if an accompanying small child can be entertained elsewhere by another member of staff for a time while wounds are cleaned and dressed, the chances of the woman feeling that she can talk of the major problems she has within her marriage are greatly increased.

In this situation a woman needs time to recover physically and time to think over her situation from a distance; she needs a refuge. Sometimes a friend or family member can help, but this carries a high risk of reprisals from the man as it is relatively easy for him to find his wife's whereabouts. Whatever subsequent action the woman decides to take, the nurse must respect, as women with violent partners are likely to return several times before finally ending the relationship. Information and contact with women's refuges should be available through the department.

For example, shelter is offered by the Women's Refuge Movement and most large towns now have such a refuge. Many women do not realize that there is an alternative to returning home to the prospect of further beatings; however, confidentiality is essential.

Whenever children are involved the health visitor should be informed. The children too may be victims and require removal to a safe environment, using legal powers, particularly if the mother intends to return home. Violence of such force as to put the mother in hospital is highly likely to also include her children as its victims.

Recent articles challenge A & E nurses to consider why they are reluctant to intervene. By not doing so one may be guilty of collusion, endorsing the myths and beliefs of domestic violence as acceptable. Indeed, Ingram (1994) challenges nurses to become proactive in their communication with women they suspect are being abused, whilst Henderson and Erikson (1994) urge nurses to reflect upon their own attitudes from a moral and ethical perspective, using the theory of beneficence as a framework for their care. By doing so the women will feel able to return to the department. Research demonstrates that women with violent partners tend to leave them and return to them several times before being able to leave them for good.

Rape and Sexual Assault

'What I felt most strongly was the look in his eyes which completely negated my existence as a human being. I was no longer a person, I was only an object, *his* object.' This description by a rape victim illustrates the psychological impact of rape upon an individual. Sexual assault is any attempt by one individual to coerce another into any form of undesired sexual contact with or without penetration either of which may lead a woman to the door of an A & E department.

The London Rape Crisis Centre has shown that in 47% of rapes the assailant is known to the victim. Sexual assault and rape in particular are emotive issues widely reported by the media, particularly where unusual circumstances prevail, i.e. age or gang rape. Why rape occurs is not clearly understood although Roberts (1989) suggests the act requires a victimizer and victim. She goes on to propose a correlation between men's contempt of women and women's passivity, at least in relation to the role portrayed by the media. Roberts also indicates that there may be an association between male aggression against women who fail to conform to the aggressor's notion of femininity. It is questionable whether there is sexual satisfaction for the male, the aim being humiliation of the victim. Social class is not a discriminatory factor; however, class and education may be associated with those prepared to disclose the crime. For this reason statistical data about occurrence is of little benefit. Women who attend the A & E department may well have been the victim of additional physical violence, therefore the immediate physical care is of paramount importance.

Where staff suspect rape they should offer peace and privacy, avoiding assumptions that 'she asked for it' because of the woman's appearance or location of incident, for these are judgements which are inappropriate for a nurse to make. Only the victim can make an allegation of rape to the police. If she chooses to do so the police will attend with a police surgeon to organize and participate in the collection of forensic material, for example semen and swabs for analysis. Ideally the optimum place for this intimate examination is in a location away from the busy areas of the A & E department. Units now offer 'suites' where intimate consultation and examination can occur.

After rape many women feel dirty and contaminated and have a great desire to wash themselves. This should be discouraged until after the forensic examination as vital evidence may be destroyed in this way. Whilst the woman is in the department a female member of staff should be continually available for psychological support. The nurse should be prepared to listen, in addition to being able to provide contact names and telephone numbers for future counselling needs. The victim may demonstrate a range of emotions and fears reflecting the impact of the trauma upon her, including self-blame and guilt. The fear of pregnancy and sexually transmitted disease are more tangible anxieties than the anticipated reactions of partners, family and friends. Apprehension about being believed by hospital staff, loved ones, the police and possibly a jury will enhance feelings of isolation and desperation. Whatever the circumstances there is no justification for sexual crimes against any individual. Rape is no longer recognized as a purely female phenomenon—the victim may be male.

Trauma and the Pregnant Woman

Pregnancy is a state of normal health. Despite this fact, however, many A & E nurses feel very anxious when confronted by a pregnant woman who has suffered trauma because of the specific ways that trauma can affect the pregnant woman. On admission always ask for the clinic card as this will provide a wealth of information.

Blunt Trauma

a. *Placental separation (abruptio placenta).* This is the second most common cause of fetal death; maternal death is the most common. The uterus will be very painful and tense in this situation.
b. *Uterine rupture.* Unfortunately fetal death and hysterectomy is the usual outcome.
c. *Pelvic fractures.* This is the most common serious fracture in pregnant women.
d. *Rupture of liver and spleen.* The gravid uterus acts as a shock absorber and protects many of the abdominal organs from trauma. However, in pregnancy the liver and spleen become distended and displaced making them more vulnerable to injury.
e. *Placenta praevia.* Whilst not associated with specific trauma, any separation of a low-lying placenta may cause torrential blood loss and is potentially fatal for the mother.

Penetrating Trauma

This is usually the result of gunshot or knife wounds and therefore relatively rare in the UK. Nevertheless it is possible given that pregnancy does not exempt a woman from the risk of assault. The gravid uterus protects the woman's abdominal organs very effectively, though at the expense of the fetus.

Abortion and Premature Labour

Trauma may lead to a spontaneous delivery. If pregnancy is greater than 24 weeks' gestation, then neonatal assistance should be sought.

Maternal Shock

A woman's plasma blood volume increases by as much as 50% during pregnancy with associated haemodilution. Serious bleeding with pooling in the abdominal cavity can occur, hidden by the gravid uterus. The increased blood volume of the woman means that she can lose up to a third of that volume before any signs of hypovolaemic shock appear. The normal response of compensating by shutting down the blood supply to non-vital organs means that the fetus is at great risk in maternal shock, for even in pregnancy, the uterus is non-vital.

Assessment of the Pregnant Woman after Trauma

The usual signs indicating abdominal trauma may be masked or complicated by pregnancy. Stretching of the abdominal wall means that guarding and rigidity are often absent. They are, therefore, unreliable indicators. The increased blood volume associated with pregnancy leads to a situation whereby hypotension and tachycardia may only become apparent when the woman has lost a third of her blood volume.

Any complaint of pain should be taken seriously by the nurse who should ask the patient to describe the pain. Vaginal bleeding is obviously a very significant sign. Monitoring of the fetal heart rate for the tachy/bradycardia will indicate fetal distress and the potential need for emergency delivery by Caesarean.

The psychological state of the woman, together with that of her partner or other friends and relatives, should be monitored closely throughout what may be an extremely distressing experience.

Intervention

Resuscitation should proceed along the standard line described earlier, except with the addition of the basic principle that the life of the mother takes precedence over the fetus.

The woman should never be kept in a supine position as the pressure from the uterus causes compression of the vena cava resulting in hypotension and fetal hypoxia. By placing the woman in the lateral position blood flow will increase to vital organs and the uterus. The fetal heart should be monitored using a portable sonic aid. If the fetal heart is not audible then an ultrasound scan will confirm viability. Any signs of fetal distress will indicate that delivery should be precipitated immediately. The nurse should be aware of non-verbal actions as these may increase the anxiety of the woman and her partner. The woman and partner's psychological state is likely to be eased by being provided with up-to-date accurate information in an empathetic manner. The midwife on call or the maternity unit should be contacted immediately.

If spontaneous delivery does occur in A & E remember that childbirth is a perfectly normal event that women have been managing to perform successfully throughout the history of humankind. The woman should be allowed to give birth in whatever position she finds most natural, wherever she feels comfortable, i.e. chair, floor with mattress. She may or may not have made plans for delivery and anxiety will be increased with the realization that she may not attain her personal goal in the environment she had envisaged.

Vaginal Bleeding

Most women between the menarche and the menopause experience vaginal bleeding at approximately monthly intervals. What actually happens to individuals varies enormously. For some women a normal period occurs every 3 weeks and lasts 8 days. For others it occurs every 8 weeks and lasts 3 days.

In assessing the patient who attends A & E complaining of vaginal bleeding, the nurse needs to discover the following:

1. Date of last menstrual period.
2. Normal frequency and heaviness of periods.
3. Why is this bleeding different?
4. Is there any pain, and if so, its location, type and duration.
5. Is there a possibility of pregnancy?
6. Psychological state of patient.
7. Baseline vital signs.

The interview should be conducted in strict privacy, especially if the nurse is dealing with an adolescent/teenager accompanied by her parents. Pregnancy testing equipment should be available in the department.

If the pregnancy test is positive, it is usual to admit the patient to the care of the obstetric or gynaecological medical teams, depending upon the stage of the pregnancy. Keep the woman comfortable and dry. Any material passed vaginally should be kept for inspection and blood loss estimated from the number of pads used. If the patient is hypovolaemic then urgent resuscitation is required as, for example, a ruptured ectopic pregnancy can cause catastrophic bleeding.

If the pregnancy aborts in the A & E department the nurse needs to provide additional psychological support. The grieving process may have already started. Placatory comments such as 'Think of your other children' or 'There is always another chance' are inappropriate.

Finally the possibility of a criminal abortion should be borne in mind if there are any suspicious circumstances.

Concealed Pregnancy

Despite general information and open discussions about pregnancy, occasionally some women are admitted to A & E complaining of acute abdominal pains only to be told they are in labour. One may assume that this occurs to teenagers who have denied the pregnancy through fear and/or ignorance. It can potentially happen to any woman who does not expect to be pregnant, particularly if menstruation is expected to be irregular, i.e. when becoming menopausal. The woman not only has to deal with the labour but has to begin the adaptation towards motherhood that would normally occur during acknowledged pregnancy. Ideally the woman should be transferred to the local maternity unit. Whilst this is not always feasible, the midwife on call will usually attend. If delivery is imminent the best policy is one of hands off. Provided the fetal heart is established the woman in labour requires attendants who are friendly and calm during contractions, and usually the person, if any, who came with her.

Lost Tampons

This is a highly embarrassing but frequent cause of attendance at A & E, caused usually by either a faulty tampon, sexual intercourse during menstruation with the tampon in place, or an attempt to cope with a heavy period by inserting a second tampon. The result of either of these latter two events is to push the tampon high into the vagina where it cannot be retrieved.

Tact and sympathy, a Cusco's speculum, a good light source, and a pair of long-handled forceps will usually permit a female member of the nursing staff to remove the offending article promptly. In order to try to prevent a recurrence of the problem, advice should be offered about the wisdom of sexual intercourse with a tampon in place or of attempting to cope with heavy bleeding by using two tampons.

Toxic Shock Syndrome

Toxic Shock Syndrome (TSS) occurs in women, generally under 25, during menstruation, who are using high absorbency tampons. It is believed that the high absorbency of the tampon dries the normal protective secretions of the vagina, allowing a sudden multiplication of *Staphylococcus aureus*. Women present with flu-like symptoms followed by hyperpyrexia and hypotension, swollen mucous membranes, abdominal tenderness which may lead to delirium, renal failure and death. In 1993 the Women's Environmental Network reported sixteen confirmed and fourteen possible cases of TSS (personal communication). The non-specific nature of the symptoms and the fact that it is non-recordable in the UK makes true estimation difficult.

Vital signs need to be recorded and maintained. Removal of the tampon as soon as possible is essential, then admission may be required for monitoring and antibiotic treatment. A & E nurses have a health role in endorsing the advice on tampon packaging to use the lowest absorbency tampon wherever possible.

References

Bewley C. A., Gibb G. (1991). Violence in pregnancy. *Midwifery*, 7, 107–12.
General Household Survey (1990). London: HMSO.
General Household Survey (1991). London: HMSO.
Graham H. (1993). Women's poverty and care. In Glendiring C. and Miller J. (eds.) *Women and Poverty in Britain*. Hemel Hempstead: Wheatsheaf.
Hadley S. M. (1992). Working with battered women in the emergency department: a model program. *Journal of Emergency Nursing*, 18:1, 18–23.
Hall C. (1989a). The butcher, the baker and the candlestick maker: the shop and the family in the industrial revolution. In *The Changing Experience of Women*, The Open University, Oxford: Blackwells.
Hall C. (1989b). The home turned upside down? Working class in cotton textiles 1780–1850. In *The Changing Experience of Women*, The Open University, Oxford: Blackwells.
Hawton K., Fagg J. (1992). Deliberate self poisoning and self injury in adolescents. A study of characteristics and trends in Oxford 1976–89. *British Journal of Psychiatry*, 161, 86.

Henderson A. D., Erikson J. R. (1994). Enhancing nurses' effectiveness with abused women. *Journal of Psycho-Social Nursing and Mental Health Services*, **32**, 11–15.

Ingram R. (1994). Taking a proactive approach: communicating with women experiencing violence from a known man in the emergency department. *A & E Nursing*, **2**, 143–8.

Merrill J., Milne, Owens J., Vale A. (1992). Alcohol and attempted suicide. *British Journal of Addiction*, **87**:1, 83–9.

Mooney J. (1994). The hidden figure: domestic violence in North London. Islington Council. Centre for Criminology: Middlesex University.

OPCS (1990). Social Trends. London: HMSO.

Pahl J. (1985). *Private Violence and Public Policy*. London: Routledge Kegan Paul.

Platt S., Robinson A. (1991). Para-suicide and alcohol, a 20 year survey of admissions to a regional poisoning Rx centre. *International Journal of Social Psychiatry*, **39**:3, 159–72.

Richardson D. (1993). *Women, Motherhood and Childbearing*. Hendon: Macmillan Press Ltd. Hemel Hempstead.

Roberts C. (1989). *Women and Rape*. Hemel Hempstead: Harvester Wheatsheaf.

Smith L. J. F. (1989). *Domestic Violence: An Overview of the Literature*. HMSO Research Study 107. London: HMSO.

Social Trends (1994). London: Central Statistical Office.

World Health Organization (1993). *Psychology Report*, **72**:3, part 2, 1202.

Chapter 15

MAJOR DISASTER PLANNING AND RADIATION CASUALTIES

Major Disaster Planning

The 1980s were labelled the 'Decade of Disasters'. Disasters are characterized by their suddenness and unexpectedness, with the result that hospital plans need to be simple, flexible and integrated with the plans of all the other emergency services (Walsh, 1989). They are always subject to improvement and should be continually reviewed in the light of lessons learnt the hard way as incidents occur.

The basic principle that should run through a good plan is that people perform best, especially under stressful conditions, when they are doing the things with which they are most familiar. Thus plans should avoid major changes in work practices and departmental layout, aiming to have the department functioning like an ordinary, although very busy, day as far as possible.

A second key principle is that of flexibility and simplicity. A rigid plan that will cope with all eventualities is not possible as it is not possible to foresee all such eventualities. After all, if disasters could be predicted they could be largely avoided. Simplicity has the virtue of allowing flexibility while the simpler a plan is, the easier it is for staff to follow. The more there is in a plan that can go wrong, the more will go wrong.

Within the department, the person who should be in charge is the senior Sister/Charge Nurse on duty, in other words, the person who would normally be in charge. The place for senior management is doing what they normally do—organizing the rest of the hospital, providing extra staff where needed and supplying the A & E unit with back-up facilities such as extra equipment, trolleys and pairs of hands.

Once the alert has been received, there is a need to evacuate A & E immediately of all patients, either by sending them to wards or moving them to a holding area (e.g. out-patients clinic), in order to free staff and facilities for casualty reception. A designated disaster ward that will receive all admitted casualties is essential, not only for immediately logistic reasons, but also for long-term psychological reasons in the days and weeks after the disaster when its victims can give each other vital mutual support.

Many of the patients that attend will be very distressed and tearful, but may be suffering little serious injury. For example, of the 76 hospitalized casualties of the 1983 Harrods bombing, only 14 were admitted. In bombings patients will complain of headaches and deafness. Perforated eardrums may be common due to the blast effect.

Provision should be made for relatives of those involved to be accommodated away from the department as the large numbers that may be involved will be disruptive. Similarly the media should be catered for elsewhere, and ideally the department should be closed by the police to all but staff and disaster casualties. Routine casualties should be informed of the situation and told that they will have to wait a long time before being seen due to the disaster (assuming their clinical condition will permit such a delay) and advised to go to another hospital or their GP. The notion of attempting to operate a non-disaster A & E unit in tandem with a department on major disaster plan is clearly a non-starter and will only result in substandard care for everybody. Liaison with the ambulance service is essential so that as far as possible 999 calls may be routed to another department.

Action cards for staff which describe their various functions are an excellent idea, for it is likely to be quite chaotic preparing to receive casualties if different groups of staff are all trying to read through the same lengthy copy of the plan in an attempt to find 'their bit'.

Staff should realize that they may get no official notification of an incident occurring; the fires at Manchester Airport and Bradford City FC in 1985 were examples of this, while communication may remain non-existent with the field for hours on end, as happened in the Hungerford Massacre in 1987. More recently A & E staff at Charing Cross Hospital were reported to be 'stunned' to find a fleet of ambulances arriving with casualties from the Israeli Embassy bombing with no prior warning from the London Ambulance Service (Nursing Standard News, 1994). Casualties may just start pouring through the doors, underlining the need for a speedy response and immediate triage. This means sorting the casualties into categories so that those who need the care first get it first, and are not delayed by either less urgent cases, or more problematically, those who will die whatever care they are given. This needs considerable expertise and the senior nursing and medical staff on duty will need to be involved in this function.

The A & E unit also has a responsibility to send a team to the site of the incident. This has been carefully discussed by Salt (1989) and he has stressed that the team should be equipped with weatherproof clothing that for safety reasons is brightly coloured, including fluorescent tabards marked 'Nurse' and 'Doctor'. There should also be helmets with lights and Wellington boots in a full range of sizes. Equipment should be carried in backpacks rather than in one big trunk that may be impossible to carry near to the site of the disaster, although a back-up trunk containing reserve equipment is worth while.

The functions of the mobile team are two-fold: first to provide life-saving measures where appropriate and pain relief for patients whose evacuation is not immediately possible. Triage on site is usually carried out by senior ambulance personnel in practice. The team need equipment to secure and maintain an airway and breathing (including chest drainage), IVIs, wound dressings, space blankets and analgesia. The only surgical pack that is worth including is an amputation set and saw, together with the means to give quick-acting IV anaesthesia.

On-site triage is needed to ensure that the most appropriate casualties reach hospital first. Theoretically this may mean that patients with probably non-survivable injuries such as 80% burns or bilateral high traumatic amputation of legs should be put to one side, in order that other patients go to hospital first, and treated symptomatically with analgesia only. In practice in a civilian situation, this would be very difficult to do, but if the scale of the disaster were big enough, it would have to be done.

A second function on site is that of splitting up the case load so that the ambulances distribute the casualties among the various departments in the area. This may not be possible in a rural area where there may not be more than one department within 30 miles, but in urban areas this is possible and greatly to be desired. In the Harrods bombing, St Stephen's Hospital received 39 casualties and the Westminster Hospital 37, a good example of sharing the workload.

The incidents that occurred in the 1980s produced two types of injury that many staff have little experience of coping with: major burns and high energy missile wounds. Apart from the need to improve knowledge among both medical and nursing staff about the care of such patients, the need for a national team of staff skilled in these areas of care is now apparent. The whole question of a national disaster plan is now firmly on the agenda, and it is to be hoped that A & E staff, both medical and nursing, will campaign for an integrated national action plan to cope with the disasters that lie ahead.

Psychological first aid is important as well as the obvious physical care needed by survivors. It is crucial they start the process of coming to terms with the horrific events they have survived by being able to talk about their experiences. A & E staff should recognize this need in the survivors and they should not try to switch the subject. Haslum (1989) has stressed that much needs to be learnt about the psychological needs of survivors and the Bradford Fire of 1985 seems to have marked the beginning of serious attempts to explore this area. Nobody could have remained unmoved at the spontaneous way the people of Liverpool transformed the Kop at Anfield into a memorial to the dead of Hillsborough. Just as the much smaller community of Aberfan still bears the scar of the terrible disaster that destroyed a school full of children, so, too, the much larger city of Liverpool will remember Hillsborough for many decades to come.

Radiation Casualties

After Chernobyl, no A & E unit can afford to pretend that it may never have to deal with radiation casualties. If nurses are to understand the principles of care, they first need to know a little about ionizing radiation.

Atoms consist of a central nucleus composed of a cluster of positively charged particles (protons) and particles with no charge (neutrons), all held together by very strong forces. Surrounding the nucleus is a cloud of negatively charged particles called electrons that are almost one two-thousandth the mass of a proton and whose number equals that of the number of protons. The atom is, therefore, electrically neutral. Neutrons and protons are similar in mass, and the number of neutrons in the nucleus of a given element can vary,

Table 15.1
Summary of common forms of ionizing radiation

Radiation type	Nature of radiation	Penetrating power air	body tissue
α ray	Particle stream, each particle consists of two protons and two neutrons.	6 cm	< 1 mm
β ray	Stream of electrons.	5 m	< 2 cm
X rays	Energy released by electrons changing position in atom.	10–100 m	whole body
γ rays	Energy released by nuclear particles reorganizing position.	100 + m	whole body
Neutrons	Stream of neutrons.	100 + m	whole body

NB. The penetrating power of γ rays and neutrons is such as to make wearing lead aprons as used for radiology of little use.

giving rise to the different isotopes of that element. The chemistry of an element is defined by the number of electrons orbiting the nucleus – from one in the case of hydrogen, two for helium, through to 92 in the case of uranium—and the number of protons in the nucleus, which should be the same.

This account of atomic structure is a great simplification, but it will suffice for our purposes. The effect of ionizing radiation is to knock out an electron from an atom or molecule, leaving it with a surplus positive charge; in this state it is known as an ion. Radiation damages cells in the human body most commonly by forming water radicals—hydrogen atoms or hydrogen–oxygen atom combinations, with an electron missing. They are written as H^+ and OH^+ and are more correctly called ions. This occurs by the radiation knocking electrons out of water molecules in the cells. These radicals can chemically oxidize and destroy parts of the DNA molecule, disrupting normal functioning of the cells (Jankowski, 1982).

The effect on the human body of radiation will depend upon the energy of the ionizing radiation, the frequency with which it will ionize atoms and molecules (knock out electrons), and its penetrating power. Table 15.1 summarizes the penetration potential of the different forms of radiation that we may encounter.

In practical terms the penetrating power of α rays is such that they are unlikely to go beyond clothing or the outer layers of skin, while β rays penetrate only a few millimetres of tissue. Other forms of radiation, while causing fewer ionizing events for a given length of track, do however fully penetrate the body and therefore are able to damage rapidly dividing cells such as the cells in the bone marrow (blood-forming tissue) and in the lining of the gut.

The amount of energy in radiation is measured in Grays (old units were rads and 100 rad = 1 Gy), while the amount of absorbed energy dose in human tissue is measured in Sieverts (old units were rems and 100 rem = 1 Sv); for practical purposes 1 Gy equals 1 Sv in most cases.

In dealing with the real situation in A & E, the likely scenarios that we would encounter are that there is a patient who has been exposed to ionizing radiation, or has ingested and/or inhaled radioactive material or has radioactive material on their body, with or without conventional trauma in each case.

A person who has been exposed to ionizing radiation, but not contaminated with radioactive material, is *not* radioactive and therefore not a danger to anybody else. The damage has been done, just as somebody who has been shot is no longer a danger to anybody else: the bullet has done its damage and gone, the ionizing radiation has gone. They may be treated in the normal way in A & E, but will need special in-patient care depending on which aspect of the radiation sickness syndrome develops according to the absorbed dose. Regular blood counts are required together with antibiotics and blood transfusions, consideration being given to the need to barrier nurse the patient in view of their lowered resistance to infection.

If a person is contaminated, urgent life-saving measures must take priority over decontamination otherwise the result may be death.

The basic principles of reception and treatment in A & E are to decontaminate the patient; to prevent the spread of contaminated material around the unit by isolation and by reducing the number of staff involved to the minimum; to protect staff looking after the patient; and to obtain monitoring equipment and personnel from the hospital physics department. Protective clothing such as plastic gloves and aprons should be worn but they will not prevent radiation affecting staff; they will simply prevent skin and clothes becoming contaminated with radioactive material. Conventional injuries should be treated as far as possible in the normal way, with great importance

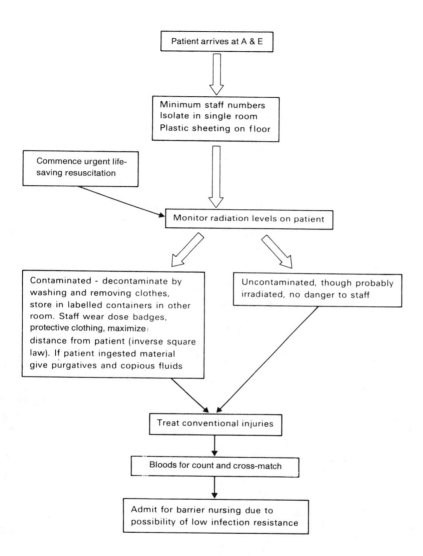

```
                    ┌─────────────────────────┐
                    │   Patient arrives at A & E  │
                    └─────────────────────────┘
                                 ⇓
                    ┌─────────────────────────┐
                    │  Minimum staff numbers   │
                    │  Isolate in single room  │
                    │  Plastic sheeting on floor│
                    └─────────────────────────┘
                                 ⇓
┌──────────────────────┐
│ Commence urgent life- │
│ saving resuscitation  │
└──────────────────────┘
                    ┌─────────────────────────────────┐
                    │  Monitor radiation levels on patient │
                    └─────────────────────────────────┘
```

Patient arrives at A & E

Minimum staff numbers
Isolate in single room
Plastic sheeting on floor

Commence urgent life-saving resuscitation

Monitor radiation levels on patient

Contaminated - decontaminate by washing and removing clothes, store in labelled containers in other room. Staff wear dose badges, protective clothing, maximize distance from patient (inverse square law). If patient ingested material give purgatives and copious fluids

Uncontaminated, though probably irradiated, no danger to staff

Treat conventional injuries

Bloods for count and cross-match

Admit for barrier nursing due to possibility of low infection resistance

NB. Inverse square law means that the intensity of radiation decreases inversely with the square of the distance. Therefore by doubling your distance from the patient, you reduce the radiation intensity to one-quarter of previous level.

Fig. 15.1   Flowchart for radiation casualties in A & E

attached to psychological support for the patient. (See Fig. 15.1 for the sequence of management.)

A & E staff may find themselves asked about civil defence planning for war. Since the monumental changes which have occurred in Eastern Europe in recent years, the threat of a nuclear war has receded. This is just as well as a series of reports by the RCN, BMA and World Health Organization (WHO), all published in 1983, concluded that to try to plan for the effects of a nuclear war is impossible as the magnitude of casualties, both conventional and radiological, would be so vast and the disruption to the infrastructure of society so great, that there would be nothing left for the survivors to do except sit and shiver in their nuclear winter and envy the dead. The scale of the problem was summarized by Openshaw and Steadman in their paper delivered to the 1983 conference of the Institute of British Geographers and quoted in the BMA report. Looking at a typical counterforce attack pattern against the UK, Openshaw and Steadman predicted over 40 million deaths.

Local authority emergency planning officers make an important contribution to planning for major disasters (Walsh, 1989). Given the clear need for a coordinated national disaster plan, it would be logical to develop their role, and that of their NHS colleagues, in line with a peacetime function, rather than maintaining the myth of civil defence against nuclear war.

The possibility of a single nuclear explosion, however, has to be borne in mind, either as a result of a tragic accident or a rogue state acting in pursuit of some megalomaniac dictator's fantasies (Iraq and North Korea are examples from the early 1990s), or even state-sponsored terrorism. A national disaster plan could usefully explore the response to a single nuclear detonation.

References and Further Reading

BMA (1983). *The Medical Effects of Nuclear War*. London: BMA

Dace M. (1987). *Radiation and Health*. London: Medical Campaign Against Nuclear Weapons.

Hartog M. et al. (1981) *Medical Consequences of the Effects of Nuclear Weapons*. Cambridge: Medical Campaign Against Nuclear Weapons.

Haslum M. (1989). The psychology of disaster. In Walsh M. (ed.) *Disasters: Current Planning and Recent Experience*. London: Edward Arnold.

Jankowski C. B. (1982). Radiation emergency. *AJN*. January, 90–98.

Nursing Standard News (1994). LAS fails to warn Charing Cross of car bomb casualties.

Nursing Times (1984). The Harrods bombing (news report). *Nursing Times*, **80:3**.

RCN (1983). *The Consequences of Nuclear War Civil Defence Planning for Nurses*. London: RCN.

Salt P. (1989). The mobile team. In Walsh M. (ed.) *Disasters: Current Planning and Recent Experience*. London: Edward Arnold.

Walsh M. (1989). *Disasters: Current Planning and Recent Experience*. London: Edward Arnold.

WHO (1983). *Effects of Nuclear War on the Health and Health Services*. Geneva: WHO.

SECTION IV

The Patient with Behavioural Problems

16   Deliberate Self-harm

17   Substance Misuse

18   The Mentally Ill Patient in A & E

19   The Difficult Problems that Nobody Else Wants

20   Sexual Problems in A & E

Chapter 16

DELIBERATE SELF-HARM

Patients attending A & E having committed acts of deliberate self-harm (DSH) or parasuicide can be among the most difficult to handle. Their acts represent in many cases outbursts of aggression which have been turned in on themselves or acts calculated to manipulate others. Either way the A & E nurse may find the aggression or manipulation that the patient is displaying focused on him or her.

The ultimate act of DSH is suicide. Over the current century the number of suicides has risen from 3121 in 1901 to average around 4600 through the 1980s with the 1989 UK figure being 4361 suicides (Chew, 1993). Suicide is more than twice as frequent in men than women, with a marked increase in suicide amongst younger men being apparent since the mid-1980s. For example, the rate per 100 000 population in men aged 15–24 climbed from 10 in 1984 to 17 in 1991 (DoH, 1992) while 17.8% of suicides in England and Wales in 1990 were male (OPCS, 1991).

One final observation about successful suicides that needs to be made is the finding by Barraclough et al. (1974) that of 100 suicides studied in depth, 90% had some sort of medical assistance within one year of their suicide and 48% within one week. In addition over 80% were receiving psychotropic drugs. These findings indicate that the idea of the 'suicide out of the blue' is not very likely—there are warning signs.

As in all cases of death in A & E, attention should focus on the living. In addition to the devastating effects of a sudden death, the knowledge that it is suicide puts an intolerable strain on the family. The nurse must be aware of this in dealing with relatives of suicide victims as an extra dimension to the grief they experience.

Drug Overdose

If we switch our attention to those patients who do not commit suicide, we are immediately struck by the size of the problem of DSH. Drug overdose is a frequently seen situation in A & E and its incidence has grown spectacularly since the law was changed in 1961 to make attempted suicide no longer a criminal offence. Knepil (1993) has however pointed out that there is no direct evidence to link these two facts in a causal way. Various sources indicate at least 100 000 patients per year are admitted with deliberate drug overdose in the UK, while the actual number seen and treated overall by GPs and A & E units is probably twice as high (Davenport, 1993; Dunleavey, 1992; Palmer, 1993). Parasuicide or DSH seems to be most frequent amongst the younger age groups and, for drug overdose, women have approximately twice the rate of men (Walsh, 1982a).

Table 16.1 shows the variation in overdose rates between different parts of the country. The incidence of overdose is found to be twice as high in the big cities as it is in the country areas, and 50% higher in London and urban areas other than the Metropolitan Areas (e.g. Manchester). This suggests strong links between living conditions, social class and overdose behaviour.

A detailed study into the city of Bristol and environs found the same pattern reproduced on a smaller scale (see Table 16.2) (Walsh, 1982b). The inner urban area of Bristol contains all the classic ingredients of the rundown inner city. Old housing, much of it in poor condition, blocks of council flats, poverty and unemployment laid the scene for mass rioting in 1980 in what have become known

Table 16.1
Geographical variation of overdose rates

Area	OD Rate per 10 000 pop.	% ODs discharged from A & E
London	22.8	31.2
Other major cities	30.9	16.9
Urban/Rural	21.8	17.4
Rural	14.7	7.5

Table 16.2
Overdose rates by areas, Bristol and Environs 1980

Area	Pop. age 18 and over	No. of overdoses	Rate per 1000 adults
Inner urban	27 842	175	6.29
Council housing	69 695	295	4.23
Flat/bedsits	36 751	113	3.08
Owner occupier	120 402	215	1.79
Dormitory towns	65 390	120	1.84
Rural	44 372	50	1.13

as the St Paul's Riots. The area where the riots occurred has an overdose rate of 14.5 per 1000 adults, more than double the whole of the inner city area.

The council housing consists of large estates on the periphery of the city where unemployment and social problems are high, while the 'flats/bedsits' area is a well-defined area of the city consisting of mostly old houses let off into flats with a high student population.

This study shows the close links between the area where people live, social class, and overdose rates. The stereotype of a bored, middle-class, middle-aged housewife is shown to be, like most stereotypes, inaccurate when considering overdose behaviour.

It remains therefore to ask why do people participate in this form of DSH? In talking to the majority of overdose patients, it quickly becomes apparent that they were not trying to kill themselves. However, within this large number of patients there is a significant number who *are* suicidal, and a trivial overdose may be a 'trial run' before a serious attempt is made. An important task in the nursing assessment is therefore to try to identify those individuals for whom there is a significant risk of suicidal intent.

A frequently found cause of overdose is manipulation of some other person or persons or simply to attract attention. Domestic disputes and relationship problems figure high in the list of reasons, the aim being to bring back a boyfriend or wife, for example, who has left or is in the process of leaving the overdose patient. Many a reluctant reunion occurs in A & E. It is frequently the case that the person themselves will raise the alarm, which is consistent with an 'attention seeking' behaviour pattern.

Palmer, however, argues that it is wrong to see DSH as attention seeking behaviour, citing Strengel (1970) who argued that it is a mistake to focus on the outcome rather than the act. This underlines the importance of not stereotyping patients and adopting a holistic approach to care. Some patients may be attention seeking, but many are not and their behaviour is underpinned by major psychological disturbance. Bent-Kelly (1992) has written critically of those A & E staff who pass judgement on patients who have committed acts of DSH without attempting to understand why the person acted the way they did. Stereotypes are no substitute for a thorough patient assessment.

Evidence supporting the view that relationship crises cause many DSH acts comes from Evans et al. (1992) in describing the work of a parasuicide team working in a large London hospital. They are of the view that the behaviour is triggered usually by a crisis that is connected to the patient's dependency needs and which the patient sees as producing an unbearable situation to which the only solution is an overdose. Painful feelings of rejection and loss are frequently involved and a desire to hurt the other person who is seen as responsible.

One very simplistic assumption to avoid is the sometimes heard opinion that a stomach washout will teach the overdose patient a lesson so that they will not do it again. Such an opinion is wrong on two counts. First nurses are not in the business of punishing patients—that is immoral and unethical—and second, behaviourist theory shows that the more attention and fuss that is made, the greater the reinforcement and therefore the more likely the person is to repeat the behaviour. If a doctor states that they wish a patient washed out to teach them a lesson, the nurse should refuse to carry out such instructions. If the doctor is so naive in his or her understanding of human behaviour and wishes to interpret the Hippocratic Oath so as to include punishing patients, then the doctor can do the washout him or herself and take the consequences.

Overdosing can, therefore, be seen largely as a coping mechanism, aimed at seeking attention or manipulating other persons or situations, though in a number of cases, real suicidal intent may be involved.

Seen as a problem-solving device, its greater frequency in the poorer areas of towns and cities becomes understandable as people there have more problems and fewer resources to deal with them.

Self-inflicted Injury

Self-mutilation frequently takes a chronic form of repeated episodes of self-laceration usually involving the forearms and varying from the superficial to the occasionally deep. It is rare for there to be any significant arterial damage because the areas attacked are often not adjacent to major arteries in their superficial portions or, in the case of the wrist, the radial and ulnar arteries are well protected by tough tendon sheaths that require considerable force to cut through. Consequently many self-inflicted wounds are easily closed by sutures or steristrips in A & E and blood loss is minimal. Deep structures are rarely damaged, and, if so, it is more likely to be a tendon or nerve than an artery.

Occasionally other areas of the body may be attacked such as the abdomen or legs, while in some very disturbed individuals, the face or genitals may be mutilated. Other forms of self-harm include self-inflicted stab wounds and swallowing objects such as safety pins.

In trying to understand why people behave in this way it has to be recognized that, as in cases of overdose, there is usually no suicidal intent but there is certainly a strong streak of low self-esteem in persons who have mutilated themselves. The aggression is often very near the surface, and while it is turned in on themselves in committing the act, the nurse should remember that that aggression could easily be turned outwards if the patient is mishandled.

Assessment

Assessment is broadly similar for acts of DSH whether they be by overdose or self-mutilation.

In approaching the patient to make the assessment, the nurse must remember that the emotional cues given out by the nurse (reflecting his or her attitude) will affect the emotional state of the patient. To minimize the risk of aggressive behaviour and obtain maximum cooperation from the patient, there is a need for a very definite effort on the nurse's part to be friendly and helpful, even though the patient may be hostile, abusive or sullen and withdrawn. An attitude of 'not another overdose' may well rebound back onto the nurse and have an undesirable effect on the patient's emotions and behaviour.

The initial interview should be conducted in privacy. The nurse should aim to find out the extent of the physical damage, and the reasons and intent that lay behind the act. If an overdose has been taken, there is a need to find out what was taken, when, how many and whether the patient has vomited since. Time since overdose is relevant not only for deciding whether to try and expel any unab-sorbed drug from the body, but also for determining treatment protocols. In paracetamol overdose for example, the specific anti-dote, acetylcysteine, can be given up to 15 hours after drug ingestion to reduce the serious liver damage that can occur from ingestion of only 12–15 tablets (Younger, 1993). The significance of this is shown by the study carried out by Davenport (1993) who found 48% of overdose patients in a three-month period had taken paraceta-mol. Of the 850 deaths by poisoning which were classed as suicide in England and Wales in 1990, 101 were due to paracetamol alone and a further 155 involved paracetamol amongst a cocktail of drugs. Paracetamol was, therefore, the most common single drug involved in suicide (OPCS, 1991).

If a self-inflicted wound is present, the nurse should examine its depth, type of bleeding (arterial or venous) and assess blood loss and whether any nerves or tendons have been damaged.

Questioning should be sympathetic and carried out in such a way as to allow the patient the maximum opportunity to talk and explain the feelings and emotions behind the act in order that the suicide risk may be assessed. High-risk factors include the presence of alcohol, the absence of close family/friends, the middle to elderly age group, and an existing psychiatric problem which is under treatment. The severity of the overdose is not a reliable guide to suicidal intent. Chronic disease and recent bereavement are further high-risk factors.

If the patient is found to be very drowsy or unresponsive, then a first priority in assessment must be airway patency and other vital signs in addition to attempting to work out what was taken and when. Hypothermia cannot be ruled out if the patient has been lying unconscious for many hours. The vasodilator effect of alcohol would increase this risk and alcohol is found commonly in association with overdose. Temperature measurement is essential. There is a high risk of vomit being inhaled in such cases so that in addition to assessing the patency of the airway, respiratory rate is an important parameter.

Tricyclic antidepressants (e.g. amitriptyline and Anafranil) in overdose have an antiparasympathetic effect which among other effects can cause life-threatening cardiac arrhythmias. A patient who has taken an overdose of tricyclic antidepressants should, therefore, have a 12-lead ECG performed as part of their assessment, and be monitored subsequently.

Throughout the assessment particular attention should be paid to the level of consciousness as a deterioration can endanger the airway. Alcohol greatly increases the effect of drugs such as the benzodiazepines (Valium, etc.) and the barbiturates in decreasing consciousness and may have a significant role to play alone, when the drug taken does not itself produce early impairment in consciousness (e.g. aspirin).

Nursing Intervention

Close and frequent observation is required to monitor vital signs and consciousness, and also to detect any further attempts at self-harm. A discreet check for potentially harmful items or other tablets should be carried out and any such objects quietly removed.

If there is a chance of recovering undigested drugs or chemicals from the stomach then a stomach washout may be performed to prevent their absorption. An alternative and less distressing procedure involves giving a dose of syrup of ipecac (30 ml) together with several glasses of water to drink; emesis should occur within 30 minutes. This procedure should not be followed where the patient's level of consciousness is impaired due to the risk of inhaling the ensuing vomitus.

If it is more than 4 hours since ingestion of the drug, there is little point in either course of action as the drug will have passed on into the intestines and been absorbed into the blood. Exceptions to this general rule are the tricyclic antidepressants which because of their parasympathetic blocking effect may stay in the stomach for more than 8 hours, and aspirin which also may be retained in the stomach for more than 12 hours (Paynter, 1993).

If a washout is to be performed, a minimum of two staff are needed. The procedure should be carefully and realistically explained, the nurse mentioning that while it is unpleasant, especially in the passing of the tube during which the patient will experience a gagging sensation, it is not painful and that with the patient's cooperation, the whole procedure can be completed in 5 to 10 minutes. False teeth should be removed, the foot of the trolley elevated to minimize aspiration risk, and the patient positioned on their left side, with a nurse at the head of the trolley with a rigid wide-bore suction catheter (e.g. a Yankaur) ready for use.

The washout tube should be well lubricated with water soluble jelly and passed over the back of the tongue. It will usually fill with gastric contents upon entering the stomach, informing the nurse of its successful placement. The nurse should observe the patient's colour and breathing during insertion as the only other place that a tube that size could go is into the airway, a fact that would be quickly apparent.

A small quantity of lukewarm water should be placed in the funnel at the end of the tube which is then elevated above the level of the patient to allow it to drain under gravity into the patient's stomach. This is then syphoned off by lowering the funnel below the level of the patient. If this first cautious procedure is successful, then the washout should be continued using a funnel full of water each time until the water returning is clear. Encouragement should be given to the patient throughout the procedure. This will help gain cooperation which will make the procedure easier and safer.

If the degree of coma is such that the patient has lost their gag reflex, a washout should only be performed if the patient's airway has been secured by intubation.

McMaster et al. (1993) consider that there is little to choose between gastric lavage and induced emesis—both are equally ineffective. In reviewing the literature, Davis (1991) has indicated that induced emesis was preferred to gastric lavage, unless the patient presented within one hour of overdose or the airway was threatened. She went on to point out the advantages of using activated charcoal which can absorb a large quantity of the drug, thus preventing its absorption into the blood stream as it is retained in the gut. It may best be administered by nasogastric tube as many patients find it very unpalatable. The normal ratio of charcoal to drugs is 10:1.

Occasionally the patient refuses both ipecac and a washout. It is the patient's right to do so, and while every attempt should be made to make the patient cooperate by persuasion, no attempt should be made by force, and if the patient states that they are leaving the A & E department, they should not be forcibly detained. Only in extreme cases, where there is a real risk to life, is attempting to treat the patient against their wishes justified.

An interesting discussion of the ethical and legal issues has been provided by Davis (1993) who points out that the suicidal but competent patient could legally be left to die. In practice, doctors and nurses feel professionally obliged to intervene even though detaining a patient against their will in A & E entitles the person to sue for damages as a result of the battery committed upon the person. The key to the problem is the competency of the patient to make rational decisions when all the facts have been explained.

Patients who have practised self-mutilation may attempt further acts while in the department. Physical intervention is not recommended; talking quietly to try to defuse a potentially violent situation is the best way to proceed. The nurse should explain that there is no benefit from such acts and point out that the wounds will be treated appropriately if the patient is willing to allow the staff to help. However, it is very dangerous for the staff and for the patient to engage in a physical struggle as the result may be to produce accidentally a far worse wound than the one that the patient would have inflicted on their own. In addition, the nurse would be rewarding any attention-seeking motivation that may lie behind such behaviour, thereby increasing the likelihood of further episodes of the behaviour.

If the patient is threatening self-harm with a more serious implement than a piece of glass for example, the best way forward is to talk to the patient and to try to let him or her express their feelings in words rather than in deeds, paying particular attention to what has been said about emotions. Physical intervention is the last resort in such a situation and, if necessary, it should be planned so as to have the maximum degree of surprise and sufficient concentration of force so that the patient is overwhelmed and separated from the implement before they realize what has happened.

The suggested guidelines for handling the patient who has taken an overdose and wishes to leave the department also apply to the person who has committed self-mutilation.

The nursing interventions around those patients who have practised DSH can therefore be seen to be of a conservative, supportive nature—safeguarding the airway, observing closely, offering psychological support where needed, but remembering the high risk of aggression that is present should they turn their self-directed anger outwards, especially as there is usually significant alcohol intake in these cases.

Evaluation

Data relating to how DSH patients evaluate their care is scarce but an interesting study by Dunleavey (1992) of seventeen such patients is available. She found the patients talked of the nursing staff being cold and distant leaving the patient feeling isolated, so much so that Dunleavey felt their interaction lacked any therapeutic quality; it merely extended the misery of the patient. Staff who respond in a stereotypical way, relying on negative first impressions, will contribute to this type of patient evaluation. It is to be hoped A & E staff will seek a more desirable outcome and aim for care that is holistic and reflects the social and emotional trauma that frequently lies behind DSH or parasuicide.

If the patient talks to the nurse about the events that led up to the DSH episode, we may recognize our intervention as being successful, and further self-harm or outbursts of anger are much less likely to occur. The psychological support offered has been effective. One final check on the nursing care of patients who have practised DSH is the attitude of the staff towards the next patient who has taken an overdose. If the attitude is one of 'Not another overdose, what a nuisance they are' then the care given is likely to fall short of what is required.

References

Bent-Kelly E. (1992). Too busy for trivia. *Nursing*, 5, 32–3.
Chew R. (1993). *Compendium of Health Statistics 1992*. London: Office of Health Economics.
Davenport D. (1993). Structures support at a time of crisis. *Professional Nurse*, **June**, 558–62.
Davis J. (1991). A consideration not to be overlooked. *Professional Nurse*, Sept 1991, 710–14.
Davis J. (1993). Ethical and legal issues in suicide. *British Journal of Nursing*, 2, 777–80.
Department of Health (1992). *Health of the Nation*, London: HMSO.
Dunleavey R. (1992). An adequate response to a cry for help? *Professional Nurse*, Jan., 213–15.
Evans M., Cox C., Turnbull G. (1992). Parasuicide response. *Nursing Times*, **88**, 34–6.
Knepil J. (1993). Paracetamol overdose. *Professional Nurse*, Sept., 792.
McMaster B., Brian D., Pimblett A. (1993). The selection of treatment for

self-poisoned patients in A & E. *Accident and Emergency Nursing*, 1, 132–8.

OPCS (1991). *Mortality Statistics England and Wales 1990*. London: Government Statistics Service.

Palmer S. (1993). Parasuicide: a cause for concern. *Nursing Standard*, 7, 37–9.

Paynter M. (1993). Gastric lavage in A & E. *Nursing Standard*, 7, 32–3.

Strengel E. (1970). *Suicide and Attempted Suicide*. Harmondsworth: Penguin.

Walsh M. H. (1982a). Patterns of drug overdose. *Nursing Times*, 78, 275–8.

Walsh M. H. (1982b). Drug overdose—the national picture. *Nursing Times*, 78, 1158–9.

Younger J. (1993). Understanding paracetamol. *British Journal of Nursing*, 2, 1027–30.

Chapter 17

SUBSTANCE MISUSE

The nurse will not be long in A & E before realizing that alcohol is a major causative factor in attendances, especially at night. In addition, there is now a marked increase in the use of various other drugs ranging from solvents to heroin. Effective care planning in A & E requires some background knowledge of who uses drugs and why and of the social setting within which drug use occurs.

From the outset it is important that the A & E nurse avoids the twin traps of stereotyping and making judgements about patients who attend A & E as a result of substance misuse. The use of terms such as 'alcoholic' or 'drug addict' should be avoided as they are value laden and judgemental. It is better to talk of a dependence upon various substances which may have physiological, psychological and sociological dimensions.

Some of the key aspects of physiological dependence according to Johns (1990) are tolerance, neuroadaptation and withdrawal states. Tolerance refers to the need for ever bigger doses of a drug to produce similar effects which in turn means that regular users can tolerate doses that would be lethal to others. This is caused by the ability of the brain to adapt to larger doses which leads to the term neuroadaptation. Withdrawal of the drug leads to decompensation and rebound symptoms which tend to be the opposite of the drug's main effects.

The psychological aspect of substance misuse may be understood by considering operant conditioning (p. 23) in which reinforcement of behaviour occurs if there are pleasurable or beneficial effects for the individual concerned. There is however no evidence for any personality type who might be particularly prone to substance misuse. How the individual perceives their situation might influence the ability to withdraw successfully from substance use, for example a 'learned hopelessness' view that things are beyond the person's control will make action to give up drug use unlikely to succeed.

Users may associate certain stimuli with the pleasures of use; the chance offer of a drink or the sight of a needle and syringe may suffice to restart the person's habit.

Finally the sociological dimensions of substance misuse must be considered. In different societies there may be widely varying views about the same drug. Islamic and western societies for example have very different views about cannabis and alcohol. The presence of a multi-million pound advertising industry actively encouraging people to smoke and drink in the UK cannot be ignored in any discussion of substance misuse. On a smaller scale, the role of peer group pressure and the social norms of the individual's environment all play a part in substance use behaviour.

These factors come together to produce a wide range of substance use behaviours which have been summarized as lying on a continuum which has three phases. There is an initial experimental stage which if seen as having beneficial effects may lead to the recreational stage in which the user still has control over drug use, but which may have by now become a regular feature of life. The final phase in this career is reached as control is lost and drug use becomes compulsive, taking over the person's whole life regardless of consequences. This model is supported by Preston (1992) who is critical of the traditional medical model approach which sees substance misuse in disease terms. As Johns (1990) points out there is little support for a disease model either from research findings or clinical evidence, yet it remains a popular model for explaining substance misuse.

It is against this background that the A & E nurse should try to understand the patient presenting with alcohol or other drug related problems, rather than media hype and the prejudiced views of stereotypes such as 'Skid Row alcoholics' and 'drug addicts'.

Alcohol Abuse

Paton (1994) suggests there are 4 million heavy drinkers in the UK of whom 800,000 are problem drinkers and 400,000 are alcohol dependent. Paton (1994) quotes a figure of 2 billion pounds as the annual cost to society of alcohol consumption. Alcohol's role in violence is borne out by the work of Yates et al. (1987) who studied patients presenting late at night to two A & E units in Manchester. They found 78% of patients after midnight were inebriated while 60% of assault victims had positive blood alcohol readings even over the whole 24-hour period.

The main effect of alcohol is as a depressant, not a stimulant as is commonly thought. Thus, in large quantities, it causes drowsiness and diminished level of consciousness, while in moderate amounts removal of inhibitions is experienced. Apart from increasing the risk of violence and accidents this also increases the risk of unprotected sex occurring, with the problems of unwanted pregnancy and sexually transmitted diseases such as AIDS following in train.

In the A & E department, there are two types of alcohol-related problems. First, there is the patient who has some significant other pathology (e.g. a lacerated wrist or a drug overdose) but who is also under the influence of alcohol, and second, there is the person whose problems are solely related to alcohol. This person may be either inebriated or alcohol dependent and demanding admission to a psychiatric unit.

In assessing a patient, whichever of these two categories they fall into, there is a need to ascertain how much they have drunk and how this compares to their normal drinking pattern, how much control they have over their physical and emotional behaviour, and how much insight they have into their present situation. Finally, there is a need to know how long it is since their last drink.

A frequent injury seen in drunk people is severe laceration of the arm from falling on glass. Unfortunately the patient is rarely cooperative enough to permit a thorough examination of the wound, and certainly cannot receive an anaesthetic. In such cases it is best to concentrate on first aid measures to stop the bleeding and if possible loosely to close the wound and wait for morning when the patient will have sobered up enough to be able to go to theatre for proper examination and exploration of the wound with repair of damaged structures as appropriate. If the patient insists on walking out of the department, this should be allowed; they invariably return in the morning with a hangover, but prepared to cooperate in most cases.

Alcohol makes the assessment of head injuries very difficult as one of the key signs is altered consciousness, which could be produced by the alcohol as much as by trauma (Fleming, 1991).

Patients are frequently brought to A & E in a collapsed state due to alcohol intake. In such a situation, their airway must be the first consideration, not only because they may become unable to protect it for themselves, but also because they are highly likely to vomit if they have been drinking heavily. They should be thoroughly examined for other injury, especially head injury. If they are to be kept in the department for some time for observation, it is recommended that they be kept on a mattress on the floor rather than on a trolley. There is less risk of them falling off a mattress and injuring themselves than there is of falling off a trolley.

The effect of moderate to heavy alcohol intake can be to produce aggression. It is important to first of all recognize that it is alcohol that is responsible for aggressive behaviour in an individual rather than other causes such as a psychotic state or a stress reaction, as this will influence the handling of the situation.

Sometimes more sober friends or relatives can be prevailed upon to calm the situation. Whatever happens, the nurse should not respond to shouting or abuse and must keep in control of the situation at all times. Usually the best approach is to enquire politely what the problem is and how the person can be helped; this will often defuse a potentially explosive situation. It is futile to become drawn into an argument with a drunk person as the powers of logic are one of the first casualties of alcohol, and an argument can quickly escalate into violence.

Patients, with alcohol problems will occasionally present in A & E asking to see a psychiatrist for 'drying out'. The usual approach of the psychiatric services is that they will only consider a patient for admission if the person is sober and therefore able to exercise clear judgement. If the patient in A & E is under the influence of alcohol, it is unlikely that the psychiatric service will admit them. They are best advised to present to a GP in a sober condition with their request, although if sober in A & E there is no reason why an admission should not be arranged there and then for detoxification and treatment. Conversely, many alcohol dependent patients go through a stage of not wanting any help. The person has to recognize there is a problem first, for themselves, before help will be sought, therefore attempts at persuasion are futile in themselves, however well intentioned the nurse may be (Shepherd, 1991).

At the end of the day, however, despite a 'low profile' approach, it may not prove possible to help a patient under the influence of alcohol, and if they refuse to leave the department when asked, then the solution is to call the police and have the person removed. Nursing staff should not have to act as 'bouncers' in situations such as these.

The Opioids

In the last decade there has been a dramatic increase in the supply of these drugs, especially heroin, to the illegal market in the UK and consequently in the number of dependent individuals. The problems associated with their use can be divided into three groups: the direct effects of heroin itself, side effects associated with illegal injection practices, and the abstinence syndrome.

Direct Effects of Opioid Injection

Heroin produces a euphoric feeling. However, like most drugs, it requires a progressively larger dose to produce the same effect as tolerance develops. There is therefore a risk of accidental overdose leading to coma and respiratory arrest. The greater part of a heroin injection will be excreted within 24 hours and is detectable in the urine as morphine glucuronide (Madden, 1990).

Furthermore, the heroin bought on the street is impure, having been diluted with additives as the pushers try and increase their share of the profits by making each quantity go further. The result is that what the addict thinks is the normal dose may only be 50% heroin, with the result that if the addict were accidentally to obtain some pure heroin, there would be an overdose by a factor of two. Accidental overdose is therefore a common hazard of narcotics abuse.

The overdosed patient will usually be in an unresponsive state, comatose with pin point pupils and severely depressed respirations, if not frank respiratory arrest. A further tell-tale sign that should be looked for is the presence of injection sites, although these need not be present if the patient had inhaled heroin which is an alternative to injection. This involves heating heroin in a metal spoon and inhaling the fumes and is known as 'chasing the dragon'.

Any patient brought to A & E, aged 15 to 40 years, in a collapsed or comatose state, with no apparent cause, should alert the nurse to the possibility of heroin or other drug overdose, and the first steps in assessment should be to check the respiratory effort of the patient and the pupil size before looking for evidence of injection sites. Overdoses outside this range of ages can occur, but they are much less likely. Great care should be taken in undressing the patient as he or she may have used needles and syringes about their person, posing a hazard of accidental needle stick injury.

The immediate aim of intervention is to clear and maintain the airway, and if necessary institute positive pressure ventilation. The patient will need an IV injection of the specific antagonist for the opiate group of drugs, naloxone (usually Narcan 0.4 mg). This will produce a dramatic change in the patient's condition in a matter of minutes, bringing them to a state of consciousness, although they may be a little confused for a few minutes. However, as the half life of naloxone is only an hour, and its peak effect much shorter than that, the respiratory depressant effect of many narcotics is in practice much longer, and the immediate improvement that is observed from naloxone administration may only be transient. It is essential, therefore, that a very close watch be kept on the patient for some time, and several further injections of naloxone may be required depending upon the clinical condition of the patient.

The situation may arise where the patient does not wish to stay for observation. In this case, whoever is with the patient should be informed that the drugs given to counter the effect of the heroin will wear off after a while and the patient may again become comatose. They should be told to keep a close watch and if necessary ring for an ambulance should this occur.

Other Effects of Opioid Injection

Most people are now aware of the risk of HIV or hepatitis B transmission from the use of shared injecting equipment, whatever the drug that is being used. The problem is particularly acute in Scotland where the rates of drug-induced HIV infection per million population are: Edinburgh 786, Dundee 487 and Glasgow 147 compared to a figure of only 60 for London (Kennedy et al., 1992). The difference between Edinburgh and Glasgow is particularly puzzling, as Kennedy et al. (1992) point out that Glasgow has the largest population of intravenous drug users in Scotland, estimated at 9500, which is two to three times the number in Edinburgh. The relationship between IV drug use and HIV is therefore more complex than might appear to be the case.

Nurses working in A & E should observe universal precautions against blood-borne infection at all times. Any patient could be an IV drug user and any patient could be HIV positive. The importance of avoiding stereotyping patients cannot be underestimated in this regard. It would be helpful if the A & E nurse is aware of local needle exchange schemes and other sources of advice and help for IV drug users such as methadone maintenance schemes. These schemes are controversial. Their aim is harm reduction by prescribing the person an oral opioid substitute, methadone, in the hope of helping the person move away from the chaotic drug culture and into regular contact with helping agencies. Additionally, avoiding IV injection greatly reduces the risk of HIV and hepatitis B infection. Intravenous drug users may also present with abscesses around injection sites and septicaemia amongst other side effects of injection.

Withdrawal Syndrome

The withdrawal syndrome is caused by the withdrawal of the drug after the body has become physiologically dependent upon it. The typical picture in the case of heroin is one of sweating, stomach cramps, vomiting, headaches and tachycardia.

In this situation, the dependent user is desperate for heroin and may well present in A & E. Extreme caution is required in handling the person as the desperation can easily lead to violence against members of staff.

Under current legislation and guidelines, however, the prescription of drugs to users is strictly limited to certain doctors specializing in the field. It is not, therefore, the place of A & E departments to be prescribing drugs for dependent users no matter how desperate they may appear. Advice should be given about registering with a GP in order to obtain a referral to either a drug treatment centre or to a psychiatrist with an interest in the field. If a person refuses to leave when refused drugs, the police should be called to deal with the situation. In practice, a user will usually be able to obtain drugs if turned away from A & E.

Cocaine

Cocaine is a highly dangerous drug capable of producing profound dependence and its illicit use is expanding dramatically as a stimulant and euphoric agent. It used to be thought of as the Rolls Royce of the drug scene but the market is now being flooded with large quantities at much lower prices. The most recent development is the appearance of 'crack', a highly addictive, concentrated and purified form of the drug which is smoked.

Hallucinogenics

The effect of these drugs is to produce hallucinations as well as bizarre sensations and feelings, such as being able to hear colours and feel sounds. The best known drug is LSD (lysergic acid diethylamide), although there are other substances such as the so-called magic mushrooms that grow wild in the UK and contain psylocybin as the active ingredient, but whose effects are less potent than LSD. A very powerful agent not found much in the UK is phencyclidine (PCP) or 'Angel Dust'.

The use of LSD declined considerably after the 'Swinging Sixties' and their associated psychedelia but has increased again in recent years. LSD is usually taken in the form of a tablet and usually in a group situation in order that anyone who is on a 'bad trip' may be talked down. However, the effects of the drug may be so alarming and disturbing that the users' behaviour constitutes a danger to themselves and possibly others. It is then that the patient ends up in A & E.

The patient's behaviour will often be totally unreasonable and unpredictable as the sensory input will be bizarre and deranged. The need is for a secure environment where the patient may be safely detained without injury; for example, a bare cubicle with a mattress on the floor. If behaviour is disturbed, sedation is required; experience has shown that what is needed is a quick-acting IV injection (e.g. diazepam 10 mg) and a long-acting IM injection such as chlorpromazine (100–200 mg). Considerable physical restraint may be needed in the first instance to give the IV sedation, and this should only be attempted when there are enough pairs of hands available to do the job safely.

After sedation the patient should be left to sleep off the effects of the drug, under observation, with particular attention being paid to airway and breathing. The patient should also be assessed for injuries that may have been sustained while under the influence of the LSD, as these can be most readily treated at this stage.

Cannabis

Cannabis may be smoked or incorporated into food and eaten. If smoked, its effects appear within minutes. If eaten, it takes approximately one hour to produce its effect. After use, the general feeling is one of mild euphoria and well-being although this is heavily influenced by factors such as the group situation and the users' expectations.

There is little evidence to suggest that smoking cannabis is harmful in the short term, although the occasional patient may present in A & E after their first use of the drug complaining of feeling unwell. It is likely that this feeling is more associated with the anxiety of the individual about the drug experience, than the drug itself. After a short period of observation, such persons can usually be discharged with reassurance.

The drug may be injected, sniffed or smoked and acts as a central nervous system stimulant. Effects include agitation, exaggerated reflexes, tachycardia, ventricular arrhythmias, hypertension and hallucinations. Convulsions and coma may occur in overdose. Sedation with intravenous diazepam may be needed as emergency treatment and, if severe cardiac effects are present, IV propranolol may be required (BNF, 1993).

Ecstasy

This drug has appeared since 1990 and is very popular with young people engaged in late night parties, 'raves' and club scenes. Its correct pharmacological name is methylenedioxymethamphetamine (MDMA) and it is a hallucinogenic amphetamine. Preston (1992) summarizes the effects of the drug as producing initially a mild euphoria followed by sensations of serenity. Stamina is enhanced along with the sensual experiences associated with sex, while visual distortions and heightening of perception are also present.

It appears that whilst the majority of users experience few long-term ill effects, a minority have severe and potentially fatal reactions. Preston (1992) and Jones and Dickinson (1992) describe the presenting signs of a severe reaction as convulsions and collapse, dilated pupils, hypotension, tachycardia, hyperpyrexia and death from respiratory failure associated with disseminated intravascular coagulation (DIC). Such reactions have been recorded amongst established users which suggests this is not some sort of allergic reaction and that the effects of the extreme heat and activity associated with dancing and the 'rave scene' combine with the toxic effects of the drug to lead to this fatal outcome.

The signs that should alert the A & E nurse to an Ecstasy-induced collapse include admission from a late night party/disco of a previously fit young person who has collapsed for no apparent reason. Tachycardia, hypotension and signs of hyperpyrexia (e.g. sweat-soaked clothing, elevated temperature) are all important indicators as would be any evidence of clotting disorder such as abnormal bruising. In a thorough discussion of the Ecstasy problem, Jones (1993) emphasizes the importance of early recognition of hyperthermia in A & E and prompt nursing action to cool the patient or at least reduce the rate at which temperature is rising. Urgent treatment is needed with admission to ITU indicated for ventilatory support. The prognosis is not good however if DIC becomes established.

Amphetamines

These stimulant drugs are popular on the drug scene, used either alone or in conjunction with other drugs. Klee (1992) has reported an increase in their use, particularly by injection which is a worrying trend given the HIV and other risks associated with IV drug use. The risk of HIV transmission is potentially greater with this group as Klee's research indicated that they were significantly more sexually active than a matched group of heroin users and 71% of her sample reported that they had not used condoms during casual sexual encounters.

The user may go for several days without sleep whilst injecting amphetamines and be brought to A & E eventually in a collapsed state. Regular use leads to serious behavioural disorders such as aggression, hallucinations, profound mood swings and paranoid delusions, making such individuals very difficult to handle in A & E. Other drugs such as barbiturates and cannabis may be used to deal with the symptoms that occur after a period of usage. Barbiturates have a respiratory depressant effect, making monitoring of respiratory rate particularly important in any patient who is suspected of attending in a collapsed state after amphetamine usage.

Solvent Abuse

The inhalation of substances for mind-altering reasons has a long history that extends back from the adolescents of today through to the likes of Sir Joseph Priestley, who discovered nitrous oxide in

1776 (N_2O inhalers included Coleridge, Southey and Wedgwood), and back to the Ancient Greeks.

The first solvents to be widely abused were different forms of glue in the USA in the 1960s, the habit spreading to the UK in the 1970s. The substances used are now many and varied, but are mostly based on organic solvents (e.g. toluene, benzene and butane) ranging from glue to nail polish remover, from polystyrene cements to hair spray, and from oven cleaners to petrol. Aerosols are also abused for the effects of the propellants (freons).

A study by Sansum (1984) of a group of solvent abusers referred to a drug treatment centre in the West Midlands found that the mean age was 14, 92% of the group was male, 50% of the group came from broken homes, and although in a multiracial area, none were of Caribbean origins. Her findings are fairly typical of reports from other parts of the country.

The substances are inhaled from a plastic bag (crisp packets are commonly used) held to the face. However, more dangerous practices include placing the bag completely over the head to get a stronger effect (and increasing the risk of death from asphyxiation) and spraying aerosols directly into the mouth which can cause laryngo-spasm and death. The number of deaths from solvent abuse has averaged over 100 per year since 1985, with the most recent year for which figures are available, 1990, seeing 149 deaths, the highest on record (Social Trends, 1993).

Mild intoxication is achieved within the first few minutes and can last up to 30 minutes. With careful usage, a user may achieve a 'high' lasting as long as 12 hours. Intoxication is an appropriate word to use in describing the experience felt by many abusers and their behaviour is similar to that of an adult who is drunk. However, there may also be hallucinatory experiences which can lead to extremely dangerous behaviour.

Any adolescent brought to A & E found collapsed or behaving strangely should be suspected of being under the influence of inhaled solvents. In assessing the patient, the clues to look for are redness around the mouth and nose, a smell of solvent, the presence of plastic bags/crisp packets in the pockets or the actual substance itself, and changes in behaviour such as an unsteady gait, aggressiveness, slurred speech and inappropriate emotional responses.

The possibility of adolescents in the department sniffing while actually waiting with a friend should also be borne in mind as their behaviour can cause considerable problems. The changes in behaviour described already should be watched for, and frequent visits to the toilet are highly suspicious indeed. The substance involved can usually be smelt on the person concerned.

The aim is to prevent harm to the individual; therefore, airway care is the first priority, coupled with detention in a place of safety, if there are hallucinations. Sedation may be necessary. It is important to involve the GP and the boy's family as soon as possible. The family's social worker, if it has one, needs to know as well. Finally, some parents may be unaware that their son is indulging in solvent abuse, so the knowledge should be broken to them tactfully to prevent a hostile rejection of offers of help. Solvent abuse has been found to affect children of all social classes, so the nurse should beware of the trap of falling into stereotyping and overlooking the likely cause of an adolescent's behaviour simply because he appears to be from, for example, an upper-class background.

The difficult area of children using drugs has been discussed by Harding-Price (1993), who points out that the Children Act gives children the right to refuse treatment even though under 16 years of age. The nurse may also find that the young person or child may refuse to consent to parents being told of the problem. The Northern Drug Services Child Care Group have drawn up a set of criteria to cover this difficult dilemma which would allow nurses and others to work with the child without parental consent. Harding-Price stresses the importance of the child's best interests, his or her ability to understand fully the situation and the probability of harm coming to the child without intervention, as the key principles upon which these criteria are founded.

References

BNF (1993). *British National Formulary*. London: BMA/Royal Pharmaceutical Society of Great Britain.

Fleming J. (1991). Alcohol-induced head injury. *Nursing Times*, **87**, 29–31.

Harding-Price D. (1993). A sensitive response without discrimination: drug misuse in children and adolescents. *Professional Nurse*, April, 419–22.

Johns A. (1990). What is dependence? In Ghodse H., Maxwell D. (eds), *Substance Abuse and Dependence*, London: Macmillan Press.

Jones C. (1993). MDMA: The doubts surrounding Ecstasy and the response of the emergency nurse. *Accident & Emergency Nursing*, **1**, 193–8.

Jones C., Dickinson P. (1992). From Ecstasy to agony. *Nursing Times*, **88**, 28–30.

Kennedy D., Emslie J., Goldberg D. (1992). HIV infection and AIDS: epidemiology and public health aspects. In Plant M., Ritson B., Robertson R. *Alcohol and Drugs: The Scottish Experience.* Edinburgh: Edinburgh University Press.

Klee H. (1992). A deadly combination. *Nursing Times,* **88,** 36–8.

Madden S. (1990). Effects of drug dependence. In Ghodse H., Maxwell D. (eds), *Substance Abuse and Dependence,* London: Macmillan Press.

Paton A. (1994). *ABC of Alcohol,* London: BMJ.

Preston A. (1992). Pointing out the risk. *Nursing Times,* **88,** 24–6.

Sansum G. (1984). Glue sniffing: a study. *Nursing,* **2,** 714–15.

Shepherd A. (1991). Dealing with dependency. *Nursing Times,* **87,** 26–9.

Social Trends (1993). London: HMSO.

Yates D. et al. (1987). Alcohol consumption of patients attending two A & E departments in the north west of England. *Journal of the Royal Society of Medicine,* **80,** 486–9.

Chapter 18

THE MENTALLY ILL PATIENT IN A & E

The A & E unit frequently sees mentally ill patients, some of whom may be very disturbed and who have lost touch with reality. Sometimes they are brought to A & E by friends or family; often they are brought by the police or ambulance service after acting in a bizarre way in public. The possibility of drug usage and cultural differences should also be borne in mind as explanations of the person's behaviour. The closure of large mental hospitals with inadequate community support services has led to significant numbers of mentally ill people presenting at A & E in a very dishevelled condition because they are living rough as there is nowhere else for them to go.

There are many other patients with less obvious psychiatric difficulties who frequently present in A & E. Atha et al. (1989) have shown how such people may be identified and helped by the development of a community psychiatric nursing service within the A & E unit. Patients engaging in deliberate self-harm may be helped by the setting up of a special 'parasuicide team' which works closely with the A & E department (Evans et al., 1992). It is important that A & E staff fully appreciate their involvement in caring for people with mental health problems.

It will be useful, therefore, to look at some of the common types of behaviour that the mentally ill patient may exhibit, along with the conventional medical diagnosis. The nurse, however, is not trying to make a psychiatric diagnosis in A & E, but rather assess the behavioural problems displayed by the patient in order to plan care which will help the patient and prevent disruption of the department. It is also essential to assign a priority for the patient to be seen by the casualty officer (triage).

Schizophrenia

Schizophrenia is conventionally described as a profound disorder of thought associated with disturbance of mood, perception and behaviour. Rather than thinking of this as a single disorder, Barker (1993) suggests it is better to view schizophrenia as a group of psychotic disorders with a range of presentations and possible causes.

The person's mood is said to be characterized by a poverty of feeling, conversation typically being in a flat monotone with the mood colourless, bland and emotionally dull. There is also said to be an inappropriate effect, i.e. disharmony, between what a person says and how they say it.

Perceptual disturbance is associated with hallucinations, usually auditory as the person hears voices telling them what to do next or giving a running commentary on events that are happening to the patient. There may be more than one voice audible to the patient. The patient becomes concerned with self, withdrawing from the outside world to live in their own world.

The thought processes become disorganized, illogical and disjointed, leading to the classical thought block where a person stops in mid-sentence, their thoughts having seemingly run into a brick wall. Woolly thinking sometimes characterizes schizophrenia; the patient will go 'all the way round the houses' in giving a simple explanation or answering a simple question.

Delusions creep into the patient's thoughts which may be paranoid or result in the person thinking that he is Christ or God. Another commonly seen phenomenon is that of ideas of reference where the person thinks there are hidden messages contained in newspapers or TV programmes, for example.

As a result of such profound disorganization of the mental processes, there is often very bizarre and inappropriate behaviour on the person's part, or they may become withdrawn and inert leading to confusion with depression. Violence may occur in response to what the voices that they hear tell them.

The incidence of schizophrenia is almost one in a hundred, and some two-thirds of patients in mental hospitals are sufferers. The age of onset is typically late teens to early twenties and it can occur in people of any intellectual level or social class. There are many theories attempting to explain schizophrenia—

some genetic, some environmental. Others look for biochemical explanations.

Depression

Everybody at some time or another has a 'low' in life; for some people though their lows are much deeper than others, so low that all is black and despair and there is no point to life. It is a short step from there to the decision to end life—suicide. Such lows are depression in the psychotic sense of the word.

It is a state characterized by the mood of despair. Associated with this mood are physical changes such as loss of appetite and weight together with inability to sleep; early morning wakening is typical. Some patients will talk of their despair, others will not; there are feelings of helplessness, hopelessness and guilt. Impotence and amenorrhoea are possible.

Mania and Manic Depression

The manic individual suffers from excessive elation of mood, irritability, flight of ideas, talkativeness and hyperactivity, all of which combine to produce extreme and bizarre behaviour. There may also be grandiose or persecutory delusions and auditory hallucinations.

It is possible for the extremes of mania and depression to be combined in the same patient who may function normally for long periods with full insight into their illness, before plunging into deep depression or becoming manic, either way requiring urgent treatment.

Anxiety States and Phobias

Anxiety is a natural feature of life that we all experience, acting often in a beneficial way in motivating us to work hard for an exam because we are anxious that we may fail or in making us careful in crossing the road.

However, anxiety can build up for some people to pathological levels, with no apparent cause or focus. Such anxiety is called free floating and may lead to acute panic attacks where the person is convinced that they are seriously ill or about to die. Patients may be brought to A & E in the grips of an acute anxiety attack, exhibiting signs associated with sympathetic nervous system stimulation such as tachycardia, palpitations, sweaty palms and a rapid respiratory rate.

This change in respiration can produce serious biochemical changes due to the lowering in blood CO_2 levels that occurs with overbreathing; this in turn upsets the pH balance making the blood more alkaline which in turn upsets the calcium balance causing muscle spasm (tetany) and tingling in the fingers. There is a characteristic carpopedal spasm of the fingers and abdominal cramps that are associated with hysterical hyperventilation. Their effect is to make the patient even more anxious and therefore more likely to hyperventilate. The solution is to try to calm the patient with reassurance and to encourage them to use a rebreathing bag to increase the CO_2 levels to normal as they rebreathe their own exhaled CO_2. After about 15 minutes, their respiratory rate will be back to normal and the muscle cramps will have abated.

If a person's anxiety is not free floating and instead is attached to some specific object (usually by classical conditioning), then a phobia is said to exist. The most likely phobic state that the A & E nurse may see is agoraphobia—fear of being outdoors—when a phobic patient has a panic attack and is brought to A & E as a result.

Assessment

The nurse will usually be the first point of contact for the patient with the department. Remembering the importance of first impressions, the A & E nurse should greet the patient in a friendly and sympathetic manner. A nursing assessment is required to assign a priority to the patient to see the casualty officer, and to decide which is the best environment in which the patient may be looked after within A & E and who are the best persons to be with the patient during this time.

The first step is to sit the patient down in a quiet room with just the receiving nurse present. The offer of a cup of tea may help relax the patient and if he or she wishes to smoke then they should be allowed to do so. Introduce yourself so that the patient knows who you are and that you are trying to help. Try and sit slightly to one side rather than square on to the patient—this is less threatening—

and make sure your distance is not so close as to intrude on the personal space of the patient (threatening?) or too far away (disinterested?)—a metre is usually an appropriate distance.

The amount of stimuli in the environment should be kept to a minimum as this may exacerbate the patient's misperception problems or overwhelm somebody who is already feeling overwhelmed by life in general.

Seeking eye contact is an important first step in commencing a therapeutic relationship, followed by a friendly gesture such as the offer of a handshake. The nurse should try to get the patient to talk about their problems, if possible gently keeping them on the subject if they try to wander. It is futile to argue with delusions and hallucinations. This will only provoke anger and aggression in the patient, so the approach should be a non-committal one, no matter how far-fetched the story told by the patient. It is best simply to say you cannot hear the voice the patient hears rather than deny its existence.

Body movements are useful indicators for the observant nurse. Hyperactivity and agitation characterize a manic state while fidgeting, restlessness, facial grimacing and Parkinsonian movements are among the side effects of the powerful phenothiazine drugs used in the treatment of schizophrenia and, if observed in a person, might give a useful clue to their previous medical history. A dishevelled appearance suggests the person has been living rough and underlines the need for the assessment to include a social history. Has he recently been discharged from a mental hospital?

Once the nurse has engaged the patient in speech, useful information may be gained from the manner in which the patient talks. A straight refusal to speak suggests withdrawal from the outside world. A reluctance on the part of the person to initiate speech, which is then slow and hesitant, is associated with depression. Not surprisingly, the opposite situation, an uninterruptable flood of speech, is associated with manic states.

The content of the person's speech will tell us much about their thought processes. Pressure of speech and leaping from idea to idea suggest a manic thought process while despair, worthlessness and guilt indicate the person is probably depressive. Psychotic illness such as schizophrenia is characterized by disordered thought and this is reflected in the speech of the person, it being vague, woolly and halting and incorporating looseness of association, e.g. if the patient is a virgin, so is the Virgin Mary, therefore the patient is the

Virgin Mary. Thought block manifests itself by the patient stopping suddenly in the middle of a sentence, their mind a blank—in the midst of thought, there is no thought. The chaotic state of their thoughts leads the person to move randomly between unconnected statements. In addition, the person may describe delusions and hallucinations, and may be seen conversing with the voices that they can hear inside their head.

Orientation in time and space should be assessed together with how much insight the person has into their illness. If the person does not think they are ill, they are unlikely to want to go to hospital, and there is nothing mad about that.

It remains to try and find out something of the person's life history—where they are from, whether they have been ill before, what their family background is, and so on. Some persons may be known to the local psychiatric service already, others may be presenting with illness for the first time, while others may have come from afar, which should make the nurse alert to the possibility of psychiatric Munchausen's syndrome (see p. 293).

After the initial assessment, the person's family should be interviewed also if they are present, and they should be involved in the person's care throughout their stay in the department, provided that meets with the approval of the patient.

During the assessment, the nurse should also consider the possibility that the patient's behaviour may be due to drugs. This possibility should tactfully be raised with the patient and evidence of drug taking should be looked for. Solvent abuse, LSD, psylocybin and alcohol withdrawal (delirium tremens) can all lead to hallucinations. Stimulants such as amphetamines and cocaine can produce acute psychotic states, while the new drug Ecstasy can produce psychological effects ranging from mild anxiety to outright psychosis (Jones, 1993).

In prioritizing the patient, the nurse should remember that acute psychotic conditions do not lend themselves to waiting for lengthy periods—the patient may abscond, cause serious disruption to the running of the department, or inflict serious harm on themselves.

Intervention

The safety of the patient and the staff are the paramount concerns. There should be a quiet, separate room, with minimal stimulation where the patient may be kept. This room should be carefully furnished to avoid providing ready-made ammunition to a very disturbed patient and should have windows that cannot be opened fully so that the patient cannot leave or attempt to leave via that route. Continual observation of the room from outside should be possible, and the patient should not be left alone at any period. If the family are not able to stay with the patient, a nurse should be assigned to this task, and as far as possible the same nurse should stay with the patient throughout their stay in the department, in order to give a feeling of security and to try to build up some sort of relationship.

After the patient has been seen by the medical staff, admission may be arranged to a psychiatric bed. The A & E department is, therefore, assessing the patient and carrying out a holding action until admission can be arranged and therapy commenced. Should violence look likely, the nurse should act in accordance with the principles laid down on p. 296.

Many people arrive at A & E departments in an acutely disturbed state, noisy and behaving in a very bizarre fashion, but leave quietly an hour or so later for a psychiatric hospital and treatment, simply because the nursing staff sat and talked with the patient, in between medical assessments. Force or drugs are not used, the secret being simply to let the patient talk and say what they want to say. The nurse need neither agree (and thereby collude with the patient's delusions) nor disagree (and provoke aggression), but simply allow the patient the opportunity of self-expression. It is worth considering that patients today who are labelled as schizophrenics would in another time and place have been hailed as great prophets and holy people due to their visions and ability to hear God talking to them.

In concluding the chapter we need to look at the situation in which the patient will not cooperate, and treatment/detention in hospital against the patient's will is called for. This requires invoking a section of the Mental Health Act 1983, and Table 18.1 summarizes the sections of the Act most likely to be used in A & E.

As can be seen from a study of Table 18.1, the A & E department may receive patients brought by a member of the police force, under section 136, due to their behaviour in a public place. Alternatively departments may receive a patient whose physical health requires treatment before their mental health, under section 135. Such patients are usually elderly and living alone, suffering from malnutrition, hypothermia and gross neglect.

The other section of the Act most likely to be applied is section 4,

Table 18.1
Summary of Mental Health Act 1983

Legislation	Criteria	Application	Medical Recommendations	Effect
Section 4. Admission for assessment in an emergency. [NB Section 24 of the Mental Health (Scotland) Act 1984 is similar in effect.]	Admission for assessment required as a matter of urgent necessity.	Nearest relative or Approved Social Worker (ASW) of Pt. must be seen by applicant during the 24 hours before application is made.	One written recommendation by any doctor, but if possible, one with previous knowledge of the patient.	Pt. detained for a max. of 72 hours unless 2nd medical opinion given and received by hospital management in that period. Provisions of Part IV on consent to treatment do not apply.
Section 136. Mentally disordered persons in public places.	If a PC finds a person in a public place who appears to be suffering from a mental disorder and is in immediate need of care or control.	A Police Officer	Nil	Person can be taken to place of safety to be interviewed by ASW or doctor, e.g. A & E or Police Station. Maximum 72 hours.
Section 135. Warrant to search for and remove patient.	There is reasonable cause to suspect that a person believed to be suffering from a mental disorder has been ill-treated or neglected, or is unable to care for him or herself and lives alone.	ASW to a JP (on oath)	Nil	PC, ASW and doctor can enter patient's premises and remove him or her to a place of safety. Maximum 72 hours.

Section 2. Admission for assessment.	Mental disorder warranting detection in hospital for assessment and treatment. The patient ought to be detained in interests of own health and safety or for the protection of others.	Nearest relative and ASW who must interview Pt.	Two doctors, one of whom must be approved under Section 12. Doctors not to be from same hospital.	Patient detained for maximum of 28 days. Part IV applies for treatment without consent.
Section 3. Admission for treatment.	Mental illness or severe impairment, psychopathic disorder or mental impairment of a nature or degree which makes medical treatment in hospital appropriate.	As for Section 2, but ASW cannot make an application if the nearest relative objects.	As for Section 2.	Patient detained for maximum of 6 months, renewable for a further 6, then for 1 year at a time.

Adapted from *A Practical Guide to Mental Health Law*, MIND (1983).

where the patient is in A & E and the decision is taken that for their own protection and well-being they must be taken into psychiatric care against their will. However patients may also attend A & E from a psychiatric hospital, who are detained under section 2 or 3 already, due to injuries or illness.

Part IV of the Act establishes several categories of treatment, each with specific legal safeguards, which can be administered to certain patients without their consent, e.g. ECT or drug therapy. Part IV does not apply to various types of patients, including all involuntary patients and those detained for 72 hours or less. Before treating a patient, therefore, the A & E department needs consent, which if withheld by the patient, means that the department should check carefully with psychiatric colleagues that it is permitted to administer treatment under Part IV, before proceeding against the patient's wishes.

The A & E nurse should be familiar with the various provisions of the Mental Health Act 1983 as it affects A & E, and should always have a readily available supply of section papers, particularly section 4. A & E nurses in Scotland should also be aware of the Mental Health (Scotland) Act 1984 which regulates treatment in that country (Killen, 1993).

Many patients presenting in A & E will not however be suffering from a major psychotic disturbance, but will be anxious, lonely and unhappy—this is particularly true in the night. Listening and the use of counselling skills may make a valuable therapeutic contribution to the individual's well-being and should be just as much a part of the A & E nurse's repertoire as resuscitation and other technical skills.

Evaluation

If a mentally disturbed patient has gone through the department with the minimum of fuss and into the appropriate treatment facility, the care given may be evaluated as successful. However, if there has been violence, it is important to look at what happened, and why, to see if there was a failure of care or whether in the end the patient was just so disturbed that violence was inevitable. If the patient has absconded from A & E, this also needs critical examination in order that the reasons for such a failure may be identified. If it was because there were not enough nurses on duty to keep adequate watch on the patient, then questions have to be asked of management whose responsibility it is to staff the unit. If, however, the person in charge on that shift failed to detail a nurse to stay with the patient, even though sufficient nurses were available, then that person's awareness of what is involved in the care of psychiatric patients is called into question, and perhaps with it the department's attitude to those with mental health problems.

References

Atha C., Salkuskis P., Storer D. (1989). More Questions Than Answers, *Nursing Times* 85: 15, 28–31.

Barker P. (1993). Major mental health problems. In Wright H., Giddey M. (eds) *Mental Health Nursing*, London: Chapman & Hall.

Evans M., Cox C., Turnbull G. (1992). Parasuicide response. *Nursing Times*, **88,** 34–6.

Jones C. (1993). MDMA: the doubts surrounding Ecstasy and the response of the emergency nurse. *Accident & Emergency Nursing*, 193–8.

Killen J. (1993). The Mental Health Acts: the UK and Eire. In Wright H., Giddey M. (eds) *Mental Health Nursing*, London: Chapman & Hall.

Chapter 19

THE DIFFICULT PROBLEMS THAT NOBODY ELSE WANTS

Most A & E departments have their share of 'regulars', the frequent attenders who are constantly turning up, often because nobody else can think of what to do with them. They include the itinerant travellers, those who are alcohol/drug dependent, those with Munchausen's syndrome, the homeless, and people suffering from psychopathic personality disorders that do not benefit from psychiatric treatment.

It is worth looking at some of these problem areas in detail, as the difficulties that some of these individuals can cause are out of all proportion to the numbers involved.

NFA . . . The Person With Nowhere To Go

The 1980s witnessed a major increase in homelessness, particularly among the young. Factors such as the decline of rented accommodation and the policy of discharging large numbers of patients from long-stay mental hospitals without providing sufficient community resources have contributed to this worrying trend. Gough et al. (1994) also point out that this is a result of a deliberate government policy of doing nothing about the problem by refusing to build more public housing or change the benefit system. There is now a large section of the community with no home of their own except a night shelter, hostel, squat, local authority bed and breakfast accommodation or, perhaps, just a cardboard box. For these people, A & E is their main source of medical help.

Alcohol abuse is a major problem that affects some people within this group. The prognosis for the 'Skid Row' alcoholic, drinking the day away with fellow dossers on the waste and parklands of towns and cities, is very poor indeed.

The dossers form a hard core of A & E regulars. Students often ask 'Surely something can be done for these people?' Society answers by locking them in prison for short sentences due to their drunken behaviour in public, which can often be quite aggressive. Most of the agencies involved with dossers, however, admit that this is a waste of time, not benefiting the individuals concerned and merely adding to the overcrowding problems in gaols.

There is no easy answer to the problem of drunken vagrancy. Cook (1975) after many years working with alcoholic vagrants in London writes: 'One certainly has the feeling . . . that Skid Row has the capacity to absorb any amount of research and social work endeavour, and to remain untouched by it. There is in the Skid Row air as it were a notion of defiance and hopelessness either part of which (or the combination of which) makes reaching out to and helping individuals . . . extremely difficult.'

The use of arguments, such as 'Surely you would be better off if . . .', to try to persuade a vagrant to seek help is considered by Cook to be useless on many occasions due to this air of defiance, this desire to stay outside and fight the system. Nurses' practical experience in A & E unfortunately tends to confirm Cook's pessimistic view.

The A & E nurse will encounter the dosser when he (the majority of dossers are male, although there are homeless women too) is ill as he is very unlikely to have a GP, when he has fallen over drunk causing injuries to himself such as scalp lacerations, or when a member of the public dials 999 for an ambulance for a dosser who has passed out in a public place.

A full assessment should be carried out on reception in A & E, paying particular attention to level of consciousness and airway. Head injury is a common problem, but due to the effects of alcohol extremely difficult to assess. Full level of consciousness and pupil observations should be carried out at regular intervals. It is important also to check for hypothermia, especially in winter.

If there are no immediate interventions needed, the patient is best laid for his own safety on his side on a mattress on the floor, under observation until he has slept off his alcohol sufficiently to leave.

Aggressive behaviour is unfortunately common due to the alcohol and is best dealt with in the usual way (see p. 296), with the police being called to evict the patient if, for example, upon sobering up somewhat, he decides to refuse to leave even though fit. A & E departments are not night shelters for vagrant alcoholics; once a person is fit to go, then they must go.

Although this may seem a hard policy on a cold night in February, the nurse should ask what exactly would be achieved by allowing somebody to stay the night in A & E simply because they said they had nowhere else to go. An alcoholic who has sobered up after a binge in the local park is suffering from far deeper social, psychological and economic problems than a free night in A & E can solve. A more constructive long-term approach is to try to forge links with the local voluntary services working in the field, and with the DHSS and the Social Work department of the hospital so that advice about helpful points of contact with these agencies may be given. There is something of the stick and carrot approach about this, but it is the best long-term solution given the state of the personal social services at present and the multiple problems that are associated with the vagrant alcoholic. Shadoobuccus (1988) offers some insights into the multiple problems of caring for the homeless alcoholic.

Psychopathic Disorder

'Psychopath' is a term often bandied about in general conversation but usually, like the term schizophrenic, in a totally inappropriate way. However, within the mental health care field there is much debate about its meaning and little agreement. An approximate consensus is offered by Barnes and Frisby (1992) who talk of a person who consistently acts against social norms without showing any recognition of the seriously deviant nature of his/her behaviour, but who is not obviously mentally ill.

Such individuals often live turbulent and troubled lives, satisfying their needs by a whole range of strategies varying from obtaining their objectives by simply hitting somebody over the head and taking whatever they want, to manipulating an individual (or the system) for their own ends. Their mood can change from one of apparent contrition and regret to extreme aggression and violence in an instant, the constant factor being a desire to get their own way regardless of anybody else and what is right or wrong.

What sort of problems do psychopathic individuals cause in A & E? The more manipulative and passive psychopaths may take drug overdoses and practise DSH. Often they attend A & E in an apparently distressed state claiming that if they are not admitted to a psychiatric ward immediately they will commit suicide. Attention-seeking behaviour is indulged in freely, such as taking their overdose or cutting themselves in front of a queue of people.

The more aggressive psychopath turns up in A & E often with injuries associated with a fight and frequently under the influence of alcohol or else demanding drugs. Their potential for violence is high, especially when they realize that they are not going to get what they want. Disruptive behaviour is common and mental illness is frequently claimed.

In dealing with such a disturbed individual, the first step is to recognize that they are not suffering from a psychotic state which has deprived them of insight. They are fully aware of what they are doing and consequently are fully responsible for the consequences of their actions in A & E. Disruptive behaviour should be dealt with firmly and promptly by asking the person to desist. If they refuse, the danger is that by making too much fuss, the nurse will be merely rewarding the behaviour and thereby leading to its likely repetition. The aim is to deny them the attention that they crave, even if they are swallowing Valium tablets two at a time in front of the queue. They know exactly what they are doing and must take the consequences (usually little more than a long sleep) and attempts to restrain them physically would only lead to staff getting hurt.

Limits have to be set for such individuals for the protection of other patients in the department whose treatment may be adversely affected by disruptive acting out behaviour. The limits of acceptable behaviour should be clearly stated at the beginning of the attendance (e.g. no shouting, running around the department or intruding into certain areas) and if the person goes beyond those limits, they should be removed from A & E by the police. Female nurses are just as likely as male nurses to be punched or kicked by aggressive individuals.

Munchausen's Syndrome

This syndrome was first recognized in 1951 by Asher and according to Enoch and Trethowan (1979) consists of individuals 'who obtain admission to hospital with apparently acute illness supported by a plausible but dramatic history which is later found to be full of falsifications. They are subsequently discovered to have attended and deceived staff at many other hospitals and frequently to have discharged themselves against medical advice, often following arguments while under investigation or following a surgical operation.'

Such is the highly mobile nature of these individuals that it is almost always to A & E that they present and, unless picked up early, they can consume great amounts of time and energy (and money) having their 'illnesses' treated.

The following five broad categories may be recognized in Munchausen's syndrome on presentation:

1. *The Acute Abdominal Type.* They will manifest acute abdominal symptoms, and some may swallow objects such as razor blades and safety pins in order to obtain the surgery and hospitalization they crave. In well-documented cases individuals have obtained well over 100 admissions and laparotomies numbered in double figures.

2. *The Haemorrhagic Type.* This is characterized by complaints of bleeding from various orifices: haematurea (coupled with renal colic in order to obtain pethidine), haemoptysis and haematemesis are common. Self-inflicted wounds with needles or razor blades are commonly used to provide the blood to make the samples realistic, e.g. a finger is nicked so that drops of blood can be squeezed into a urine specimen or the back of the tongue may be cut to lend colouring to haemoptysis.

3. *The Neurological Type.* This type of the syndrome is characterized by very convincing (and some not so convincing) epileptic fits or complaints of migraine.

4. *The Cardiac Type.* This type is characterized by a very convincing display of central chest pain that shows considerable knowledge of medical textbooks. Many such patients know that IV diamorphine is administered for chest pain, hence their behaviour.

5. *The Psychiatric Type.* Imitating various forms of mental illness in order to gain admission to psychiatric hospitals is another manifestation of the syndrome.

Some patients maintain a consistent story; others will change their symptoms as they travel. In trying to understand these people, we should not expect a single simple answer. In some cases obtaining drugs is undoubtedly a major feature (e.g. the chest pain type and those feigning renal colic), but there is much more to it than this. They are often attention-seeking, very immature and psychopathic in personality. For others admission to hospital is a way of escaping from the demands of having to cope with the real world outside.

In many Munchausen's patients there appears to be a strong streak of masochism. This fits well into the abdominal type of the syndrome, as they undergo repeated self-induced wounding and may also practise self-mutilation. It has been found that tolerance to unpleasant diagnostic procedures may be high, and their pain thresholds are also high. It is difficult to explain their desire for mutilation, be it by the hand of the surgeon or (sometimes) their own hand, without including a masochistic element in their personality.

The following list of observations should alert the nurse to the possibility that the patient is suffering from Munchausen's syndrome.

1. Any patient presenting alone, who is non-resident in the catchment area of the hospital, who has no apparent injury.
2. A vague reason for being in the area that cannot be readily substantiated, e.g. a long-distance lorry driver says he has left his lorry at a lorry park.
3. If a discreet search of their clothing and effects reveals inconsistencies in their story such as a different name or address from that given, or evidence of having come from a different part of the country from that which they have stated. There may be evidence of their last port of call such as hospital name tags inside clothes and pyjamas, or evidence of being on the road such as shaving equipment or a change of underwear in a jacket pocket.
4. If the person is known to the A & E department in their previous locality. Check that there is such an address or GP as that given in the area.
5. If there are signs of recent IV sites or cut downs. Multiple abdominal scars should rate a very high probability of Munchausen's, if points 1 and 2 are found to be present.
6. If the patient's description of their symptoms is just a little too perfect or textbookish. In practice very few people ever have all the symptoms in the textbook for any given illness.
7. If the patient's manner and behaviour, especially when they think they are not being observed, gives cause for suspicion.
8. If the patient asks for analgesia by the name of a drug.
9. If there is a circular about the person in your department.

What is the course of action when little or no physical signs of illness can be found, and the staff are reasonably sure of the diagnosis of Munchausen's syndrome? The basic health problem here is undoubtedly a mental one; however, experience has shown that when offered psychiatric help (except in the case of the psychiatric type), the patient will often abscond and move on to try elsewhere.

There are differing opinions about whether to confront the person in A & E with their diagnosis. It is the author's belief that they should be confronted and informed that all hospitals in the area will be circulated at once with their descriptions and details. This should be done over the telephone immediately for your local A & E departments. The rationale that lies behind this policy is that while they are resistant to most forms of psychiatric help that have been tried, the best chance is to deny them the attention that they seek by ensuring that they are discovered as soon as possible in other areas, thereby removing the rewards that the individual gets from their abnormal behaviour. Experimental evidence suggests that this is the most effective way of suppressing unwanted behaviour as has been referred to before in this book (see p. 23). In addition it will also save the hard-pressed NHS considerable time and money. Enoch and Trethowan come to similar conclusions in their detailed review of the problem, hoping for a decline in the behaviour by denying the rewards that are associated with it.

Such a policy requires cooperation between departments on a national scale to exchange information on these sad individuals. Computer technology could lead to the development of a central registry with each A & E department having access via a terminal. The scale of the problem, given the itinerant nature of these people, is national; therefore the solution should reflect this characteristic of the problem. Meanwhile departments are recommended to ensure maximum distribution of information concerning Munchausen's patients they come across.

Violence and Aggression

The origins of aggression and violence in the human species are the subject of much debate. One group of theories suggests that aggression comes from within, that it is an integral part of the human condition. Freud postulated that there was a basic aggression drive within all humans that was an instinct. This view was however rejected by later theorists in the Freudian tradition who developed a frustration–aggression hypothesis based on the idea that preventing a person from obtaining a goal leads to frustration and the focusing of aggression on to the blocking object.

An alternative view of aggression sees it as a learned response no different from any other, so that together with violent actions, it is learned by observation and imitation. The more they are rewarded, the more they will be reinforced and consequently the more likely they are to recur. Bandura's classic experiments (1979) showed how children learned to be violent and the reader is referred to Schachter's work (see p. 17) for a discussion of the emotional behaviour that is involved in aggression.

Violence occurs in many different settings and with many different types of actors. The following list enumerates just some of them.

1. Domestic/family violence.
2. Associated with organic disease, e.g. post-head injury or hypoglycaemic state.
3. Associated with psychosis, e.g. schizophrenia.
4. Due to the effects of drugs, e.g. hallucinogenics and alcohol.
5. Professional violence, the mugger or the soldier.
6. Groups such as football hooligans.
7. Sexual violence, rape.
8. Individual loss of control—violence in response to a situation, heavily influenced by role playing and stereotypes.

The victims of all these types of aggression and violence, and their perpetrators, end up in A & E. An understanding of the psychological processes that are involved in aggressive and violent behaviour will help us to help our patients, and prevent us from being counted among the next victims ourselves.

It is very rare for violence to erupt spontaneously without any warning and reason. There are opportunities, therefore, for intervention before violence occurs which will allow nurses to defuse the situation and lower the temperature.

A major cause of aggression in A & E, compounding any of the situations listed above, is a patient's unrealistic expectations. The classic one that most A & E nurses will be familiar with is the length of the queue to see the doctor.

Research by the author supports this view. A patient satisfaction questionnaire showed that the one thing liked least about A & E for 55% of respondents was the wait, followed by the waiting room environment for another 21% of patients. In this study 54% of patients were dissatisfied with their waiting times. When these patients were interviewed as they registered in A & E, 20% expected to be treated within the hour and a further 35% within 2 hours. In fact only 7% were treated within the hour and a further 27% within 2 hours. When patients were asked about expected diagnostic tests and treatments, only 47% were approximately correct in their expectations. This data was gathered from a sample of 200 adult ambulatory patients at a large city centre A & E department and illustrates how unrealistic many patients' expectations are. Investigation of patient complaints about A & E by Hunt and Gluckman (1991) confirmed that waiting times were the main problem but also showed there was another major criticism, that of staff attitudes, particularly when patients felt staff were not interested in them or did not take them seriously.

Good communication with patients will therefore remove a great deal of frustration stemming from unreal expectations and also improve staff–patient relationships. A triage nurse system provides an important first point of contact, a visual display of approximate waiting times gives valuable information to the patient and, above all, good communication with the patient can avoid many unpleasant situations by preventing misunderstandings.

Departments should think about the provision of facilities to keep people amused while they are waiting; toys, magazines, piped radio, a TV or a video (well secured to the wall!), a public phone and a drinks machine would all be desirable. Generally nurses should look at the waiting environment provided in A & E and ask if it is really satisfactory—especially if patients have to wait there for 3 or 4 hours with a painful injury.

If, however, you are confronted by an aggressive individual, what then? There are several things that you can do to prevent the situation from getting out of hand. First, keep your voice to its normal pitch and volume. When shouted at, it is easy to shout back, but don't. It only raises the temperature immediately. There is nothing wrong with telling yourself repeatedly to control yourself; it is a feedback mechanism that works.

Body positioning is critically important. Stand just a little more than an arm's length (the patient's arm) away. This is far enough to give you the chance to escape any sudden grab or punch, but not so far away as to suggest disinterest in the patient's problem. Standing too close, on the other hand, crowds the person's individual space and is very threatening, so try to keep this arm's length distance between you and the patient at all times.

Your posture should be slightly oblique to the patient. Standing square on is very confrontational, especially if you have your arms in the traditional nursing position of folded across the chest.

The correct stance, according to Moran (1984), is with one leg slightly behind the other. The back leg should be the dominant one and should be straight with your weight fully on it, while the leading leg should be slightly flexed at the knee. This position poses minimal threat, but coupled with the distance you have placed between yourself and the aggressor, gives you the best chance of avoiding a kick or a blow.

Moran points out that in this particular situation, eye to eye contact can be construed as very provocative and should therefore be avoided. He recommends that the nurse should concentrate their attention at a point about level with the second shirt button down. This still conveys interest and gives you the best chance of seeing a punch or grab with your peripheral vision while not threatening the aggressor with direct eyeball to eyeball contact. (See Figs 19.1–19.3.)

Finally you should be aware of any suspicious bulges in jacket pockets that may be potential weapons such as bottles, and of any potential weapons in the immediate environment of the patient. Do not carry pointed scissors and, whatever sort you do use, keep them well out of view. They have been used on a number of occasions to assault nursing staff. The practice of wearing a stethoscope draped around the back of the neck should be frowned upon as it makes it very easy for an assailant to restrain a nurse in a potentially life-threatening manner.

Verbal contact with the patient will often allow the situation to be brought under control. Try to avoid an immediate confrontational attitude—a them and us situation. Explain that you are there to try to help. What can you do? What is the patient's problem? Kinkle (1993) recommends the nurse to follow a strategy of 'verbal venting', allowing the patient to say their piece without interruption, even if there is a strong urge to defend verbally another member of staff who is coming in for serious criticism during such an outburst.

The person should be interviewed individually if possible, without friends and relatives who are often the cause of more trouble than the patient. When a group of rowdy individuals brings one of their mates to A & E, the best policy is to ask the rest to leave. They will accomplish nothing in the department except be disruptive and endeavour to impress each other with acts of bravado, depending on the pecking order in the group. Such behaviour is well documented in studies of group violence. Allowing such a group to remain in the department will only lead to trouble; therefore they should be asked to leave and if they refuse, the matter referred to the security service or the police.

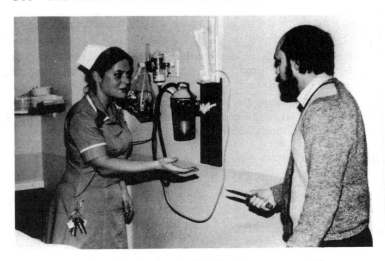

Fig. 19.1   The patient in A & E with a weapon. The wrong approach: the nurse has allowed the patient to get between her and the outside of the cubicle. She is holding out her hand demanding the knife and she is making eye to eye contact. This is confronting and threatening to the patient and may cause him to respond violently and he may use the knife to inflict serious harm.

One of the most effective ways of defusing a situation is simply by passing on information. People are far less likely to get angry if they know what is going on, how long they will have to wait, and why.

However, there are some situations in which, despite all these measures, violence still erupts or, to be more precise, passes from being verbal to physical. In many cases, the patient will smash some physical objects, throw a chair at a wall or window, but then become calmer again having 'let off steam' as it were. Therefore, if a patient indulges in an outburst against property, they are best left to break whatever it is they have in mind (within reason) as probably that will be the end of the episode and if you do intervene the result will be a violent struggle in which you will become the object of the person's aggression. Broken windows are easier to repair than broken staff nurses' arms.

The police should, however, be contacted and asked for assistance, for the staff may yet become the objects of the person's violence.

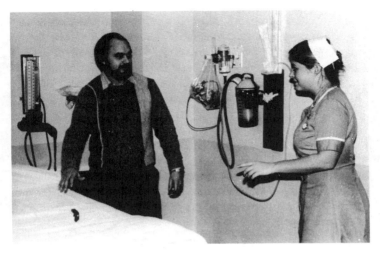

Fig. 19.2   The right approach. The nurse is keeping to the outside of the cubicle and is asking the patient to place the weapon on neutral territory before attempting to remove it. She is keeping at a safe distance (arm's length) and avoiding eye to eye contact.

Furthermore, prosecution for serious damage to hospital property should be the policy of the department.

If the person challenges a male member of staff to a fight, going perhaps through the ritual of removing the coat, issuing threats and insults, then violence is less likely to occur, provided the situation is handled correctly. Allow the person to have a 'moral' victory by backing off. The ritual having been fulfilled (Mungham, 1977; Marsh, 1975), physical contact is unlikely. While the patient is boasting of his victory and swaggering around the department, the police can be on the way. Remember it's usually the winner of the last battle that wins the war.

At the end of the day, however, a direct assault on a member of staff may occur. When intervention is needed (as in such a situation), the basic premises of military strategy still hold good, i.e. concentration of force in time and space coupled with the element of surprise. This means that you should ensure sufficient pairs of hands to do the job (ideally at least 4 people), plan the move to be simultaneous so as to overwhelm the person, and if possible distract his attention or come from the rear. This way the risk of injury to

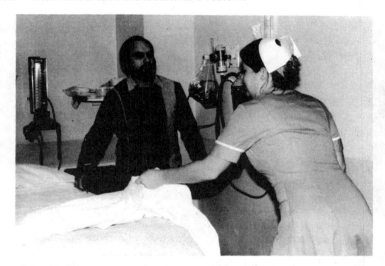

Fig. 19.3 If attacked with a weapon, the nurse should try to smother it with a blanket or anything else available, while retreating rapidly to safety and calling for help.

staff and patient is minimized. Although the situation in which direct physical intervention is required is unpredictable and, therefore, hard and fast rules cannot be made, the nurse would do well to adhere to these basic principles.

A final comment on aggression and violence in A & E—all incidents should be documented, and there should be in-service training for all A & E nursing staff in the skills required to handle aggressive patients.

References

Bandura K. (1979). In Hilgard E., Atkinson R., Atkinson R. C. (eds) *Introduction to Psychology*. New York: Harcourt, Brace, Jovanovitch, pp. 322–3.

Barnes C., Frisby R. (1992). Personality disorders. In Brooking J., Ritter S., Thomas B. (eds) *A Textbook of Psychiatric and Mental Health Nursing*. Edinburgh: Churchill Livingstone.

Cook T. (1975). *Vagrant Alcoholics*. London: Routledge & Kegan Paul.

Enoch M. D., Trethowan W. H. (1979). *Uncommon Psychiatric Syndromes*. Bristol: John Wright and Sons.

Gough P., Maslin-Prothero S., Masterson A. (1994). *Nursing and Social Policy*. Oxford: Butterworth-Heinemann.

Hunt M., Gluckman M. (1991). A review of 7 years' complaints in an inner city A & E department. *Archives of Emergency Medicine*, **8,** 17–23.

Kinkle S. (1993). Violence in the E. D. *American Journal of Nursing*, July, 22–4.

Marsh P. (1975). Understanding aggro. *New Society*, 3 April.

Mitchell R. G. (1983). *Breakdown: Commonsense Psychiatry for Nurses*. London: Nursing Times Publications.

Moran J. (1984). Response and responsibility, *Nursing Times*, **80,** 28–31.

Mungham G. (1977). The sociology of violence. *New Society*, 13 Oct.

Shadoobuccus H. (1988). Nursing care of the homeless alcoholic. *Nursing*, **3,** 52–3.

Chapter 20

SEXUAL PROBLEMS IN A & E

Sexually Transmitted Disease

Patients sometimes present at A & E, often in a very distressed condition, thinking that they are suffering from some form of sexually transmitted disease. It is essential to know something of the more common types and their presenting symptoms in order that an assessment of the patient's problems may be made.

Table 20.1 shows the numbers of people attending clinic in 1989 according to the main types of sexually transmitted disease (STD). There has been a reduction in numbers from 1986 levels, for example gonorrhoea fell by 44% and NSGI by 20%. The anxiety that is produced by any sort of condition affecting the genitalia is shown by the fact that 22% of attendees in Table 20.1 required no treatment.

Patients usually come to A & E when the local department of genito-urinary medicine is closed, and very often refuse to give details of their complaint to the receptionist, either out of embarrassment or because they cannot find the words to express their problem, without resorting to vulgar terms which they are often unwilling to use in front of the receptionist.

The department should have a policy to the effect that if a patient does not wish to disclose the nature of their complaint, rather than have a receptionist pursue the matter to their embarrassment, a member of the nursing staff (preferably of the same sex) should be asked to talk to the patient.

In assessing the patient, privacy is important, and the nurse should try to set the patient at their ease and then ask them to explain the nature of their problem. Many people are not familiar with the medical words used to describe sexual function and anatomy, therefore the language used may involve slang and some rather crude terms. It is important to obtain a description of the

Table 20.1
New cases of STD, 1989, in thousands

Disease	Male	Female	Total
Syphilis	1.3	0.5	1.8
Gonorrhoea	13.8	9.0	22.8
Herpes simplex	9.8	9.3	19.1
Non-specific genital infections (NSGI)	79.9	45.3	125.7
Candidiasis	9.8	48.6	58.5
Others needing treatment	57.1	48.3	105.4
Others not needing treatment	73.9	56.8	130.7
Total*	301.9	280.8	582.8

*NB Grand total not sum of above due to different categories in use.

Source: DoH (1991) Health and Personal Social Services Statistics

symptoms—how long they have been present for and how they relate to the patient's sexual behaviour over the last 4 weeks. If the patient has been monogamous during that period, the clear implication is that their partner has not, which can have a very damaging effect on their relationship. As in other illnesses, the psychological and social sides of the problem must not be overlooked, and great care and sensitivity is required in talking, for instance, to a married woman who has suddenly developed a vaginal discharge, two weeks after her lorry driver husband has returned from a trip to Europe.

The two most common complaints that will be heard are a discharge (vaginal or urethral) or ulceration of the genitalia. The significance of these complaints is as follows:

1. *Urethral discharge in males*. This is almost always pathological and can be broadly classified into either gonococcal or non-gonococcal, the most common non-gonococcal causes being *Chlamydia trachomatis, Trichomonas vaginalis* and *Candida albicans* organisms. If uncircumcized males are suffering from Candida infection, they will reveal the site of the infection clearly upon retraction of the foreskin. However the origin of the discharge in the other conditions is not so easily located. If the discharge is of a gonococcal origin, it should be noted that this disease is far more common in homosexual than heterosexual men (Donaldson and Donaldson, 1993).

A useful test is to ask the man to pass 60–120 ml of urine into a glass container, and then to finish off passing his urine into another glass container. If there is infection of the anterior urethra, the first specimen will be hazy, containing threads or specks of pus, while the second specimen will be clear. If, however, they are both hazy this indicates that the infection involves other parts of the urinary tract, e.g. cystitis or nephritis.

2. *Vaginal discharge*. This can be either pathological or non-pathological. Some degree of discharge from the vagina occurs in all women, the amount varying along a continuum. It is important to ascertain, therefore, what the normal discharge is like and why this condition is different. The woman should be reminded that a normal vaginal discharge may increase and be only noticed premenstrually, at time of ovulation or when using the contraceptive pill or an IUD. A discharge therefore does not automatically imply a disease process.

If the discharge is pathological in origin, the most likely cause is *Candida albicans* (which some authorities do not consider to be an exclusively sexually transmitted disease), while other organisms that might be responsible are *Neisseria gonorrhoeae*, *Trichomonas vaginalis* and *Chlamydia trachomatis*. Cervical lesions may also produce a vaginal discharge whether they are infective (herpes or warts) or not (neoplasm, polyps).

3. *Genital ulceration*. In practice, there tend to be two types of ulcer found, ulcers that are multiple and painful (usually herpes) and those that occur singly and are painless (usually syphilis).

Diagnosis of the infecting organism on clinical findings is very uncertain, therefore careful microbiological examination and culture are required, which is why departments of genito-urinary medicine usually insist that A & E departments do not treat these cases, but rather refer them on to their clinic. It is a famous dictum that there is no such thing as an emergency in venereology, and while there may be a lot of truth in this from the physical point of view, it may not be so true from the psychological angle.

Standard policy is not to treat the patient but to tell them instead to attend the clinic the following day or the next Monday, and it is probably true to say that no physical harm will come to the patient. However, when nurses are passing this information on or reinforcing what the casualty officer has said, they need to remember that the patient will be very anxious and considerable reassurance is needed that this wait is for the best. Abstinence from sexual activity is to be strongly recommended until attending clinic when it is next open. One of the most important reasons for the patient attending the clinic rather than receiving treatment in A & E is the need for the patient's sexual partners to be traced—a role that A & E units cannot take on. Various forms of sexually transmitted disease produce no symptoms, or symptoms which can be and are ignored. For example, rectal gonorrhoea is often symptomless and, given the often multiple nature of homosexual encounters, it is therefore very important indeed to trace contacts as they may not know that they have been infected. (If symptoms do appear they consist of anal pain and discomfort, painful defaecation and a blood-stained or purulent discharge.) Oropharyngeal gonorrhoea likewise is often asymptomatic.

The reader will be aware that there are various forms of sexually transmitted disease besides those described so far (e.g. genital warts), but this is not a textbook on genito-urinary medicine. What matters is that the nurse can show sympathy and understanding for what is a very distressing condition *for the patient*, and that the nurse is able to assess that the most likely cause of the problem is sexual transmission, and therefore that the most appropriate place of treatment is not A & E but the out-patient clinic of the department of genito-urinary medicine. Telephone calls to the department in the middle of the night are another manifestation of the anxiety felt by persons who think they may have acquired such a disease. Such calls should be dealt with tactfully and with due understanding, the patient being advised to attend the appropriate clinic and abstain from sexual activity meanwhile.

AIDS

While most forms of STD can be treated and cured, the exception— AIDS—remains, and the fear of having contracted this disease is understandably likely to produce extreme anxiety. By June 1992 there had been 15 765 HIV-positive reports in men, of whom 68.6% involved homosexual exposure, 11.1% IV drug use and 6.5% heterosexual exposure. Of the 2128 female reports, 52% were as a result of heterosexual exposure and 32.6% from IV drug use. A total of 3637 men and 202 women had died of AIDS.

A patient who phones or presents at A & E in a greatly distressed state, worried that because of some casual sexual adventure he or she may have contracted AIDS, should be treated sympathetically. There is little that can be done except to emphasize the need for sexual abstinence and to encourage an early visit to the STD clinic. It will help if the unit can pass on the phone number of useful agencies such as the Samaritans, or the local Gay Switchboard.

Although AIDS is relatively rare in the heterosexual population, it does raise the question of the nurse's attitude towards homosexuality which is not a sexual problem but rather a sexual choice. (It is discussed here for lack of a more appropriate section.) A significant proportion of the population is homosexual or bisexual, and as a consequence a significant proportion of A & E patients will be gay. In many cases this probably will not be recognized, but in other situations the person may display behaviour that is more in keeping with their sexual orientation, in a way that is perfectly natural to them. This is a sexual orientation that the nurse has no right to censure.

Society still broadly disapproves of homosexuality, which places many homosexuals under great pressure. Some are more able to live with these pressures than others, while others again are just unable to come to terms at all with their homosexual tendencies, especially if they are married. The result is a great deal of stress in the lives of many homosexuals which, coupled with the often transient nature of homosexual relationships and, therefore, a lack of stability and support, may lead to a higher incidence of unhappiness and anxiety than in other sections of the population. The nurse must, therefore, lend an understanding and sympathetic ear if required by a gay or lesbian patient.

The discussion about HIV should remind the nurse of the fundamental rule that in dealing with all body fluids nurses must take great care and beware sharp objects, needles etc. to avoid the risk of accidentally contracting any blood-borne disease such as hepatitis B or AIDS. Although IV drug users and homosexuals engage in high-risk behaviour, the nurse should remember that *anybody* could have AIDS.

That emergency department (ED) nurses are very aware of the risks of HIV infection in the USA is confirmed by research carried out by Burgess et al. (1992). They found ED nurses to have the highest fear of contracting HIV from workplace infection when compared to a range of other workers such as ED doctors, prison officers and police officers. When data from doctors and nurses alone was examined, gender, years of practice and previous experience of caring for HIV-positive patients were found to have no effect on fear. A repeat of this study in the UK would be very interesting.

Genital Trauma

The sexual acts that people perform in the privacy of their own homes are their own business. However, some practices can occasionally have unfortunate consequences which lead the person, with great reluctance and embarrassment, to the local A & E department.

A common problem is that of a foreign body that has either been retained in the rectum, vagina or urethra, or damage done to any of these organs by such a foreign body.

In dealing with a rectal foreign body, the patient may admit to what is causing the problem (e.g. a carrot or a sex-aid such as a vibrator) or to what was responsible for the injuries sustained (e.g. a glass or bottle that has broken leading to lacerations of the rectum and anal area) which makes treatment much easier. However, such is the embarrassment felt that the patient may not bring themselves to admit the truth. It is essential to bear this in mind when somewhat reluctant individuals walk into A & E complaining they have not been able to open their bowels for several days or that they are bleeding rectally, or simply complaining of abdominal pain. In such cases, rupture of the bowel is possible with disastrous consequences. Laparotomy to remove the offending object may be necessary; vibrators have been known to reach the transverse colon. Severe rectal damage may be caused by practices that involve inserting the forearm into the rectum; smooth muscle relaxant drugs are used in conjunction with this practice, e.g. glycerin trinitrate.

A wide variety of foreign bodies may be removed from the vagina, with or without the woman's admission of their presence.

Urethral trauma can occur from the passing of objects such as straws or the flexible inside part of a biro. Fresh bleeding from the urethra should raise this possibility even though the patient may not admit to such a practice.

Trauma to the external genitals may be the result of sadomasochistic practices, or may be accidental. An unlikely story together with the patient's unease should make the former cause more likely in the nurse's mind, but nurses should treat the injuries at their face value, and not be too concerned with how they were caused (unless there is a possibility that they were inflicted against the person's will, in which case discreet probing when alone with the patient should be undertaken).

A common injury is the zip injury to the penis which can be exquisitely painful. Generous analgesia with Entonox will greatly facilitate freeing the penis from the zip. If swelling is present, ice packs should be applied and lignocaine gel may be of help. Wyatt and Scobie (1994) have reported on a series of 30 boys with this problem seen in A & E. Only a small proportion required a general anaesthetic, no circumcisions were required to free the zip and all recovered without any subsequent complications. This work supports the approach advocated here.

Uncircumcized males who have a tight foreskin run the risk during their first sexual encounters of the foreskin becoming so retracted that it will not resume its normal anatomical position, acting as a tight constriction around the end of the penis leading to swelling and oedema (paraphimosis). This is a very alarming condition and, as with all such sexual problems, the nurse should display great tact and reassurance in dealing with the patient. Ice packs to reduce the swelling together with the use of lignocaine gel will in most cases allow the foreskin to be manipulated back to its normal position.

Relatively minor lacerations to the penis can bleed profusely, and the patient may well limp into A & E after several hours of bleeding. Even after suturing, bleeding may occur. Ice packs and firm manual pressure are recommended, although it may take some time finally to stop the bleeding from what is a very vascular organ.

Bruising and swelling of the scrotum are often seen after accidents and are best treated with ice and a scrotal support. The nurse should be alerted, however, by the young man who says that he has severe pain but has no apparent injury as this is the classical presentation of torsion testis which, if not promptly relieved by surgery, can lead to a gangrenous testicle due to the impairment of the blood supply. This should be treated with a high priority to see the casualty officer.

One final problem that may occur, although not usually associated with genital trauma (although it may be), is the patient who refuses to undress for no apparent reason. The nurse may be dealing with a case of transexuality or transvestism. Transexuality involves a person who wishes to live like a member of the opposite sex because they consider that that is their appropriate sex. Transvestism is more in the nature of deriving pleasure from wearing women's clothes. In either case, the person's attire may not conform to their biological gender. The patient's extreme anxiety may be understood in such a situation and the nurse should ensure that as few people as possible know about the patient's predicament. This will build up the trust and cooperation that is needed to treat the injuries sustained by the patient most effectively.

Occasionally cases of genital mutilation may be seen in persons craving to be of the opposite sex, which in the author's own experience have ranged from a pair of tights tied tightly around the base of the penis and scrotum (in the hope that 'Like a wart tied with string, it would all drop off'—the result was only an agonizingly painful blue scrotum) to an attempt to shoot off, with a shotgun, the relevant piece of anatomy.

In dealing with the sort of problems described above, the nurse may have feelings ranging from surprise to complete revulsion. But a non-judgemental attitude is the key to helping the patient, which means that feelings and emotions must be kept under control and not communicated to the patient who, as can be imagined, is already in a hypersensitive condition. The sexual aspect of a patient's life is largely ignored in nurse training—perhaps another Victorian legacy of the Nightingale tradition—but in A & E this cannot be, as many of the problems that patients present with are directly sexual in origin, or can be traced at least partly to the stresses and anxieties that have been generated by sexual problems.

References

Burgess A., Jacobsen B., Baker T., Thompson J., Grant C. (1992). Workplace fear of acquired immunodeficiency syndrome. *Journal of Emergency Nursing*, **18:** 233–8.

CSO (1993). *Social Trends 23*. London: HMSO.

DoH (1991) Health and Personal Social Services Statistics.

Donaldson R., Donaldson L. (1993). *Essential Public Health Medicine*. Lancaster: Kluwer Academic Publishers.

Wyatt J., Scobie W. (1994). The management of penile zip entrapment in children. *Injury*, **25:** 59–60.

The Research Base for A & E Nursing

21   Nursing Research in A & E

Chapter 21

NURSING RESEARCH IN A & E

Why Research in A & E?

The last chapter in a book is often in the nature of a postscript. However, this book will not end with a look-back or an added-on afterthought, but rather with a look forward at an opportunity for the development of A & E nursing. That opportunity is nursing research.

One of the distinguishing features of a profession is thought to be a discrete body of knowledge distinctive to that profession. If nursing is to be regarded as a profession, then it must be based on a body of nursing knowledge, rather than on bits and pieces of knowledge taken from medicine. Certainly there is a need for close links with the various other professional groups in the health care field, and much can be learnt from them, but nursing also needs to develop its own body of nursing knowledge.

One way of acquiring nursing knowledge is simply to do what we have always done, which is to pass procedures (often with no sound basis) on from generation of nurses to generation as either revered traditions or mystical truths beyond question. But if other areas of human endeavour had followed that method, then it is likely that we would still believe that the earth is flat and at the centre of the universe and that people who talk of wheels are dangerous disruptive elements or simply mad.

Human knowledge has advanced through questioning and enquiry, through reason, investigation and experiment, i.e. research, and so it should be with nursing. That is why there is a need for nursing research, carried out by nurses, and in a specialist field like A & E, there is a need for A & E nursing research to supplement that done in other fields of nursing.

How Do You Carry Out Research?

Polit and Hunter (1991) describe two basic research designs, experimental and non-experimental. In the former case the researcher studies the effect of some action or deliberate intervention, e.g. a new wound dressing; in the latter case, no physical act is involved, but rather we are concerned to gather information about a problem or behaviour either by a survey or observation.

Another way of looking at research is to consider the method employed. We can either start off with an idea that we wish to test by research to see if we can find evidence of support or not. This idea is called a hypothesis and the method, a hypothetico-deductive method. A hypothesis cannot be said to be proven or disproven by research. Those statements are too definite given the potential for error and uncertainty that exists even in the best designed experiments. Instead we should talk in terms of a hypothesis which is supported (or otherwise) by the available evidence. The hypothetico-deductive method lends itself to either an experimental or survey design, and requires careful statistical analysis of its findings.

An alternative method is to start off not with a clear idea or hypothesis that we wish to test, but rather with an interest or problem that we wish to investigate. The researcher then sets about gathering information by observation and unstructured interviews, from which it is possible to make certain statements that the gathered evidence tends to support. This is the inductive method and has the advantage that as the researcher did not start out with a definite idea or preconceived notion there is less chance of bias creeping in along the way. Such an approach can be used to generate theories out of observation and is sometimes referred to as qualitative research.

Experimental Research

True experimental research involves a manipulation, and that which is manipulated is known as the independent variable, the observer noting the effect of this on the other variable, the dependent variable. For example, in a wound healing experiment, the type of dressing applied is the independent variable and the rate of observed healing would be the dependent variable, i.e. it depends upon the dressing.

A second ingredient of an experiment is that there must be a control, a comparison group which is not subjected to the manipulation or act that is the subject of the experiment, so that the effect of the manipulation can be fully assessed. In nursing, we could not withhold nursing care in many situations to see how our control group compared with the group upon whom we tried out our new dressing, but having a control group of subjects who receive the conventional dressing or treatment that was in practice before the new treatment under investigation, constitutes a valid control.

Randomization constitutes the third essential part of a true experiment. This means that each subject has an equal chance of being in either group, experimental or control. This is essential to eliminate bias. Where relatively small groups are used, it is essential to match certain characteristics such as sex and age, as otherwise substantial distortions can occur by chance inclusion of a disproportionate number of a certain type in a group.

In many practical situations, it is not possible to fulfil rigorously all these three criteria of a true experiment. Techniques are available to overcome the problems of lack of full control or randomization which still permit the findings of the research to have meaning. This is known then as quasi-experimental research.

Survey Research

In practice it is usually impossible to try to obtain information from every single member of the population that you wish to investigate (that would be a census), so the researcher has to use a sample of the population, a smaller group which to be acceptable has to be truly representative (contain the same proportions of characteristics as the total population in terms, for example, of sex, age and occupations) and has to be randomly selected.

The information may be gathered from questionnaires, although they have to be very carefully constructed so as not to lead the subject into answers. The wording of the question also needs careful attention as what may be obvious to the researcher phrasing the question may not be obvious to the subject trying to answer it. Another method of gaining information is the structured interview in which the researcher has a questionnaire worked out in advance and interviews the subject in order to gain the information. This eliminates misunderstanding of questions and other problems such as whether the person to whom the questionnaire was sent actually fills it in, but it does introduce an element of interviewer bias, although this can be minimized to some extent by close conformity with the questions as though it were a script. The researcher can also use existing documentation and records to gather data such as the A & E register or patient case notes. The quality of this data is only as good as the original records which raises issues of reliability in such a retrospective survey.

Qualitative Research

An alternative approach to research is concerned more with the way people behave, how they communicate and their understanding of the world. Such an approach is less concerned with testing hypotheses by the gathering of numerical data and statistical analysis. The emphasis is upon observed behaviours and verbal data gathered from in-depth interviews which may be very loosely structured. The phrase qualitative research is an umbrella term covering a whole range of research methods which fall within this tradition. It should not be seen as an easy alternative to more quantatitive methods, as the data gathering and analytical techniques used are just as demanding. The strongest research embraces both traditions, as different aspects of a problem may be amenable to different approaches.

What Can be Researched in A & E?

There is an almost infinite range of research questions that the A & E nurse can tackle. The following section summarizes some of the key areas

Quality of Service

Reference has already been made to waiting times and staff attitudes as being principal causes for complaint. The emphasis on quality has never been greater in the NHS and this has been pushed along by the Patient's Charter. Factors such as waiting times and patient perceptions of staff and treatment are therefore essential components of any department research strategy.

The use of 'tick box questionnaires' (typically involving Likert scales) to assess patient satisfaction is not however recommended as they lack discrimination. Bond and Thomas (1992) are very critical of these instruments, commenting on how a whole range of studies that have relied upon this approach all seem to have identical, very favourable, findings. This suggests something wrong with the measuring instrument as intuitively we know that not all nursing care is excellent all of the time. Research by the author in A & E confirms the tendency that people have to sometimes tick 'satisfactory' or 'very satisfactory' on a questionnaire and then talk about their A & E experience in very different tones. Interviewing patients about their care seems a more reliable method of gathering data. This could take place in A & E as French (1981) argues that there is no evidence in the research literature of a 'hospital halo effect' by which she means patients say one thing if interviewed in hospital, but might give different answers later at home.

Patients Who Walk out Unseen

This is a useful index of how well the department is functioning and also a cause for concern as such people may have significant medical problems which could have serious consequences if not treated promptly. The author could find no reference in the UK literature to following up such patients to look at outcomes, apart from my own research (Walsh, 1993a) which indicated the walkout rate could be 10%. The prime reason for walking out amongst the 48 postal questionnaire respondents (sample size 100) was the waiting time being too long. Forty-two patients had traumatic conditions and in 31 cases the condition was less than 24 hours old. Those patients who walked out had no significant difference in pain and anxiety levels from those who stayed, whilst a third made no further contact with a doctor. It is this latter group that is most worrying.

Providing Correct Staffing Levels

Close monitoring of attendance rates will reveal distinct patterns of variation. It is possible therefore to have the right numbers of staff with the right skill mix on duty as required. This improves patient care and ensures cost-effective use of the most expensive item in the NHS budget—staff.

A & E Statistics as a Guide to Wider Health Problems

The prevention of accidents is a major target in the government's Health of the Nation report (DoH, 1992). This first of all requires accurate gathering of statistics and there are various areas where official figures are hopelessly inaccurate.

Works accidents are only recorded if the person has more than three days off work as a result. Harrington and Tar-Ching Aw (1989) have been very critical of this hole in the official figures as there appears to be no record of the more frequent but less disabling works accidents. The official statistics recorded 188 442 serious works accidents in 1989 (OPCS, 1990) which is only 2% of all A & E attendances. However, Williams (1984) reported that 23.5% of trauma patients at his A & E unit were as a result of works accidents and Worth and Hurst (1989) reported a figure of 25%. Walsh (1990) found that 13.8% of all adult attendances were works accident related. These sort of figures suggest that for every officially recorded works casualty, another 10 attend A & E!

The true incidence of assault is much greater than official statistics suggest. Shepherd et al. (1988) for example found that in a study of 294 assault victims who were treated in A & E, only 23% appeared in official police statistics suggesting that the real incidence of assault is at least three times higher than official figures. The A & E nurse can reflect upon sports injury and domestic accidents as two major areas where there is not even an attempt to compile accurate central statistics.

Accident and Emergency departments have a key role to play in accident prevention work both in terms of accurately identifying the scale of the problem and targeting at risk groups. Health education work could be carried out in A & E, it could be a very constructive use of patient waiting time, while the effects of accident prevention campaigns can be best monitored through A & E records. The prevalence of other conditions can also be monitored through A & E, for example acute episodes of asthma, deliberate self-harm or changing patterns of substance abuse.

The Use made by the Public of Medical Services

The reasons people come to A & E can only be discovered by asking patients themselves. This was the basis of the author's own PhD work and revealed that patients usually have rational and logical reasons for A & E attendance. The debate about inappropriate attendance at A & E is futile, for it is not the patient who is inappropriate, it is the services provided by the A & E department that are inappropriate (Walsh, 1993b)!

Only by talking to patients can health care providers find out what is required and make provision accordingly. The development of nurse practitioner services in A & E or the health centre will take a lot of the pressure off the main A & E department and its hard-pressed medical/nursing staff.

Nursing Care in A & E

This is a huge area but opens up a whole range of possibilities. Nurse triage and the nurse practitioner concepts could revolutionize A & E but the need must be correctly identified before implementation can be carried out appropriately. Finally evaluation of such projects is essential. All three stages therefore involve research.

The research topic need not be on such a large scale. A new dressing, wound closure or casting technique may be suggested. New ways of working with other staff such as the mental health services or community nursing staff may be thought desirable. Whatever the project, it must be carefully evaluated, i.e. researched.

The scope to improve the quality of the A & E service is enormous and the preceding paragraphs suggest just a few of the areas in which nursing research could be very beneficial. Nurses should also be willing partners in collaborative research with other professional groups such as doctors or the ambulance service. Before starting any A & E research, however, the nurse must also recognize that there are problems which will be encountered along the way.

Problems Facing the Nurse Researcher in A & E

Permission and Consent

Work which involves patients must be cleared by the Trust Ethics Committee. Confidential and often very sensitive information is involved, therefore it is essential that the nurse satisfy senior nursing and medical colleagues and the ethics committee that the work is potentially beneficial, will in no way harm patients or infringe the Protection of Data Act. This can be a daunting experience, especially as ethics committees have had little experience of nursing research. The proposal must therefore be well prepared and thought out to gain approval.

The nurse must seek the consent of patients at all times and maintain confidentiality and anonymity. For example, patients should be referred to as code numbers wherever possible, while if a study was looking at the geographical distribution of patients in a town, only the street should be recorded rather than the house number.

Reliability of Recorded Data

When a retrospective study is being undertaken based upon case notes and/or register entries, the data is only as reliable as the original entries. This may lead to the loss of a considerable amount of detail.

The first stage of the author's own work illustrates the point. A study of 2000 A & E case notes was undertaken and one of the key factors was length of time since onset of condition. In 538 cases it was impossible to make any kind of statement about this variable as no information was recorded. In the second stage of the study, 200 patients were interviewed by the author and this data was recorded for all patients. A further example comes from trying to classify the cause of the injury. In the retrospective study referred to above, 5.9% of patients were assigned to the category of domestic accident, yet in the interview sample this figure was 15% with a significant drop in the general 'others' category as more detail was available.

Sampling Problems

It is essential that a representative sample be obtained. The researcher must be sure that all periods of the week are covered and also of the year if necessary (e.g. if looking at sports injuries). Are male and female patients equally represented? Are different ages of patients represented in the sample? A sampling frame therefore needs to be worked out to ensure a representative sample is obtained, otherwise it will not be possible to generalize in any meaningful way from the sample to the whole A & E population. The nurse must ensure that steps have been taken to avoid bias in drawing the sample (e.g. selecting every tenth patient) and also, if statistical analysis is to be undertaken, that the sample is big enough.

Pilot the Instrument

Whether an interview schedule or questionnaire is to be used, it must first of all be tried out to check for ambiguous questions that can be misunderstood. Data recording equipment such as a microphone and tape recorder should be checked to ensure effective functioning. Postal questionnaires are notorious for poor response rates and if used, the questionnaire should be be piloted on a small scale. If say 10 are sent out and only 1 or 2 returned, there is clearly no point in proceeding with the main study as a response rate of 10–20% is useless, because it cannot be considered in any way free from selective bias.

Ethical Problems

Confidentiality and anonymity have been referred to already. The nurse should however be careful not to pressure patients into participation as this is unethical. The patient's well-being is more important than research, therefore some patients may have to be dropped from the study because urgent intervention is needed. Careful consideration must be given to which patients are suitable whilst drawing up the sampling frame. Patients should always be given a full explanation of what is required before they participate in any way.

Bias

The nurse should consider how s/he presents him/herself to the patient as this can bias responses. A nurse's uniform might significantly alter the response as might the location of an interview. Response rates below at least 40% make postal questionnaires useless because of the selective bias that might creep in (see above).

Questions should always be scrutinized for bias or for leading towards a particular answer.

The nurse would be well advised to undertake a research methods course before actually attempting any research. Most higher education institutions have modular part-time degree programmes for nurses and other health care professionals which include at least one research course as a module. Even if not enrolling for the whole programme, the nurse is encouraged to follow one such module if s/he intends carrying out any research. It is also important that the department arranges links with a member of staff who has experience of carrying out research to support the nurse researcher. Research is immensely rewarding but it needs experience and support, particularly for the novice, to produce worthwhile results.

References

Bond S., Thomas L. (1992). Measuring patients' satisfaction with nursing care. *Journal of Advanced Nursing*, **17**, 52–63.

DoH (1992). *Health of the Nation*. London: HMSO.

French K. (1981). Methodological considerations in hospital patient opinion surveys. *International Journal of Nursing Studies*, **18**, 7–32.

Harrington M., Tar-Ching Aw (1989). Industrial accidents. *BMJ*, **298**, 14 Jan., 68–9.

OPCS (1990). *Social Trends 1989*. London: HMSO.

Polit D., Hunter B. (1991). *Nursing Research: Principles and Methods*. Philadelphia: J.B. Lippincott Co.

Shepherd S. et al. (1988). Assault: characteristics of victims at an inner city hospital. *Injury*, **19**, 185–90.

Walsh M. (1990) Social factors and A & E attendance. *Nursing Standard*, **5:9**, 29–32.

Walsh M. (1993a). Patients' views of their A & E experience. *Nursing Standard*, 7, 30–32.

Walsh M. (1993b). A & E or the GP? How patients decide. *Nursing Standard*, 7, 36–8.

Williams K. (1984). Who uses the accident service? *Injury*, **16**, 35–7.

Worth C., Hurst, K. (1989). False alarm. *Nursing Times*, **85**, 24–7.

INDEX

Abdomen,
  pain, 112–15
    assessment, 112–14(table)
    causes of, 113(table)
    evaluation, 115
    intervention, 114–15
    pathology, 113
  trauma, 82–7
    assessment, 83–4
    evaluation, 86
    intervention, 84–6
    pathology, 82–3
Abortion, 237
  criminal, 240
Abrasions, 152
  cleaning, special attention,
    158
Abscesses,
  dental, and facial swelling,
    204
  and infected wounds, 167
Adolescents, solvent abuse,
    276
Age, and accidents, 7–9
Ageing, psychology of, 28–9
Aggression, 296–302
  and alcohol, 269
  body positioning, 298
  male tendency, 8
  and patient satisfaction, 297
  and psychopathy, 293

AIDS, 307–9
  and alcohol, 268
  and sexual orientation, 308
  visual disturbances in, 189
  see also HIV infection
Airway,
  in burn victims, 176
  in critical injury, 55, 56
  evaluation, 58–9
  intervention, 56–7
  pathology, 55
Alcohol(ism), 11–13, 267–9
  and aggression, 269
  cause of accidents, 11–13, 266
  dependent patients, 290
  detoxification, 269
  and drivers, 11, 13
  health education, 50
  and homelessness, 290
  in pedestrian trauma, 12
  psychiatric services, 269
  psychological and economic
    problems, 292
  and psychopathy, 293
  in trauma, 3
  and violence, 267–8
  and women's health problems,
    232
α rays, effect on human body,
    248
Ambulance scoop, 81

Ambulance service,
    collaboration with nurses, 321
    communication with, 43
Amnesia,
    post-traumatic, 76
    retrograde, 76
Amphetamines, 275
Amputation, following fractures,
    126
Aneurysms, 113–14
'Angel dust' (phencyclidine,
    PCP), 273
Angina,
    and acute myocardial
        infarction, 89, 91
    pain due to hypoxic
        myocardium, 90
Ankle injuries,
    fracture-dislocation, 131
    plaster of Paris backslabs,
        143(fig.)
Antibiotics, treatment of
    abscesses, 169
Antiseptics, cleaning soft tissue
    wounds, 158
Anxiety,
    changes in respiration, 106,
        282
    common in old age, 223–4
    and pain, 28
    and phobias, 281–2
    reduction due to information,
        29
Appendicitis, locus of pain,
    112
Arm injuries,
    forearm fractures, 132
    plaster casts for, 145–6
    upper arm, 134
Arousal, autonomic, 16
Arrhythmias,

and assessment of chest pain,
    93
    serious, 97(fig.)
Assaults,
    sexual, 235–6
    on staff, intervention needed,
        301
    statistics, 320
Assessment,
    early, 40
    interview, 29–30
    social factors, 13
Asthma, 101, 215
Asystole,
    correct diagnosis of, 71
    recognizable by nurse, 96
Atoms, structure of, 246
Attribution theory, 20–1

Backslabs, effectiveness, 140
Bandages, 164
Behaviour, and learning, 22–7
Behaviourism, 23
    techniques, 30
Bennett's fracture, 131
Bereavement, 17–19
β rays, effect on human body,
    248
Bites, 152
Bleeding, control of, in soft
    tissue injury, 157–8
Blood,
    circulation, *see* Circulation
    psychological response to, 157
    supply, in fracture healing,
        121
Blood pressure, misleading
    normality, 66
Blood sugar, in assessment of
    impaired consciousness,
        109

Body fluids, and risk of HIV, 308
Body positioning, in dealing with aggression, 298
Bomb incidents, patients' symptoms, 244
Bones, children's, 121
Bony orbit, fracture, 184
Bowel, rupture of, 309
Bradycardia, poor prognosis in myocardial infarction, 92–3
Brain damage,
  in facial trauma, 203
  and respiratory rate, 77
Brainstem, herniation, 73
Breathing,
  assessment, 62
  in critical illness, 59–65
  in critical injury, 55
  evaluation of, 65
  flail segment, 61(fig.)
  intervention, 63–5
  pathology, 59–62
  see also Respiration
Bronchiolitis, in children, 215
Bronchitis, acute on chronic, 101
Bullets,
  abdominal trauma, 83
  tissue destroyed by, 154
Burns, 171–83
  area of, 171–3
  assessment, 176–7, 183
  children, 216
  classifications, 173
  critical pathway, 182(fig.)
  depth of, 173–4(fig.)
    assessment, 177
    Mount Vernon formula, 173

dressings, 179–81, 183
  children, 216
  self-care of, 181–3
electrical, 174, 177
elevation of limbs, 180
flamazine bag treatment, 175(fig.)
fluid loss in, 172
full thickness, 173
and infection, 176
intervention, 177–83
  airway, 177–8
  first aid, 177
  pain relief, 178
  psychological support, 178–9
IVI and fluid balance, 179
later effects, 176
oedema, 174
partial thickness, 174
pathology, 171–6
psychological effects, 175–6
special areas affected by, 174–5
superficial, 174
treatment on arrival, 181(table)
Wallace's Rule of 9, 172(fig.)
Burr holes, in treatment of head injury, 74
Bursae, 155

Calcaneum, fracture, 130
Cannabis,
  misuse, 273–4
  short term effects, 274
Cannulation, hypovolaemic shock, 71
Cardiac . . ., *see also* Heart; Chest pain, cardiac origin
Cardiac pain, 92

Cardiac arrest, 67
  in children, 69
  insufficient circulation, 65
  likely arrhythmias, 69
Care planning, 35–8
  approaches, 36
  implementation, 37
  research, 36
  standardized, 37
Carpo-pedal spasm, 103(fig.),
    104
Cartilage, common tissue
    injuries, 155
Casts, synthetic materials,
    149
CAT scans, requiring nursing
    support, 78
Cataract, due to radiation
    injuries, 186
Cellular perfusion, reduced in
    shock, 65–6
Cellulitis, dental, 205
Cerebral hypoxis, confusion due
    to, 105
Cerebrovascular accident
    (CVA), impaired
    consciousness, 108
Cervical collar, in treatment of
    spinal injury, 81
Chest, 92(fig.)
  drain, 63, 64(fig.)
  restricted expansion, in rib
    fractures, 59
Chest pain,
  cardiac origin, 89–100
    assessment, 91–8
    evaluation, 100
    intervention, 98–100
    pathology, 89–91
  central, 104
Cheyne–Stokes breathing, 62

Child abuse, *see* Children, abuse
Children, 206–19
  abuse, 210–13
    assessment, 211
    examination, 211
    sexual, 211
  accidents,
    environmental hazards, 208
    prevention, 206
  burns, 177, 216
    feelings of parents, 178
  cardiac arrest, 69
  childcare facilities, 231
  common emergencies, 213–8
  death, mothers' response,
    18–19
  development of thinking,
    208–10
  and domestic violence, 235
  ear infections, 197
  ear trauma, 195
  fears caused by classical
    conditioning, 25
  febrile convulsions, 214
  and head injury, 77
  inadequate supervision, 208
  mortality, 5
  nurses, 206
  nursing intervention, 215–8
  at risk, 212
  social deprivation and
    accidents, 207
  solvent abuse, 277
  special facilities, 206
  stages of development, 208–10
  stridor, 200
  trauma, and inner urban
    environment, 6
  and violence, 297
  violent behaviour learned by
    imitation, 25

Circulation, 65–73
  assessment, 67–8
  and care of critically injured, 55
  evaluation, 72–3
  intervention, 68–73
  pathology, 65–7
Civil defence, 250
Class, *see* Social class
Clavicle, fractures, 135
Clostridium pathogens, 152–3
Cocaine, 272
Colles fracture, 126, 133(fig.), 141
Coma,
  in deliberate self-harm, 262
  scale, 75(fig.)
Communication, 42–3
  nurse/patient, removal of frustration, 298
  networks, 43
  nurses and abused women, 235
  skills, development of, 42
Concrete operational stage of childhood development, 209
Concussion, eye injury in, 186
Conditioning,
  classical, 24(fig.), 24–5
    fears and phobias, 30
    fears in children, 25
  operant, 23
Confidentiality,
  and RTAs, 44
  and police, 43
  nursing and medical records, 44
Confusion,
  in elderly patients, 22
  and psychology of ageing, 222

Consciousness,
  assessment of head injury, 74–5
  impaired, 106–112
    assessment, 109
    evaluation, 111–12
    intervention, 109–11
    pathology, 106–9
  monitoring of
    role of nurse, 78
Consent,
  child solvent abusers, 277
  young people, 46
Contraception, 50
Contusion, and eye injury, 186
Convulsion, febrile, 214
Cornea, 191
  abrasion, 185
  epithelium, defect in, 194
  inflammation of, 186
Cot death (SIDS), 217
CPR, in critical injury, 67, 68
Crack (cocaine), 272
Cricothyrotomy, needle, 56
Crimes, and confidentiality, 44
Critical pathways,
  burns, 182(fig.)
  examples, 39(fig.), 85(fig.)
  presenting conditions, 38
  and quality assurance, 38
  respiratory distress, 114(fig.)
  standardized care planning, 37–8
  wounded patient, 168(fig.)
Croup, 200, 215
Crutches, 148
Culture,
  effect on pain, 28
  and ethnicity, 10–11
  and grief, 18

Cyanosis,
    evidence of, in assessment, 62
    late sign of respiratory
        deterioration, 63
    and severe respiratory failure,
        103

Deafness, 196
    see also Ear; Eardrum
Death,
    in children, 5, 17–19
    rates, and social class, 4,
        5(fig.)
Deep vein thrombosis (DVT),
    and assessment of chest
        pain, 104
Defibrillation, asystole not
        responsive to, 71
Deliberate self-harm, *see*
        Self-harm, deliberate
Denial,
    following death, 18
    women and domestic violence,
        233
Dental problems, 204–5
Dentures, obstruction of airway,
        56
Denver Developmental
        Screening Test, 210
Dependency, continuum of, 34
Depression, 281
    common in old age, 223–4
    manic, 281
Deprivation, sensory, *see*
        Sensory deprivation
Desferrioxamine IV, 214
Diabetes, impaired
        consciousness in, 108,
        109
Diaphragm, and abdominal
        injury, 83

Diarrhoea, and abdominal pain,
        113
Digits, fracture or dislocation of,
        136
Disaster planning, 243–6
    catering for the media, 244
    liaison with ambulance
        service, 244
    life-saving measures, 245
    needs of survivors, 246
    pain relief, 245
    patients' distress, 244
    psychological first aid, 246
    and radiation casualties,
        243–51
    triage, 245
Discharge from A&E,
    elderly people, 228
    problems following fractures,
        128
    soft tissue injury patients, 169
Discipline, moral duty of nurses,
        48
Dislocations, 119–37
    complications, assessment,
        123–9
    evaluation, 129
    see also individual joints
Doctors,
    collaboration with nurses, 321
    communication with, 43
Dolls, in child abuse assessment,
        212
Drainage, in treatment of
        abscesses, 167
Dressing(s),
    burns, 183
        children, 216
    . self-care, 169, 181–3
    check before discharging, 169
Drowning, 102

Drug(s),
  dependent patients, 290
  health education, 50
  overdose, 256–8
    assessment, 260
    attention seeking, 257
    coping mechanism, 258
    gastric lavage, 262
    problem-solving device,
      258
    and psychopathy, 292
    and relationship problems,
      257
    rates, 256(table), 257(table)
Dyspnoea,
  and respiratory rate, 103
  hoarseness in children, 200

E chart (eye test), 190
Ear, 195–7
  diseases of, 196–7
  infection, 196
  trauma, 195–6
Eardrum
  damage by pressure change,
    195–6
  perforated, deafness, 196
ECG, 69, 95(fig.)
  and and assessment of chest
    pain, 93
  components, 94
  performed by nurses, 94
Ecstacy (hallucinogenic
    amphetamine)
  long-term effects, 274
  short-term effects, 274
Education,
  development of nursing role,
    38
  health, 48–50
    first aid, 49

  prevention of illness, 48
  vital part of self-care, 50
  social factors in care planning,
    14
Elbow,
  dislocation, 134
  injuries, 134
  pulled, 134
Elderly patients, 220–9
  assessment, 226–7
  confusion due to sensory
    deprivation, 22
  discharge from A&E, 228
  falls, 224
    fractures caused by, 225
    and head injury, 225
  fractures,
    due to falls, 225
    femoral, 129
    problems with discharge
      from A&E, 128
    psychological aspects, 124
  fragile skin, 153
  hypothermia, 228
  intervention, 227–9
  living alone, 10
  mobility, 225
  need for stimulating sensory
    environment, 223
  nose bleeds, 198
  population, increase in, 7
  stereotypes of, 20, 224
  understanding, 115
Electrical burns, 174, 177
Elevation,
  of burnt limbs, 180
  pain relief in fracture patients,
    125
  reducing swelling, 167
  self-care of soft tissue injury,
    169

Emotion,
    atmosphere in A&E, 16–17
    theories of, 16–17
    upsetting long term memory,
        27
ENT, 195–204
    specialist referrals, 200
Enuresis, induced, in drug
        overdose, 262
Environment, 14, 29
    and class, 6
    and childhood accidents, 208
    inner urban, effect on child
        trauma, 6
    and sensory deprivation, 21–2
    stimulating, for elderly
        patients, 223
Epilepsy,
    and impaired consciousness,
        108, 109
    stigma attached to, 214
Epithelium,
    corneal,
        damage to, 191
        defect in, 192
    partial thickness burns, 174
Erythema, 174
Ethics,
    conflicts in nursing, 47
    duty of accident witnesses, 48
Ethnicity, and culture, 10–11
Extinction, behavioural, 23
Eye complaints,
    assessment of visual acuity, 190
    drops and ointments, 193
    inflammation, 188
        common causes, 189(table)
    injuries,
        assessment, 188–91
        car windscreen, 187(fig.)
        chemical, 185–6

corneal abrasion, 185
evaluation, 194
foreign body, 185
irrigation, 192, 194
non-penetrating, 184–6
padding, 192
penetrating, 187
psychological effects, 191,
    194
radiation, 186
intervention, 191–4
pathology, 184
trauma to surrounding
    structures, 184–5

Face,
    and dental emergencies, 201–5
        intervention, 203–4
    and fractures, 202(fig.)
    injuries, assessment of, 201–3
    trauma, 201
        and brain damage, 203
Falls, in elderly people, 224, 225
Family(ies),
    circumstances, and care
        planning, 34
    disintegration of, and health, 4
    emotions following trauma, 17
    suicide and grief, 255
    support following SIDS, 217
Fear(s),
    avoidance of creating, 30
    and pain, 28
Femur, fractures of, 136
    in elderly patients, 129
Fibula, fracture of, 130
First aid,
    health education, 49
    psychological, 246
Fits, and impaired
        consciousness, 108

Flail segment, 61(fig.)
Flamazine, in treatment of
    burns, 175(fig.), 179,
    180
Foot injuries, 130
  plaster of Paris backslabs,
    143(fig.)
Forceps,
  to clear airway, 56
  for lost tampons, 240
Forearm, *see* Arm
Formal operational stage of
    childhood development,
    209–10
Foundation for the Study of
    Infant Deaths, 217
Fracture(s), 119–37
  Bennett's, 131
  causes of, 119
  in children, 121
  Colles, 126, 133(fig.), 141
  complications, 123–9
  in elderly people, 225
  evaluation, 129
  healing, 121–2
  immobilization, 121
  metatarsal, 130
  pain, 124, 125
  pathology of, 122(fig.)
  patterns of, 120(fig.)
  Smith's, 132
  stress, 119
  trimalleolar, 131
  types of, 119–20
Free recall curve, 26(fig.)

Gas gangrene, 153
Gastric lavage,
  accidental poisoning in
    children, 213
  drug overdose, 262

Gauze,
  antibiotic inpregnated, 164
  paraffin inpregnated, 164
  plain dry, 163–4
Gender, and accidents, 7–9
Genitals,
  mutilation, 311
  trauma, 309–11
  ulceration, 305, 306–7
Glasgow coma scale (GCS), 75
Glaucoma, acute, 189
Goals,
  socially attainable, 14
  time limit for evaluation, 36
Gonorrhoea, symptomless, 307
GPs,
  ear treatment, 196
  psychiatric referral in alcohol
    abuse, 269
Grief, 17–19
  components of, 18
  description, 18
  following SIDS, 218
  following suicide, 255

Haematoma, in fracture healing,
    121
Haematurea, test for, 84
Haemothorax,
  and pneumothorax, 59
  chest drain, 63
Hallucinations, 280
Hallucinogenics, 273
Halo brace, 82
Hand,
    immobilization of, plaster of
      Paris setting, 142(fig.)
  injuries, 136
Head injury, 73–9
  and alcohol, 268
  assessment, 74–7

in children, 77, 208
in elderly patients, 225
evaluation, 79
intervention, 77–9
minor, 78
pathology, 73–4
wound dressing, 164
Health,
affected by unemployment, 5
effects of stress on, 6
women's problems, 230–41
Health education, 48–50
first aid, 49
prevention of illness, 48
as vital part of self-care, 50
Health visitors,
children and domestic
violence, 235
physical development in
children, 210
Hearing, deterioration with age,
221
Heart,
attacks, fatalities, 91(fig.)
block, recognizable by nurse,
98
front view, 92(fig.)
see also Cardiac . . .; Chest
pain, cardiac origin; ECG
Hepatitis B, risk from opioid
injection, 271
Herpes, infection of pinna, 196–7
Hip,
dislocation, 136
injuries, 136
Histoacryl, wound closure, 163
HIV infection,
nurses' dealing with body
fluids, 308
risk from amphetamine
misuse, 275

risk from opioid injection, 271
visual disturbances in, 189
see also AIDS
Homelessness,
A&E regulars, 290
head injury, 291
hypothermia, 291
increase in, 290
Housing,
council, and drug overdose,
257
and road traffic accidents, 6
Human Needs Model, 35
Humerus, fractures of, 134
Hyperventilation, hysterical, 102
calming techniques, 106
Hyphaemia, 194
Hypothermia,
deliberate self-harm, 260
elderly people, 221, 228
Hypovolaemia
in abdominal trauma, 82, 83,
86
blood loss, 157
burnt patients, 171
causing shock, 71
correction by fluid, 171
in penetrating injury, 157

Imitation,
behaviour in nursing, 25
violent behaviour in children,
25
Immobilization, of fractures, 125
Impetigo, 197
Incontinence, impaired
consciousness and, 110
Individualized care
effects of stereotypes, 20
and primary nursing, 35
and psychology, 29–30

and social factors, 13–14
Injuries,
    crush, 152
    degloving, 152
    self-inflicted, 259–64
Intermittant Positive Pressure
        Ventilation (IPPV), 57
    and intubation, 58(fig.)
    patient not breathing, 63
    respiratory arrest, 59
Intubation,
    in coma, 262
    and IPPV, 58(fig.)
    maintaining airway, 57
    requiring nursing support, 78
Intuitive stage of childhood
        development, 209
Ipecacuanha poisoning in
        children, 213
Ischaemic heart disease (IHD)
    cause of chest pain, 89, 93
    regional mortality , 90(fig.)

Joints, injury to, 151

Keratitis, due to radiation, 186
Knee injuries, 135
    plaster of Paris backslabs,
        144(fig.)

Labour, premature, 237
Laceration, 152
    pretibial flap, 154(fig.)
Language problems, effective
        intervention, 30
Law,
    and the nurse, 43–8
    treatment against patient's
        will, 46
Le Fort facial fracture, 202(fig.),
        203

Leg injuries,
    plaster casts, 146–7
    lower leg, 130
Little's area, 198
Local authorities,
    children at risk, 212
    emergency planning officers,
        250
Long leg cylinder, 147
LSD hallucinations, 273
Lumbar vertebra, whiplash, 79–
        80
Lung, trauma, respiratory
        impairment, 61

Malleoli, fractures of, 131
Mania, 281
Mastoiditis, causing ear pain,
        196
Medical Anti-Shock Trousers,
        72
Melolin, burns dressings, 179
Memory, 26–7
    long-term, 27
    short-term, 27
    theory, 30
Menière's disease, causing
        vertigo, 197
Menstruation,
    toxic shock syndrome, 241
    women's health problems, 239
Mental Health Act, 286–7(table)
Mental hospitals, 279
Mental illness, 279–89
    anxiety, 288
    assessment, 282–4
        drug taking, 284
        patient's life history, 284
    counselling skills, 288
    cultural factors, 279
    delusions, 283

and drug abuse, 279
evaluation, 288–9
hallucinations, 283
intervention, 284–8
loneliness, 288
police intervention, 285
patient/nurse relationship, 285
violence in, 288
Metacarpal fractures, 136
Migraine, causing vertigo, 197
Misperception, *see* Perception
Mobility, elderly people, 225
Modelling, learning by, 25
Models of nursing, 33–5
Moral issues, *see* Ethics
Mortality, *see* Death
Motorcycles, role in RTAs, 7
Mount Vernon formula (depth of burns), 175
Munchausen's syndrome, 293–6
masochism in, 294–5
psychiatric help, 295
self-mutilation in, 295
Muscle,
injury to, 151
loss in ageing, 221
Muslim naming system, 11
Myocardial infarction (MI)
acute, and history of angina, 91
and bradycardia, 92–3
differentiated from angina, 89
Myocardium,
damage limitation, 99
hypoxic, and angina pectoris, 90

Neck injuries,
airway obstruction, 56
and spinal damage, 80–81, 199
whiplash, 82
Needle exchange schemes, 271
Negligence, legal view, 47–8
Nose, 197–9
bleeds, 198–9
trauma, 197–8
Nurses,
role of, 33–51
expanded, 38–9
Nurse practitioners, 41–2
development of role, 42
research into, 321
role in soft tissue injury, 151
and triage, 41–2
Nurse researchers, problems of,
bias, 323–4
ethical, 323
permission and consent, 322
piloting, 323
reliability of data, 322
sampling, 322–3

Obesity, health education, 50
Oedema, pulmonary,
care of respiratory distress patients, 100
fatal effects of, 61
Oesophagus,
objects in throat, 199
perforation of, 200
Olecranon process, fractures of, 134
Ophthalmitis, sympathetic, complicating eye injury, 187
Opioids, 270–2
injection of,
effects, 270–1
non-direct effects, 271–2

overdose, 270
Orientation,
   following head injury, 76
   reality, *see* Reality orientation
Osteoarthritis, changes with age,
   221
Osteomyelitis,
   fracture complications, 123–9
   risk from skull fracture, 74
Osteoporosis, changes with age,
   221
Otitis externa, causing ear pain,
   196
Otitis media, treatment of, 196
Otorrhoea, evidence of skull
   fracture, 77
Oxygen, circulatory problems,
   68

P wave (ECG), 94
P-Q interval (ECG), 94
Paediatric services
   child abuse, 212
   see also Children
Pain,
   assessment of breathing, 62
   expression in different
      cultures, 29
   problem for assessment, 30
   psychology of, 30–1
   reduction due to information,
      29
   relief,
      abdominal pain, 114
      chest pain, 99
      fractures, 125
   soft tissue injury assessment,
      155
Paracetamol, 260
Paralysis, flaccid, spinal injuries,
   80

Parasuicide, 255
   and mental illness, 279
   most frequent in young
      people, 256
   and women's health problems,
      232
Parents,
   consent of, 46
   guilt over burnt children, 178
   perception of danger, 208
   single
      linked with poverty, 207
      stereotypes, 210
      stress, 231
   stereotyping, 210
Patella,
   dislocation, 135
   fracture, 135
Patients,
   critically ill, 89–115
   critically injured, 55–87
   factors in common, 3
   goals, and individualized care,
      35
   psychology, 16–32
   satisfaction, and aggression,
      297
   treatment against will of, 46
Pelvis, fracture, 136
Penis, zip injury, 310
Perception,
   assessment of patient, 19
   person, research into, 19
Peritoneum, lavage, 84
Peritonitis,
   and abdominal injury, 83
   locus of pain, 112
   recognizable by nurses, 84
Personality disorder, 290
Phencyclidine (PCP, 'angel
     dust'), 273

Phobias,
    and anxiety, 281–2
    avoidance of creating, 30
Physiology,
    changes in ageing, 220,
        221–2
    and substance dependence,
        266
    and substance misuse, 266
Pinna,
    infections, 196–7
    injury, 195
Planning,
    emergency officers, 250
    major disasters, 243–6
Plaster of Paris,
    alternatives to, 149
    application, 138–50
        basic principles, 138–41
        constriction, 139–41
        movement during, 139
    backslabs, 142–4
        for ankle and foot injuries,
            143(fig.)
    bandage application,
        140(fig.)
    casts,
        for arm injuries, 145–6
        Colles, 145
        discharging patients with,
            147–9
        for leg injuries, 146–7
        patient exercises, 148
        Scaphold, 145
    limb padding, 138–9
    limb positioning, 141–2
    moulding, 139
    self-care, 148
    setting time, 141–2, 148
    tissue swelling, 140
    water temperature, 139

Pneumonia,
    and acute respiratory distress,
        in children, 215
    and generalized chest pain,
        104
Pneumothorax, 60(fig.)
    chest drain, 63
    pathology of breathing, 59
    spontaneous, 101
Poisoning, accidental, in
        children, 213
Police,
    communication with, 43
    evidence, 45
    good working relationship
        with, 43, 46
    physical violence in A&E,
        300
    rape allegations, 236
    statistics, 320
Poverty,
    caused by single parenthood,
        9
    caused by unemployment, 9
Pre-conceptual stage of
        childhood development,
        209
Pregnancy,
    abortion, 237
    concealed, 240
    maternal shock, 237–8
    premature labour, 237
    trauma in, 237
        assessment of women after,
            238
        blunt, 237
        intervention, 238–9
        penetrating, 237
    unwanted, due to effects of
        alcohol, 268
    vaginal bleeding, 239

Pressure sores,
  and A&E trolleys, 227
  in elderly fracture patients,
    129, 226
Primary nursing,
  advantages, 35–6
  and individualized care, 35
Principles, ethical, *see* Ethics
Psychiatric hospitals, 288
Psychiatry, and alcohol, 269
Psychology, 16–32
  of abdominal trauma, 86
  of ageing, 28–9, 220, 222–4
  of alcoholism, 292
  of battered women, 234
  of bleeding patient, 157
  of breathing difficulties, 63,
    105
  of burns, 175–6, 178–9, 183
  of child abuse, 211
  of elderly people, 226
  essential for nursing, 16
  of eye complaints, 191
  first aid, 246
  impact of rape, 235
  and individualized care, 29–30
  of respiratory distress, 63, 105
  of self-harming patients, 263
  of sexually transmitted
    disease, 305
  of shock, 68
  of spinal injury, 81
  of substance misuse, 266
Psychopathic disorder, 292–3
  and aggression, 293
  and alcohol, 293
Pulmonary embolism (PE), 101
Pulse oximetry, 105
Pyrexia, intervention in
    impaired consciousness,
    110

Q wave, pathological,
    recognizable by nurse, 95
QRS complex (ECG), 94
Questionnaires, research 317

Radiation,
  atomic structure and, 247
  casualities, 246–50, 249(fig.)
    and major disaster planning,
      243–51
  contamination, 248
  decontamination, 248
  effect on human body, 247
  ionizing, common forms of,
    247(table)
  sickness, in-patient care,
    248
Radius, fractures of, 133(fig.)
  distal, 132
  head, 134
  mid-shaft, 132
Rape, 235–6
  role of police, 236
Rashes, common, 156(table)
Reality orientation,
  effectiveness of, 111–12
  elderly people, 227
  treatment of impaired
    consciousness, 110
Recall, improvement of, 26
Records, confidentiality, 44
Refuges, women's, 10, 234
Reinforcement, in operant
    conditioning, 23, 24
Research, 315–24
  designs, 316
  experimental, 316–7
  into quality of service, 318–9
  into staffing levels, 319–20
  into walkouts, 319
  methods, courses in, 324

public use of medical services,
321
qualitative, 318
survey, 317–8
Respiration,
assessment, 103
changes in, and anxiety, 282
in shock, 67
rate, and brain damage, 77
see also Breathing
Respiratory distress, 100–106
acute, in children, 214–5
assessment, 102–4
critical pathway, 114(fig.)
evaluation, 106
intervention, 104–6
pathology, 100–102
principle causes, 100–102
Resuscitation, 238
circulatory, and surgical
intervention, 86
European Council Guidelines,
70(fig.)
mouth-to-mouth, 68
Retina, detached, 194
Rhinorrhoea, evidence of skull
fracture, 76–7
Rib, fractures, 59
Road traffic accidents (RTAs),
8(fig.)
casualties, 12(fig.)
and confidentiality, 44
and older housing, 6
young people, 7
Rule of 9 (burns), 172, 176

Scaphoid fracture, 131
Schizophrenia, 280–1
and violence, 280
paranoid delusions in, 280
Self-care,

of abscesses, 167
of burns dressings, 181–3
in elderly people, 228
health education, 50
plaster casts, 148
role of nurses, 33–5
of soft tissue injury, 169
Self-Care Demands, 34
Self-esteem, low, and self-
inflicted injury, 259
Self-harm, deliberate, 255–65
assessment, 259–64
emotional trauma, 264
evaluation, 264
nursing intervention, 261–3
and psychological disturbance,
258
and psychopathy, 292
questioning of patients, 260
and relationship crises, 258
social trauma, 264
and stereotyping, 258, 264
in young people, 256
Self-mutilation, 259
physical intervention by
nurses, 263
Sensori-motor stage of
childhood development,
209
Sensory deprivation, 21–2
in elderly patients, 223
risks of, 22
Sensory input, importance of,
22
Sepsis, caused by pathogens,
153
Sexual problems, 304–11
sympathy for, 307
Sexually transmitted disease
and alcohol, 268
embarrassment of patient, 304

new cases, 3–5(table)
psychological and social
    problems, 305
Shock,
    cardiogenic, 66
    causes of, 71
    chest pain assessment, 92
    classification of, 66(table)
    hypovolaemic, 66, 76,
        in burns, 171
        in fractures, 123, 124
    pathology of, 65
    vasogenic, 66
Shoulder,
    dislocation, 128, 135
    girdle, 81
    injuries, 135
SIDS (cot death), 217
Siderosis bulbi, 188
Sikh naming system, 11
Single parenthood, *see* Parents,
    single
Sinusitis, eye pain in, 189
Skin condition, circulatory
    problems, 67–8
Skull,
    bleeding within, 73
    fracture, 74, 76
Sling, high arm, 165(fig.)
Smith's fracture, 132
Smoke inhalation, 101–102
Smoking,
    health education, 50
    women's health problems, 232
Snellen Visual Acuity Test, 190
Social class, 4–7
    and environment, 6
    and health, 3
    mortality rates, 4, 5(fig.)
    overdose rates, 257
    use of English, 30

Social deprivation, and
    childhood accidents, 207
Social Services, and child abuse,
    212
Social status, in elderly fracture
    patients, 124
Social workers, communication
    with, 43
Sociology,
    of ageing, 220, 224, 226
    of sexually transmitted
        disease, 305
    of substance misuse, 266, 267
    of trauma and illness, 3–15
Soft tissue injuries, 151–70
    assessment, 155–7
    closed, 154, 167
    evaluation, 169
    infection, 151, 167
    intervention, 157–69
    pathology, 151–5
    wound cleaning, 158
    wound closure, 159–63
    wound dressing, 163–4
Solvent abuse, 275–7
    adolescents, 276
    children, 277
    social factors, 276
Spalding effect, 61
Speech, in assessment of mental
    illness, 283
Spinal cord, vulnerability to
    injury, 79
Spine injuries, 79–82
    assessment, 80–81
    and head injury, 78
    intervention, 81–2
    pathology, 79–80
    threat from neck injury,
        199
Sprains, 154

ST segment, elevated, recognizable by nurse, 95
Stabbing, 83
Statistics, 320
Status epilepticus, medical intervention, 110–11
Stereotypes,
    awareness of nurses, 30
    dangers in nursing, 20
    of deliberate self-harming patients, 264
    of elderly people, 20, 224
    of parents, 210
    in substance misuse, 266
Steristrip, 159, 162(fig.)
Stitches, suturing soft tissue wounds, 159
Stomach washout, 258, 261
Stress,
    effect on health, 6
    physical and psychological symptoms, 232
    of single parenthood, 9
    and women, 231–2
Stridor, 62
    in children, 200
Substance misuse, 266–78
    withdrawal syndrome, 272
Substance use behaviours, 267
Sudden Infant Death Syndrome (SIDS), 217
Suicide,
    and deliberate self-harm, 255
    and depression, 281
    and grief, 255
    paracetamol, 260
    and psychopathy, 292, 292
    prevention of, 47
    see also Parasuicide
Surveys, retrospective, 318

Survivors, psychological needs of, 246
Sutures,
    soft tissue wound closure, 159
    techniques, 160–1(fig.)

T wave (ECG), 94
    inversion, recognizable by nurse, 96
Tampons,
    lost, 240–1
    and toxic shock syndrome, 241
Teeth, problems, 204–5
Tetanus, 152
    characteristics, 153
    vaccination, 164–7
Thigh injuries, 136
Throat, 199–201
    trauma, 199–200
Thrombolytic therapy, treatment of cardiac problems, 99
Thumb, base of, fracture, 131
Tibia, fractures of, 130
    tibial plateau, 135
Tissue, soft, *see* Soft tissue injuries
Toes, fractures and dislocations of, 130
Tonsils, and objects in throat, 199
Toxaemia, and impaired consciousness, 108
Toxic shock syndrome, 241
Tracheotomy, and airway obstructions, 56
Trades unions, legal problems, 47
Training, nurse,
    for handling violence and aggression, 302

sexuality ignored in, 311
Transexuality, 310
Transvestism, 310
Trauma, scoring systems, 86–7
Travellers, as A&E regulars, 290
Treatment, refusal of, 47
Triage,
    chest pain patients, 99
    reduction in walkouts, 41
    research into, 321
    role of nurse, 40–1

Ulna, fracture, 132, 133(fig.)
Ultra-violet light, eye injuries,
    186
Unemployment,
    cause of poverty, 9
    effect on health, 5
Universal Self-Care Demands,
    34
Urethra,
    discharge from, 305
    trauma, 309
Urine,
    detection of opioid injection,
        270
    haematurea test, 84
    patients in shock, 67

Vagina,
    bleeding from, 84, 239–40
    discharge from, 305, 306
Vasoconstriction, mechanisms
    against shock, 66
Ventilation, requiring nursing
    support, 78
Ventricular ectopics (VEs), 98
Ventricular fibrillation (VF), 96
Ventricular tachycardia (VT),
    97
Vertigo, 197

Violence, 296–302
    and alcohol, 267–8
    and children, 235, 297
    domestic, 233–5
    group, 299
    patients with weapons,
        300(fig.)
    and schizophrenia, 280
    towards women, 9
    verbal, 300
Vision, deterioration with age,
    221
Vomiting, and abdominal pain,
    113

Walkouts, 41
    reduced by nurse
        practitioners, 42
War,
    civil defence planning, 250
    nuclear, disaster planning,
        250
Wheezing, 102
Whiplash, 82
    spinal injury, 79
Women,
    battered, 233–5
        age at commencement, 234
        communication with nurses,
            235
    changing employment
        patterns, 230–1
    dependency on men, 230
    education, 230
    families and A&E, 9–10
    health problems, 230–41
    and stress, 231–2
    trauma and pregnancy,
        236–9
Women's Refuge Movement,
    234

Women's refuges, 10, 234
Work accidents, statistics, 320
Wrist injuries, 131
    plaster of Paris backslabs, 144(fig.)

X-rays, requiring nursing support, 78

Young people
    consent, 46
    nose bleeds, 198